SAMUELS

— & —

ROPPER'S

NEUROLOGICAL CPCs

FROM

THE NEW ENGLAND
JOURNAL OF MEDICINE

SAMUELS
— & —
ROPPER'S

NEUROLOGICAL CPCs
FROM
THE NEW ENGLAND
JOURNAL OF MEDICINE

Martin A. Samuels, MD

Chair, Department of Neurology
Brigham Women's Hospital
Professor of Neurology
Harvard Medical School
Boston, MA

Allan H. Ropper, MD

Executive Vice-Chair
Department of Neurology
Brigham Women's Hospital
Professor of Neurology
Harvard Medical School
Boston, MA

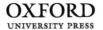

OXFORD
UNIVERSITY PRESS

OXFORD

UNIVERSITY PRESS

Oxford University Press is a department of the University of Oxford.
It furthers the University's objective of excellence in research, scholarship,
and education by publishing worldwide.

Oxford   New York
Auckland   Cape Town   Dar es Salaam   Hong Kong   Karachi
Kuala Lumpur   Madrid   Melbourne   Mexico City   Nairobi
New Delhi   Shanghai   Taipei   Toronto

With offices in
Argentina   Austria   Brazil   Chile   Czech Republic   France   Greece
Guatemala   Hungary   Italy   Japan   Poland   Portugal   Singapore
South Korea   Switzerland   Thailand   Turkey   Ukraine   Vietnam

Oxford is a registered trademark of Oxford University Press in the UK and certain other
countries.

Published in the United States of America by
Oxford University Press
198 Madison Avenue, New York, NY 10016, United States of America

© Oxford University Press 2013

Library of Congress Cataloging-in-Publication Data
Samuels, Martin A.
Samuels and Ropper's neurological CPCs from the New England Journal of Medicine / Martin Allen
Samuels, Allan H. Ropper.
p. ; cm.
Neurological CPCs from the New England Journal of Medicine
Includes bibliographical references and index.
ISBN 978-0-19-992751-7 (pbk. : alk. paper)
I. Ropper, Allan H.   II. New England journal of medicine.   III. Title.   IV. Title: Neurological
CPCs from The *New England Journal of Medicine*.
[DNLM: 1. Nervous System Diseases–diagnosis–Case Reports.   2. Nervous System
Diseases–diagnosis–Collected Works.   3. Nervous System Diseases–pathology–Case Reports.
4.   Nervous System Diseases–pathology–Collected Works.   5. Neurologic Manifestations–Case
Reports.   6. Neurologic Manifestations–Collected Works. WL 141]
362.1968—dc23
2012020639

The science of medicine is a rapidly changing field. As new research and clinical experience broaden
our knowledge, changes in treatment and drug therapy occur. The author and publisher of this
work have checked with sources believed to be reliable in their efforts to provide information that
is accurate and complete, and in accordance with the standards accepted at the time of publication.
However, in light of the possibility of human error or changes in the practice of medicine, neither
the author, nor the publisher, nor any other party who has been involved in the preparation or
publication of this work warrants that the information contained herein is in every respect accurate
or complete. Readers are encouraged to confirm the information contained herein with other
reliable sources, and are strongly advised to check the product information sheet provided by the
pharmaceutical company for each drug they plan to administer.

9 8 7 6 5 4 3 2 1
Printed in the United States of America
on acid-free paper

To Clinical Neurology
and
The Giants on Whose Shoulders We Stand

Raymond D. Adams
Charles D. Aring
Joseph Felix Babinski
Jean Martin Charcot
C. Miller Fisher
Joseph Foley
Norman Geschwind
William Gowers
Henry Head
John Hughlings Jackson
Gordon Holmes
Pierre Marie
H. Houston Merritt
Fred Plum
E. P. Richardson
Maurice Victor
Thomas Willis
S.A. Kinnier Wilson

FOREWORD

On my desk, carefully piled, were the most recent seventeen weekly issues of the *New England Journal of Medicine* (*NEJM*). Thirteen issues had listed on the cover "Case Records of the Massachusetts General Hospital". Case Records have been published regularly in the *NEJM* since 1923 when the *NEJM* was still known as the Boston Medical and Surgical Journal. This amounts to more than four thousand, six hundred issues, and near that number of Case Records of the Massachusetts General Hospital. It has only been in recent years that Case Records have not been printed in every weekly issue.

In the past thirty-plus years, two eminent neurologists, Dr. Martin A. Samuels and Dr. Allan H. Ropper, have often been invited to take on the role of clinical discussant of Case Records. In fact, they are the two most frequent clinical discussants ever. All of the cases they have discussed displayed neurological dysfunction, and in many of these an associated medical disorder lurked. Such cases suited Drs. Samuels and Ropper to their own liking, given that they are both board certified in internal medicine and also in neurology. They have specialized their practices, their teaching and their clinical investigation in neurology, but have never forgotten or strayed from their roots in internal medicine.

The eighteen Case Records brought together in this volume are highly instructive, and cast light on how to go about sorting and sizing up unusual and difficult cases. These case discussions also showcase an impressive display of clinical knowledge on the parts of both Dr. Samuels and Dr. Ropper. These two giants in neurology and in medicine at large contribute to many other publications. For instance they are the co-authors of Adams and Victor's *Principles of Neurology*. But this collection of their well done discussions of eighteen Cabot Cases will stand as a shining example of how to go about analyzing difficult clinical cases.

Arthur K. Asbury MD, FRCP
Van Meter Professor of Neurology Emeritus
University of Pennsylvania Perelman School of Medicine
3400 Spruce Street
Philadelphia, PA 19104–4283

FOREWORD

In Raymond Adams' *Foreword* to the book "Neurologic Clinicopathologic Conferences of the Massachusetts General Hospital" edited by Benjamin Castleman and E.P Richardson, Jr., and published just about 45 years ago, he remarks that, through the end of the nineteenth century, Neurology was taught to medical students largely by the demonstration of patients in the clinic. With the coming of the twentieth century, that practice was expanded in one important pedagogical innovation – the case method of teaching, espoused by Drs. Walter B Cannon and James Jackson Putnam, respectively, Professors of Physiology and of Neurology at Harvard Medical School. The case method of teaching became the technique employed in the "Cabot Cases" published since 1923 in *The Boston Medical and Surgical Journal* (now *The New England Journal of Medicine*) and has continued from that time to the present. The basic structure of the neurologic CPC included the detailed clinical discussion of the case and diagnosis, followed by the presentation of the neuropathologic findings. The choice of the fifty cases discussed in the span between 1938 and 1956, chosen for that volume was guided by selecting examples where the clinical analytical acumen of a distinguished staff, or invited neurologist allowed for the anatomic localization of the lesion (largely in the absence of radiologic information) and a final clinical diagnosis; a second criterion was the inclusion of a broad spectrum of the various classes of neurologic disease so as to demonstrate the most up-to-date understanding of the neuropathology and pathophysiology of the disease entity.

These principles have not changed in current compilation entitled *Neurologic CPCs from the New England Journal of Medicine*, by Martin Samuels and Allan Ropper (clinical discussants in each one of the cases) where they present a series of eighteen cases over the past forty years, giving a historical continuum to the earlier volume. What is particularly noteworthy about this monograph is the demonstration that careful and informed clinical analysis by an expert neurologist is still of utmost importance in reaching a diagnosis (however buttressed by the armamentarium of sophisticated imaging techniques). Furthermore, from the range of neurophysiologic and neuropathologic (biopsy or autopsy), and molecular diagnostic techniques presented by the faculty discussants, the extraordinary expansion of knowledge in laboratory diagnosis is amply illustrated. These advances emphasize the importance of continued research efforts in the laboratory so as to augment, on the one hand, diagnostic accuracy, and on the other, basic understanding of neurologic diseases. The cases chosen illustrate a broad range of neurologic illness including neoplasm, infectious and parainfectious inflammatory diseases, degenerative diseases, vascular and neuromuscular disease.

This time-honored tradition of the CPC continues at the Brigham and Women's Hospital through weekly sessions faithfully attended by Drs. Samuels and Ropper where a detailed case presentation is followed by clinical discussion before medical students and neurology residents and faculty. The neuroradiologic and neurophysiologic findings are then presented, and finally there follows a demonstration of the neuropathologic findings in a formal conference format, or at brain cutting. In that tradition, this volume will be welcome reading to any medical student, clinician, or pathologist interested in the methods of clinical and pathological analysis in neurologic diagnosis.

Umberto De Girolami, MD
Professor of Pathology,
Harvard Medical School
Neuropathologist, Brigham and
Women's Hospital,
Boston, Massachusetts

FOREWORD

When I was a first-year medical student, one of my favorite professors advised me to always read the *New England Journal of Medicine's* CPC to help build my knowledge base and diagnostic skills. Following this sage advice, I would eagerly grab the Journal when it arrived each week and immediately flip to the CPC. During this first year, the names of the diagnoses were indecipherable (yet alone correctly identifying them), but by the time I graduated, I could follow the discussions and occasionally find my way to the answer along with the discussant (although not as often as the medical students depicted in the Boston audience apparently).

Many neurologists move away from these CPCs as their careers progress and as training in internal medicine fades more into the rearview mirror. However, for the majority of us who still spend time in the hospital, these CPCs have transformed into a weekly tour of systemic disorders that are, in many cases, rarely encountered by us and serve as a reminder of their important relationship to neurologic diseases. We all feel a particular sense of excitement when a neurologic case or expert neurology discussant is selected as it illustrates to the larger medical community those always fascinating aspects of the nervous system and allows one of "our folks" to shine, demonstrating to all how we neurologists think.

Samuels and Ropper's Neurological CPCs from the New England Journal of Medicine is a wonderful tour of these neurologic CPCs, updated with important perspectives that allow one to view these disorders through the lens of modern pathophysiology and treatment. The commentaries provided also pull back the curtain on the inner workings of the CPC – quips that were removed, one-upmanship that emerged, and tales of the giants of medicine who participated in these discussions and contributed to the understanding of these important disorders. The discussants here are predictably marvelous in their thought process and neurologic approach, but what remains astonishing is the sheer breadth of central and peripheral nervous system diseases that are covered, serving as a fantastic neurologic review for a broad range of readers ranging from medical students to the most seasoned of practicing neurologists.

In the end, my professor was probably right in that everyone should take the time to read these CPCs on a weekly basis regardless of their specialty. As a neurologist though,

I cannot imagine a more perfect journey through "our" CPCs as the one that Martin Samuels and Allan Ropper are about to take you on...enjoy.

S. Andrew Josephson MD
Vice-Chairman and Associate Professor
Director, Neurohospitalist Program
Medical Director, Inpatient Neurology
University of California, San Francisco

PREFACE

Until the advent of systematic anatomy and pathology, doctors were literally in the dark, dependent on mystical views of disease dominated by astrology, theism, and unsubstantiated concepts of the causes of disease (e.g., the wrong mixture of the basic four humors: blood, plegm, black bile, and yellow bile). It is probable that human dissections were performed by some Arab and Greek physicians early in the common era, but preservation techniques were virtually unknown, making systematic study of tissue difficult or impossible.[1] It was not until the 19th century that microscopic pathology became practical and was popularized by Rudolf Virchow. Early pathologists, like Virchow, were practicing physicians who checked their diagnoses and improved their skills by performing autopsies on their own patients. Analysis of biopsy results, genetic tests, and imaging information were added later, of course, but served a similar purpose.

The practice of carefully analyzing case records and correlating the results with pathological findings was popularized in the United States by Richard Cabot, Harvard Medical School class of 1892, who apparently found that most physicians practicing early in the 20th century paid little attention to the autopsy results on their patients. Cabot found a powerful advocate for his method, Walter B. Cannon, Harvard Medical School Class of 1900. Cannon apparently had a roommate who was studying at the Harvard Law School, where the case method was already a well-established tradition, having been in place at least since the 1870s. Cannon proposed that detailed case histories should be placed into the curriculum in order to enliven the lecture-based medical education of the time. In 1915, Cabot arranged for a stenographer to record the case histories and their discussions and in 1924 this feature, known as the "Case Records of the Massachusetts General Hospital," began appearing as what has been the most recognizable feature of The *New England Journal of Medicine*.[2]

Over the course of the 20th century the Cabot Cases became known to virtually every doctor as the *New England Journal* "Clinico-Pathological Conference" (CPC). Many loyal readers would turn first to the CPC and try to make the diagnosis from the title alone. Matching wits with the experts (and the mysteriously almost always correct medical students) was a hobby of several generations of young doctors. Many fantasized about the apparently formal yet spontaneous discussion in which arcane truths seem to virtually spill from the mouths of the erudite discussers.

Those of us "in the know" realized that the discusser was carefully chosen and given the clinical summary several weeks before the exercise. Images could be reviewed in advance with all-knowing and friendly radiologists. We all know that the students had looked up the pathology, thus accounting for their uncanny accuracy. Behind the scenes during much of this era were Bill and Betty McNeely. Bill produced the formal yet elegant "protocols." Betty recorded the events on an old reel-to-reel tape recorder and then transcribed them, not unlike the stenographer of Dr. Cabot's time. During breaks, Betty could be found outside of the auditorium having a smoke. A roughly edited version would be delivered to the discussers (clinician and pathologist) a few weeks later, adjusted ever so slightly and then published with very little if anything removed from the often long and flowery discussions. To Betty's credit, no diagnosis was ever changed, so there were some missed diagnoses; but clearly the object of the game was to produce an elegant discourse demonstrating the process of diagnostic reasoning.

Efforts at humor had to be very subtle or they would be expunged. On one occasion the speaker revealed that he had inadvertently learned the diagnosis in advance. In another, the discusser found a paper in the literature describing the very case, complete with all the illustrations planned to be used by the pathologist. Once, a renowned neurologist declared that there was no such thing as a differential diagnosis: only a correct diagnosis preceded by list of incorrect diagnoses. Many discussions were spiced with the history of the condition, including its putative role in history, as with the porphyrias' influence on the American Revolution.

The current volume was inspired by a prior compilation of the neurological CPCs of the *New England Journal of Medicine*, edited by the late Edward P. Richardson, Jr., former chief of neuropathology at the Massachusetts General Hospital. We have been fortunate not only to have been exposed to Dr. Richardson's teachings but also have discussed the largest number of Cabot Cases. Here we have reprinted them, added some unpublished material from the archives, and added a brief commentary, which is meant to bring a more modern perspective to each disorder and its discussion. These cases cover a wide range of conditions of the nervous system and demonstrate a way of thinking that the authors believe remains the basis of refined clinical medicine.

In the 21st century, the value of the CPC has come into question. In recent years, the discussions have no longer been weekly; they are also shorter and more structured than in the past and largely devoid of historical perspective or medical humor. Some have argued that the old CPCs were stilted and encouraged a type of medicine that modern society could not afford, filled as they were with myriad studies, blood tests, and images. Our view is very much the opposite. In the 20th century, the case method was discovered, discarded, and rediscovered. The "inventors" of modern case-based medical education are largely unaware that the same idea occurred to Cabot and Cannon just about a century ago. The traditional values of medicine—marked as they are by dedication to the patient, careful history taking, and a broad knowledge of medical science as it applies to the patient at hand—has never changed and never will. The CPC method is a patient-centric, dignified, evidence-based, cost-effective, continuously improving method for learning the practice of medicine.

Judge for yourself. We hope you enjoy this volume.

MAS

AHR

1. Von Staden H. The discovery of the body: human dissection and its cultural contexts in ancient Greece. Yale J Biol Med 1992; 65: 223–241.
2. Ballaro B. Mystery Theater. Harvard Medicine 2005; 85: 12–17.

TABLE OF CONTENTS

SAMUELS

— & —

ROPPER'S

NEUROLOGICAL CPCs

FROM

THE NEW ENGLAND
JOURNAL OF MEDICINE

A 51-Year-Old Man with Neck Pain

FORAMEN MAGNUM MENINGIOMA
CPC 29-1979

PRESENTATION OF CASE

A 51-year-old right-handed man was admitted to the hospital because of neck pain.

Three years earlier he experienced aching pain in the left nuchal region. Evaluation, including x-ray films of the neck, led to a diagnosis of cervical arthritis with osteophytes at multiple levels. The administration of anti-inflammatory agents and cervical traction gave little relief. Sixteen months before admission the pain intensified. A cervical myelographic examination was reported to show a ventral extradural abnormality at the C3-C4 level and possibly at the C6-C7 level. Eleven months before entry anterior-disk removal and decompression were performed at the C6-C7 level, with only slight relief of pain for the next six weeks. During the succeeding months there was an increase in the severity of the pain, with occasional "burning" sensations in both shoulders and arms and in the fingertips. Temperature sensation decreased in the right hand, and weakness developed in the right arm and leg. The patient retired from his position as an insurance executive because of his disability. Nine months before admission he began to experience occasional diplopia on glancing to the left, and his speech was slightly thick. Weakness progressed in the right leg, and he was unable to stand up from a squatting posture.

Eight months before entry he returned to his local hospital. An edrophonium chloride test was reported to be positive, but subsequent neostigmine methylsulfate tests were negative. He was discharged on pyridostigmine bromide. One month later he returned to the same hospital because of the cervical pain and a nonspecific febrile illness. After recovery from the fever another cervical myelographic study disclosed a ventral extradural abnormality at the C5-C6 level; no defect was seen at C3-C4. A muscle biopsy revealed no abnormality; tests of thyroid function were negative. Pyridostigmine bromide was discontinued, and within a week the diplopia and dysarthria decreased; the neck pain persisted.

Six months before entry the patient was first seen at this hospital. Evaluation showed bilateral end-point nystagmus; ocular movements were full, and the other cranial nerves were intact. There was moderate weakness of the right arm, particularly of the upper portion, without fasciculations. A decrease in pinprick and cold sensation was demonstrated distal to the base of the neck and over the right shoulder and arm; the left shoulder and arm, trunk and lower parts of the body were spared. The tendon reflexes were +++ and symmetric; Babinski and Hoffmann reflexes were present bilaterally. Review of the initial cervical myelographic examination revealed ventral extradural abnormalities at C3-C4, C5-C6, and C6-C7, with osteophytic encroachment on the spinal canal at each of these levels; the defect at C6-C7 was not demonstrated on an examination performed postoperatively; contrast material was seen as high as C2. Two weeks later an extensive posterior laminectomy was performed at his local hospital. In the immediate postoperative period a right hemiparesis appeared; the cervical pain was not relieved. Motor function in the right extremities gradually improved with physical therapy, but severe, burning pain persisted in the posterior cervical region and affected the left hand; codeine and meperidine were required for relief. The patient gradually became able to walk with assistance but could not arise from a chair without help. Two weeks before entry he returned to the same hospital, complaining of severe neck pain and urinary hesitancy. Another cervical myelographic examination showed no interruption in flow of contrast material up to the C2-C3 level; small anterior defects were again seen at C5-C6 and C3-C4. A marked increase in weakness of the right extremities followed the procedure, accompanied by paresthesia in the left shoulder, arm and trunk. He was readmitted to this hospital.

A lumbar laminectomy was performed at the age of 31 years because of a ruptured intervertebral disk, with left sciatic pain. There was no family history of neurologic disease.

The temperature was 37°C, the pulse 80, and the respirations 18. The blood pressure was 120/80 mm Hg.

On examination the patient appeared despondent and chronically ill. The general physical examination was negative. Neurologic examination disclosed limitation of neck motion in all directions. End-point nystagmus was present on horizontal gaze, more prominently on gaze to the left. The gag reflex was diminished bilaterally; the uvula rose slightly on the right side. The tongue was midline, with fasciculations that were more conspicuous on the left side. The sternocleidomastoid and trapezius muscles were weak, especially on the right side. There was marked atrophy, with weakness of the right suprascapular, infrascapular, deltoid, biceps and triceps muscles, the wrist flexors and extensors and the intrinsic muscles of the hand; the right scapula was winged. Minimal weakness of the intrinsic muscles of the left hand was also observed. Pinprick and thermal sensations were diminished in a hemicape distribution from C2 to T5 on the right side. Hypalgesia and thermal hyperesthesia were observed over the left side of the neck and shoulder. Touch, vibratory and position senses as well as response to double simultaneous stimulation were intact on the neck, shoulders and arms. The tendon reflexes were +++ and symmetric except that the right-ankle jerk was ++++, with clonus, and the left-ankle jerk was absent. Bilateral Babinski signs were observed. The patient could stand but needed assistance in walking; he dragged the right leg.

The urine was normal. The hematocrit was 39.6 per cent; the white-cell count was 6000, with 54 per cent neutrophils. A serologic test for syphilis was negative.

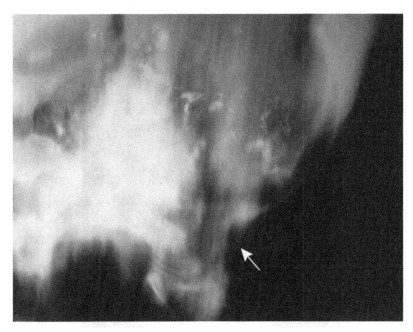

FIG 1 Pneumoencephalogram, Lateral View of the Posterior Fossa, Showing a Soft-Tissue Mass below the Foramen Magnum Posteriorly (Arrow).

Codeine and amitriptyline HCl were administered. Pain persisted, with little relief. On the seventh hospital day polytomograms of the cervical spine showed that the anteroposterior measurement of the foramen magnum was 36 mm; at the C1 level the anteroposterior measurement was 19 mm, and at C2, 14 mm. The remainder of the spinal canal was enlarged by a previous posterior laminectomy that extended from C3 to C6; there was an anterior fusion at the C6-C7 level. Minimal osteophyte formation extended posteriorly from the inferior portion of C3, and anterior osteophytes were seen at the C4-C5 level. A posterior-fossa and upper cervical pneumoencephalographic examination (Fig. 1) revealed a soft-tissue mass that extended caudally along with the contour of the cerebellar tonsils through the foramen magnum to the level of the upper margin of the lamina of the first cervical vertebra; the mass was dorsal to the spinal cord, and a separate contour of the tonsils was not seen. The spinal cord beneath the C1 level was not clearly defined. The fourth ventricle was in a normal position, and air entered the cisterna magna. The cerebrospinal fluid was clear and colorless and contained 2 red cells per cubic millimeter; xanthochromia was graded 1 on a scale of 10; the glucose was 74 mg, and the protein 175 mg per 100 ml; a culture yielded no growth of micro-organisms.

On the 11th hospital day the patient was unable to lift his right hand off the bed in the supine position; he could elevate his right heel 15 cm for 10 seconds. On the 14th hospital day a computed tomographic (CT) scan of the brain (Fig. 2), performed after the administration of contrast material, disclosed a small low-absorption area with a density value in the range of cerebrospinal fluid in the center of the spinal cord at the level of the foramen magnum; the remainder of the posterior fossa was normal.

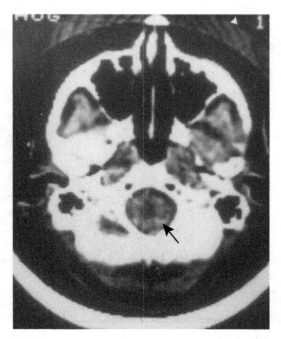

FIG 2   Computed Tomographic Scan of the Cranium at the Level of the Foramen Magnum, Revealing a Low-Absorption Area in the Center of the Upper Cervical Canal (Arrow).

A bilateral vertebral angiographic examination (Fig. 3 and 4) revealed no displacement of the tonsillar hemispheric branches; a tumor stain was present in the upper cervical region posterior to the cord. On the next day examination disclosed dissociated sensory loss for pain and temperature from C1 to T5 bilaterally. The bladder was distended, and he was unable to void. Catheterization yielded 440 ml of foul-smelling urine; ampicillin was begun. The temperature rose to 39.4 and fell promptly to 37.2°C. An x-ray film of the chest revealed no abnormality.

An operation was performed on the 18th hospital day.

DIFFERENTIAL DIAGNOSIS

Dr. Martin A. Samuels[*]: The principal interest in this case is not in the differential diagnosis since it is obvious that the patient had a tumor in the region of the foramen magnum. Of greater importance are the lessons learned from the course of the illness as well as several theoretic issues regarding upper cervical myelopathies.

This patient's illness began with pain in the neck, which in retrospect clearly resulted from an intraspinal tumor. It is well known that severe pain in the neck, which often radiates to the shoulders, hands or occipital region, is frequently the

[*] Associate in medicine (neurology), Peter Bent Brigham Hospital; chief, Neurology Section, Veterans Administration Hospital, West Roxbury, Massachusetts; assistant professor of neurology, Harvard Medical School. Currently Chair, Department of Neurology, Brigham and Women's Hospital.

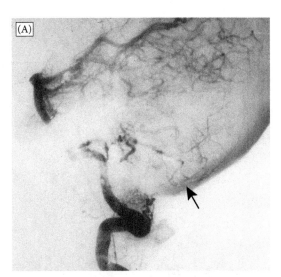

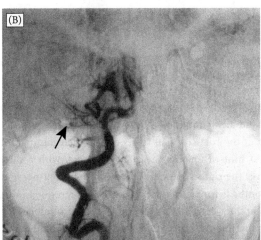

FIG 3 Anteroposterior (A) and Lateral (B) Views from the Right-Vertebral Angiographic Study, Showing a Normal Position of the Tonsillar Branches of the Posterior Inferior Cerebellar Arteries (Arrows).

major complaint of patients with a lesion at the level of the foramen magnum. It is not surprising that the attending physicians thought initially of a cervical radiculopathy, which is a much more common cause of neck pain than a neoplasm. However, when conservative measures failed to alleviate the symptoms, alternative diagnoses had to be considered. During a myelographic study 16 months before admission, the contrast material was not carried high enough to evaluate the region of the cervical–medullary junction. Instead, unimpressive anteriorly placed extradural defects were seen at C6-C7 and C3-C4, and a diskectomy, performed at C6-C7, failed to give benefit.

In fact, the patient's difficulties increased, and he entered the second phase of the illness, that of extramedullary myelopathy, with weakness developing in the right

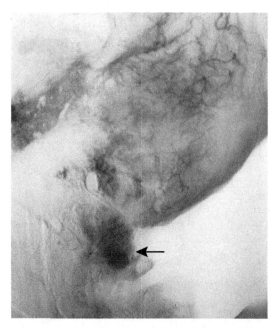

FIG 4 Left-Vertebral Arteriogram, Late Phase, Lateral View, Demonstrating a Tumor Stain in the Upper Posterior Cervical Canal (Arrow).

arm and leg. In the typical case of upper cervical extramedullary compression the contralateral leg and arm should be affected in that order because of the progressive compression of the corticospinal tracts due to their lamination.[1,2] In addition, there was the first hint of an intramedullary process, with a dissociated sensory loss beginning over the right shoulder. The signs of cranial-nerve dysfunction that emerged nine months before admission could have been due to direct involvement of cranial nerves in their extramedullary course or hydrobulbia. In either event, the combination of a myelopathy and cranial-nerve palsies should have drawn attention to the cervical–medullary junction. The second myelographic examination, performed seven months before entry, also failed to demonstrate that area. As a result, the attending clinicians were misled by the unimpressive anterior extradural defect and what seems almost certainly to have been a falsely positive edrophonium test. Anticholinesterases were later abandoned when they failed to alleviate and perhaps even worsened the patient's condition. Studies to exclude primary muscular disease with tests of thyroid function and a muscle biopsy were negative and reflect the confusion caused by the incomplete myelographic examinations.

The third phase of the illness began six months before admission, when for the first time there were unequivocal signs of an intramedullary process with a dissociated sensory loss over the right shoulder and arm, and the tendon reflexes were hyperactive, with bilateral Babinski signs. The right hemiparesis that appeared after the posterior laminectomy further suggests an intraspinal tumor, which often produces striking worsening of the myelopathy after the subarachnoidal space has been violated. The reason for such a change is unclear, but herniation of the mass may cause vascular embarrassment to the cord as a result of fluid shifts after removal of the cerebrospinal fluid below the mass. In this case the postoperative deterioration may well have been due to infarction of the cord for that reason. The third myelographic examination, performed just before transfer to this hospital, again resulted in deterioration, suggesting the presence of an intraspinal mass above the level of the lumbar puncture. Also, the study was once again carried only to the C2-C3 level.

On admission to this hospital there was an undeniable intramedullary syndrome with a dissociated sensory loss over the trunk, several cranial-nerve abnormalities and lower-motor-neuron weakness of all the muscles innervated from C5 to T1 on the right side. The reflexes were hyperactive, with Babinski signs.

Several findings are particularly noteworthy. First of all, lower-motor-neuron weakness of muscles innervated by roots well below the caudal extent of an upper cervical lesion is well known, having been described in 1913 by Oppenheim[3] and subsequently by many others. Whether this finding reflects myelomalacia due to vascular obstruction or hydromyelia remains unsettled. In this case the latter mechanism may have been operative. Liveson, Ransohoff and Goodgold[4] performed electrophysiologic testing on a patient with a foramen-magnum meningioma and showed denervation in all the muscles of an upper extremity, the roots for which, of course, were well below the caudal extent of that tumor.

Cranial-nerve abnormalities, which are well known manifestations of lesions in the region of the foramen magnum, are generally thought to result from cranial extension of the process. However, the cause of these abnormalities is usually an anterior mass that has interrupted cranial nerves, particularly IX through XII, as they pierce the dura en route to the jugular and hypoglossal foramens. A posterior mass could not produce cranial-nerve abnormalities by this mechanism, although torque forces on the medulla might account for them. In this case the long history of pain in the neck suggests that the tumor began intraspinally and extended cranially, a so-called spinocranial tumor, rather than the reverse. A second explanation for the cranial-nerve findings is hydrobulbia, which may also have been present in this patient.

A third possibility is the intramedullary syndrome, which may well have been a syringomyelic or hydromyelic complication of a lesion at the level of the foramen magnum. Intramedullary tumors have a well known association with syringomyelia, but extramedullary tumors are also accompanied by it, although far less often.[5] The term "syringomyelia" was coined by Charles Ollivier d'Angers[6] in 1827 to describe pathologic dilatation of the central canal in continuity with the fourth vehicle as a developmental anomaly. After Stilling,[7] in 1859, demonstrated that the central canal could persist in childhood and even into adult life in all vertebrates, the term "hydromyelia" was adopted for dilatation of this cavity. The designation "syringomyelia" was subsequently restricted to the presence of cord cavities unconnected with the central canal and associated with myelitis, tumors and gliosis. In 1888 Chiari[8] concluded that syringomyelia and hydromyelia were the same, recognizing their association with anatomic anomalies of the posterior fossa. In a series of papers published between 1957 and 1967 Gardner and his associates[9–13] proposed the so-called hydrodynamic theory of the development of syringomyelia, according to which cystic dilatation of the cord results from over-distention of the neural tube because of partial or complete obstruc-tion of the foramens of Luschka and Magendie. A cavity of such an origin communi-cates with the ventricular system and is often associated with hydrocephalus. In some cases, however, the cavity within the cord, whatever its cause, does not communicate with the ventricular system or the central canal. This noncommunicating syringo-myelia is seen after acute traumatic injury to the spinal cord and in association with intramedullary tumors. Therefore, hydromyelia and hydrobulbia properly refer to a communicating form of cystic myelopathy associated with obstructed outflow of the cerebrospinal fluid from the fourth ventricle of any cause, whereas syringomyelia in the strict sense of the term refers to a glia-lined cavity that does not communicate with the central canal or ventricular system and contains a proteinaceous material different from that of spinal fluid. Despite their different meanings these terms are still often used interchangeably.

In this case one could postulate the presence of a mass on the posterior rim of the fora-men magnum that produced two separate syndromes—an extra-medullary syndrome with severe pain and rigidity in the neck, followed by weakness and spasticity of the legs due to corticospinal-tract compression, and, secondly, a hydromyelia-hydrobulbia syndrome as a result of obstruction of spinal-fluid outflow from the fourth ventricle by the tumor. The second syndrome could account for the dissociated sensory loss cranial-nerve signs, lower-motor-neuron weakness and wasting of the right arm. Such a sequence of events, although rare, is known. Kosary et al.[14] reported a case of an occipital meningioma associated with an apparently communicating hydromyelia–hydrobulbia and hydrocephalus; removal of the tumor resulted in alleviation of the hydrocephalus and reduction in the size of the cord.

The only remaining task is to determine the nature of the mass in the region of the foramen magnum. The three most likely possibilities are a tumor, an arachnoidal cyst and a Chiari malformation. The early clinical course, which was dominated by the pain in the neck, suggests a tumor. The neuroradiologic procedures will undoubtedly be of help, and this is an appropriate time to examine the films.

Dr. JAMES M. DAVIS, III: The pneumoencephalograms show a soft-tissue mass that extends posteriorly below the foramen magnum (Fig. 1). It could represent cerebel-lar tonsillar herniation as part of a Chiari I malformation or a neoplasm. The cervical spinal cord is not outlined. The bilateral vertebral arteriograms (Fig. 3 and 4) were originally interpreted as normal. Subtraction views show no displacement of the ton-sillar branches of the posterior inferior cerebellar arteries below the foramen mag-num, making it unlikely that the soft-tissue mass seen on the pneumoencephalograms was composed of the cerebellar tonsils, although one occasionally encounters ton-sillar herniation without such displacement. No tumor vascularity was appreciated. A contrast-enhanced computed tomographic scan (Fig. 2), with particular reference to the foramen-magnum region, reveals a low-absorption area in the center of the upper cervical canal, which was originally interpreted as a central cavitation consistent with the diagnosis of syringomyelia but could have been normal cervical cord or a computer artifact. No abnormal contrast enhancement is seen. A review of the angiograms reveals enlarged muscular branches of the vertebral arteries, with the subsequent demonstration of a well demarcated homogeneous hypervascular stain in the upper cervical region posterior to the cord (Fig. 4). The probable diagnosis from the angiographic findings is a meningioma. Far less likely are a hemangioblastoma and a neurofibroma.

DR. SAMUELS: Did you ever perform a study with metrizamide?

DR. PAUL F. J. NEW: No. It was not available when we completed the investigative work.

DR. SAMUELS: Do you have any more rostral cuts of the CT scan to give some indication whether there was hydrocephalus?

DR. DAVIS: No.

DR. SAMUELS: In one of the lower cuts the temporal horns of the lateral ventricles appear somewhat prominent, consistent with hydrocephalus. Is the mass extradural or intradural?

DR. NEW: Intradural.

DR. SAMUELS: The neuroradiologic procedures have helped considerably in limiting the differential diagnosis. The pneumoencephalograms document the presence of an intradural, extramedullary mass in the region of the posterior lip of the foramen magnum. The angiograms demonstrate that the mass was not the cerebellar tonsils, thus excluding a Chiari malformation, and furthermore show an impressive tumor stain, suggesting that the mass was a neoplasm and not an arachnoidal cyst. In addition, I believe that the CT scan suggests hydrocephalus and may indicate the presence of hydromyelia and hydrobulbia as well. However, experience with interpretation of the CT scan in this region is very limited. Without the use of metrizamide, which helps to differentiate the cord itself from cysts within the cord, it is difficult to be certain that a cyst was not present in this case.

What type of tumor could this mass have been? In most large series meningiomas and neurofibromas account for about 98 per cent of tumors in this region, with the former being about five times more common than the latter. This fact, combined with the very prominent vascular stain seen on the angiograms, makes a meningioma the more likely diagnosis. Two small points favor a neurofibroma, however. There is a higher proportion of male patients among those with a neurofibroma, and a higher proportion of female patients among those with a meningioma, but since the overall frequency of meningiomas in this region is five times greater than that of neurofibromas, a meningioma is more likely. This tumor was posterior, whereas most meningiomas in this region are anterior or lateral to the cord and brainstem. Posterior meningiomas have been reported, however. Other neoplasms, such as lipomas, cavernous hemangiomas, cystic teratomas and metastatic tumors, are exceedingly rare in this region. Moreover, most of those tumors are epidural rather than intradural and extramedullary.[15]

This case may be of great theoretic importance since the medical literature repeatedly states that foramen-magnum tumors may simulate syringomyelia. How does this simulation occur? Is it the result of vascular insufficiency of the cord or hydromyelia? If it is the latter, by what mechanism does it occur? Since most foramen-magnum tumors are anterior or lateral, when they extend cranially they can produce palsies of the cranial nerves by interfering with their extramedullary courses. The rarer posterior tumors, in contrast, could extend into the region of the foramens of Luschka and Magendie or distort that region sufficiently to interfere with the outflow of cerebrospinal fluid from the ventricular system, producing hydromyelia, hydrobulbia and hydrocephalus, just as a mass composed of the cerebellar tonsils might do in a Chiari malformation. This hydrodynamic mechanism seems to have been in operation in this case, and if so a repeated postoperative CT scan should have demonstrated resolution of both the hydrocephalus and the hydrobulbia.

In conclusion, I think that the operation was an exploration of the foramen magnum and perhaps the posterior fossa. I propose that it revealed an intradural, extramedullary tumor, probably a meningioma, which was posterior to the spinal cord in the region of the foramen magnum and extended cranially to obstruct outflow from the fourth ventricle. Secondary communicating hydromyelia, hydrobulbia and hydrocephalus resulted.

Dr. Ernest H. Picard: I'd like to add two other differential diagnostic considerations to the types of tumor that occur in this area. A patient currently in this hospital has a chondrosarcoma in that location, and I know of another patient who had a melanoma that apparently arose primarily from the meninges in that region.

Dr. Nicholas T. Zervas: Dr. Samuels, what do you think happened to the intrinsic muscles of the hands after the operation? Would the fasciculations and atrophy disappear?

Dr. Samuels: Unfortunately, those manifestations may have resulted from death of anterior horn cells. One would hope that the progression would stop, but it seems doubtful that there would be improvement.

Dr. New: It is disappointing that the contrast-infusion CT scan failed to reveal an enhancing mass, a characteristic feature of meningiomas unless they are heavily calcified, when they are very dense on plain scans. We have subsequently studied another patient in whom an anterior tumor in the region of the foramen magnum appeared as a large mass of soft tissue in the foramen magnum on the CT scan but did not have the characteristic enhancement of a tumor.

CLINICAL DIAGNOSIS

Cervicomedullary compression, ? due to syringobulbia or tumor.

DR. MARTIN A. SAMUEL'S DIAGNOSIS

Meningioma, with cranial extension and obstruction of foramens of Luschka and Magendie, resulting in communicating hydrocephalus, hydrobulbia and hydromyelia.

PATHOLOGICAL DISCUSSION

Dr. Edward P. Richardson, Jr.: The operation was done by Dr. Crowell with the assistance of Dr. Robert L. Martuza. Dr. Crowell, will you tell us your findings?

Dr. Robert M. Crowell: We performed a suboccipital craniectomy, and removal of the posterior arch of the first cervical vertebra revealed a tumor, 3 by 1.5 cm, lying to the left of the cervicomedullary junction and causing marked compression of the spinal cord and medulla. The tumor was totally removed microsurgically, and the left vertebral artery, to which it was attached, was carefully preserved.

Postoperatively, there was slight leakage of cerebrospinal fluid for a few days, but the pain disappeared almost immediately after the procedure. Neurologic examination two months after the operation showed only slight weakness in the right upper extremity and slight sensory abnormalities in the right hand.

A PHYSICIAN: Dr. Crowell, did you find that the outlets of the fourth ventricle were involved by the tumor and that there was expansion of the cervical cord?

DR. CROWELL: The outlets of the fourth ventricle were probably obliterated by the tumor externally, and the spinal cord seemed compressed in such a way that it did not permit the existence of a substantial fluid collection within it. We considered the possibility of needling the cord to ascertain whether it contained fluid, but that seemed too risky.

DR. RICHARDSON: Dr. Kleinman will describe the tumor.

DR. GEORGE M. KLEINMAN: The tumor was circumscribed and consisted of lobules of neoplastic cells separated by fine fibrovascular septa (Fig. 5). The reticulin stain demonstrated that the fibrils were generally confined to the septa and did not penetrate between individual tumor cells. The cells were polygonal to fusiform and had eosinophilic cytoplasm and indistinct margins. The nuclei were oval, with delicate nuclear membranes, fine chromatin and one or more nucleoli. In a few areas the tumor cells formed concentric whorls; elsewhere they were stellate and finely fibrillar, giving the tumor a microcystic appearance. This appearance is characteristic of a meningotheliomatous meningioma.

The classification of meningiomas is complicated because of three features. First of all, the tumor cells vary from large and polygonal in the meningotheliomatous or syncytial type to elongated and spindleshaped in the fibroblastic type; intermediate forms are

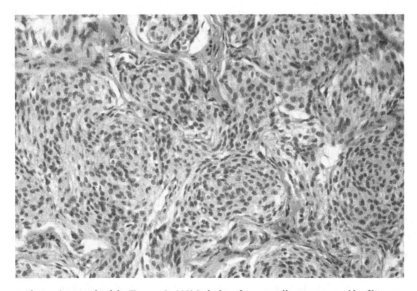

FIG 5 Photomicrograph of the Tumor. (× 320) Lobules of tumor cells are separated by fibrous septa.

referred to as the transitional type.[16–21] There is no apparent difference in the prognosis for these three types.[16,17,20] Secondly, superimposed on the various cellular patterns are several secondary alterations, such as xanthomatous changes, characterized by abundant cells with foamy cytoplasm scattered throughout the tumor, or focal areas of microcystic appearance.[16,17,22,23] There may also be foci of fibrosis and calcification, and at times metaplastic bone or cartilage can be identified.[16–21,23] Thirdly, the vascularity of these tumors varies greatly. In some cases the vessels are confined to the fibrovascular septa, but in other cases they are sufficiently extensive to obscure the nests of neoplastic cells.[16–20]

The term "meningioma" is convenient and widely accepted[16,17,20] but is not completely satisfactory since it does not designate the histologic attributes of the tumor. Cushing and Eisenhardt[21] used the term because they considered it simple, noncommittal and all-embracing. Currently, the designation indicates a meningothelial tumor, a more restrictive definition that Cushing and his associates used. For example, Cushing and Eisenhardt classified chondrosarcoma of the meninges as "chondroblastic meningioma" and believed that the "fibroblastic meningioma" was the most aggressive type. That conclusion was not substantiated by other observers, who found that the so-called angioblastic variety was the most malignant.[16,17,20,22] Subsequently, it has been debated whether some of these aggressive or malignant meningeal tumors should be classified as meningiomas or as soft-tissue neoplasms.[22,24–27] Thus, the so-called angioblastic meningiomas may include two different types of tumor[17,19,20,22,24–26]—the hemangiopericytoma, which is indistinguishable from the hemangiopericytoma of soft tissues, a locally aggressive tumor with a tendency to repeated recurrence and eventual metastasis,[26,28] and the hemangioblastoma, which is benign and histologically indistinguishable from the capillary hemangioblastoma of the cerebellum.[19,20,22,25]

Some malignant tumors of the meninges clearly belong in the meningioma group.[16,17,24,29,30] These tumors tend to infiltrate rather than compress the brain and eventually may metastasize, most often to the lungs and bone. On microscopical examination they are similar to benign meningiomas but often can be distinguished because of their increased cellularity, mitotic activity and pleomorphism.[24,29,30] A papillary arrangement of the tumor cells around fibrovascular cores has also been correlated with an aggressive behavior.[31] None of these features were present in this case, and this tumor is classified as a benign meningotheliomatous meningioma.

DR. RICHARDSON: One might wonder whether the histologic features of this tumor accounted for the fact that it did not show the contrast enhancement on computed tomographic scanning that usually occurs with meningiomas. Is that possible, Dr. New? As Dr. Kleinman has shown, it was a rather densely cellular tumor with relatively little vascularization.

DR. NEW: The contrast enhancement of meningiomas, like that of other intracranial neoplasms, is mainly due to leakage of contrast material from the tumor vessels. Tumor enhancement in general is due mainly to extravascular contrast material, and meningiomas that are not heavily calcified can be expected to enhance considerably. Well marked enhancement of meningiomas with minimal vascularity shown on angiographic study is a common finding. The lack of visible enhancement of the meningioma in this case and in the other case that I mentioned is puzzling and is not readily explained solely on the basis of computer artifacts.

ANATOMICAL DIAGNOSIS

Meningotheliomatous meningioma.

REFERENCES

1. Elsberg CA: Tumors of the Spinal Cord and the Symptoms of Irritation and Compression of the Spinal Cord and Nerve Roots: Pathology, symptomatology, diagnosis and treatment. New York, Paul B Hoeber, 1925

2. Symonds CP, Meadows SP: Compression of the spinal cord in the neighbourhood of the foramen magnum. Brain 60:52–84, 1937

3. Oppenheim H: Weitere Beiträge zur Diagnose und Differentialdiagnose des Tumor Medullae Spinalis. Monatsschr Psychiatr Neurol 33:451–93, 1913

4. Liveson JA, Ransohoff J, Goodgold J: Electromyographic studies in a case of foramen magnum meningioma. J Neurol Neurosurg Psychiatry 36:561–4, 1973

5. Poser CM: The Relationship between Syringomyelia and Neoplasm. Springfield, Illinois, Charles C Thomas, Publisher, 1956

6. Ollivier CP: De la Moëlle Epinère et de ses Maladies. Paris, Crevot, 1827

7. Stilling B: Neue Untersuchungen über den Bau des Rückenmarks. Casel, Commissions-Verlag von Heinrich Hotop, 1859, p. 13

8. Chiari H: Uber die Pathogenese der sogenannten Syrïngomyelie. Z Heilkunde 9:307–21, 1888

9. Gardner WJ, Abdullah AF, McCormack LJ: The varying expressions of embryonal atresia of fourth ventricle in adults: Arnold-Chiari malformation, Dandy-Walker syndrome, "arachnoid" cyst of cerebellum and syringomyelia. J Neurosurg 14:591–600, 1957

10. Gardner WJ, Karnosh LJ, Angel J: Syringomyelia: a result of embryonal atresia of the foramen of Magendie. Trans Am Neurol Assoc 82:144–61, 1957

11. Gardner WJ, Angel J: The mechanism of syringomyelia and its surgical correction. Clin Neurosurg 6:131–40, 1958

12. Gardner WJ: Hydrodynamic mechanism for syringomyelia: its relationship to myelocele. J Neurol Neurosurg Psychiatry 28:247–60, 1965

13. *Idem:* Myelocele: rupture of the neural tube? Clin Neurosurg 15:57–79, 1967

14. Kosary IZ, Braham J, Shaked I, et al: Cervical syringomyelia associated with occipital meningioma. Neurology (Minneap) 19:1127–30, 1969

15. Cohen L: Tumors in the region of the foramen magnum. Handbook of Clinical Neurology. Vol 17. Edited by PJ Vinken, GW Bruyn. Amsterdam, North-Holland Publishing, 1975, pp. 719–30

16. Rubinstein LJ: Tumors of the Central Nervous System (Atlas of Tumor Pathology, Fase 6, Second Series). Washington, DC. Armed Forces Institute of Pathology, 1972, pp. 169–90

17. Russell DS, Rubinstein LJ: Pathology of Tumours of the Nervous System. Fourth edition. London, Arnold, 1977

18. Ball J, Cook TA, Lynch PG, et al: Mixed mesenchymal differentiation in meningiomas. J Pathol 116:253–8, 1975

19. Burger PC, Vogel FS: Frozen section interpretation in surgical neuropathology. I. Intracranial lesions. Am J Surg Pathol 1:323–47, 1977

20. *Idem:* Surgical Pathology of the Nervous System and Its Coverings. New York, John Wiley & Sons, 1976

21. Cushing H, Eisenhardt L: Meningiomas: Their classification, regional behaviour, life history, and surgical end results. Springfield, Illinois. Charles C Thomas, Publisher, 1938

22. Pitkethly DT, Hardman JM, Kempe LG, et al: Angioblastic meningiomas: clinicopathologic study of 81 cases. J Neurosurg 32:539–44, 1970

23. Garrido DO, Kepes JJ: Histologic variants of meningiomas: interrelations between subgroups. J Neuropathol Exp Neurol 37:616, 1978

24. Jellinger K, Slowik F: Histological subtypes and prognostic problems in meningiomas. J Neurol 208:279–98, 1975

25. Horten BC, Urich H, Rubinstein LJ, et al: The angioblastic meningioma: a reappraisal of a nosological problem. J Neurol Sci 31:387–410, 1977

26. Goellner JR, Laws E Jr, Soule EH, et al: Hemangiopericytoma of the meninges: Mayo Clinic experience. Am J Clin Pathol 70:375–80, 1978

27. Kernohan JW, Uihlein A: Sarcomas of the Brain. Springfield, Illinois, Charles C Thomas, Publisher, 1962

28. Enzinger FM, Smith BH: Hemangiopericytoma: an analysis of 106 cases. Hum Pathol 7:61–82, 1976

29. Repola D, Weatherbee L: Meningioma with sarcomatous change and hepatic metastasis. Arch Pathol Lab Med 100:667–9, 1976

30. Tytus JS, Lasersohn JT, Reifel E: The problem of malignancy in meningiomas. J Neurosurg 27:551–7, 1967

31. Ludwin SK, Rubinstein LJ, Russell DS: Papillary meningioma: a malignant variant of meningioma. Cancer 36:1363–73, 1975

Perspectives and Updates

This was my first Cabot Case discussion and in it I established a clinical and didactic method that I follow to this day. The principle is to not make the case too complicated (Ockham's razor) and to avoid treating the exercise as a game. This has proved somewhat prescient, as detractors of the CPC methodology have argued that the clinical thinking demonstrated therein is stilted, overly arcane, and that it encourages excessively expensive care by seeking zebras instead of horses. As an aside, some years ago I was acting as visiting professor at the Groot Schuur Hospital in Capetown. The conference room overlooked a meadow, in which were grazing several dozen four-legged creatures with black and white stripes. Squinting out the window at this unusual pastoral scene, I declared: "horses." A chuckle erupted in the room and the senior South African professor replied: "When you hear the sound of hoofbeats, think of zebras; not horses." An important lesson: what is considered common depends on the context.

With just over 30 years of medical progress behind us, there are two aspects of this important case that are worth embellishing.

The first is the role of imaging in diagnosis. In 1979, the clinical presentation sounded like a lesion at the foramen magnum, but the available imaging techniques (myelography using air or contrast) required great skill. It was, as it were, an extension of the clinician's hands. In fact, studies of this type were often performed by neurologists, who needed a fairly good idea of what they were seeking, as the study required proper patient positioning as every part of the nervous system could not be studied at once. In this case, the error occurred when myelography was not carried high enough to image the relevant locations (the foramen magnum). Subsequently, when it *was* carried high enough, the myelography needle was not removed and the patient was not turned into the supine position to allow contrast material to settle into the location of the tumor on the posterior rim of the foramen magnum. Removing the needle and turning the patient over was not done routinely for mundane cervical spine problems as this required a repeat lumbar puncture to remove the contrast material, which was oil (prior to the development of water-soluble agents) in order to avoid arachnoiditis, a rare but serious complication of oil-based contrast materials. In the current era, the tumor would have likely been found on either a cranial or cervical spine MRI, even without the injection of the relatively low-risk metrizamide contrast material. In one sense, this marks a clear improvement based on better technology, but this approach is subject to unearthing radiological findings that have no relevance to the patient's condition (incidentalomas). Thus one problem has been replaced by another.

The second interesting aspect of this case is the denervation found in several roots to the upper extremity, well below the caudal extent of the meningioma. In the discussion, I tried to address this issue by referring to the then current views about the generation of intramedullary processes caused by lesions in the region of the foramen magnum. I went to great pains to distinguish hydromyelia (i.e., a cyst in the spinal cord emanating from the central canal and filled with spinal fluid) and syringomyelia (i.e., a cyst in the spinal cord, not in direct communication with the central canal, lined with glial cells and filled with an extracellular fluid that may not be spinal fluid). The theories of the generation of cysts within the spinal cord in various circumstances were those of Gardner (the hydrodymanic theory, which mainly addressed hydromyelia), Oldfield (which emphasized the effect of the cerebellar tonsils acting as pistons, which forced fluids from the subarachnoid space into the perivascular and interstitial spaces), and William (which argued that the differential between intracranial pressure and initraspinal pressure caused a craniospinal gradient, drawing fluid into a developing syrinx).

In recent years, the rigid distinctions among the various theories have merged into more of a unifying hypothesis. Greitz[1] has argued convincingly, using human and animal data, that the driving force behind the development of the cyst in the cord is intraspinal and that this leads to extracellular fluid accumulation. The current theory is synthetic in that it accounts for hydromyelia and syringomyelia in various circumstances, including lesions in the posterior fossa (e.g., a meningioma, as in this case, or a Chiari I malformation) or maldevelopment of the posterior fossa and cervical medullary junction (e.g., the Chiari II–Arnold Chiari malformation) in the case of spinal tumors and in post-traumatic myelopathy.

Thus Case 29-1979 was prescient in that it suggested a direction for future research which could explain a myelopathy well below the caudal extent of a lesion in the region of the foramen magnum.

Martin A. Samuels

REFERENCE

1. Greitz D. Unraveling the riddle of syringomyelia. Neurosurg Rev 2006; 29:251–63.

A 68-Year-Old Man with a Gait Disorder

PAGET DISEASE WITH EXTRAMEDULLARY HEMATOPOIESIS

CPC 23-1981

PRESENTATION OF CASE

First admission. A 68-year-old man was admitted to the hospital because of inability to walk.

There was a long history of Paget's disease of bone. Four years before admission urinary retention developed and led to the findings of a urethral stricture and benign prostatic hypertrophy. A urethrotomy was performed. An x-ray film of the chest showed a smooth, elongated paravertebral density parallel to the right cardiac border, interpreted as extraosseous Paget's disease. Two years before entry the patient returned to the hospital because of cellulitis of the left leg. Examination disclosed that the liver descended 4 cm below the right costal margin, with a vertical span of 14 cm. An x-ray film of the chest demonstrated the same paravertebral density; the heart was enlarged, and the lungs were clear; changes of Paget's disease were visible in multiple ribs, vertebras, the left clavicle and scapula, and the right humerus. A left pelvic venographic examination revealed that the common iliac vein was compressed but patent. An intravenous pyelographic examination disclosed an extrinsic impression upon the left lateral wall of the bladder by a soft-tissue density, with displacement and elevation of the distal portion of the left ureter. A barium-enema examination demonstrated a pelvic mass, 15 cm in diameter, that displaced the distal sigmoid colon to the right and superiorly. A ^{99m}Tc sulfur colloid liverspleen scan showed normal radionuclide activity within the liver; the spleen was slightly enlarged, with increased activity of radionuclide. A needle-aspiration biopsy of the mass disclosed mature fatty tissue with hematopoietic elements. Laparotomy revealed a large mass in the left side of the pelvis that appeared to erode the ischium and was attached to the posterior aspect of the pubis; microscopical examination of the excised mass showed a myelolipoma.

Calcitonin was administered because of bone pain. After the operation the patient complained of persistent leg cramps. Neurologic examination disclosed an abnormal gait attributable to bony deformities and pain. Sensation was decreased in all modalities in the lower extremities, predominantly on the left side. The tendon reflexes were ++ and equal except that the ankle jerks were absent bilaterally; the plantar responses were flexor. Phenytoin sodium was prescribed. The bony deformities extended and worsened during the next few months. Three days before admission the patient became unable to walk and was brought to the hospital.

There was a long history of cardiac enlargement, without evidence of congestive heart failure. The patient had chronic obstructive pulmonary disease secondary to longstanding abuse of tobacco, and a gastric ulcer had been demonstrated elsewhere in the past. There was no history of chills, chest pain, hemoptysis, dyspnea, or symptoms of nephrolithiasis.

The temperature was 36.8°C, the pulse 84, and the respirations 18. The blood pressure was 120/60 mm Hg.

The patient was a small elderly man with marked, extensive bony deformities of Paget's disease. The carotid pulses were ++, with a systolic bruit on the left side. The lungs were clear. The heart was enlarged, and a Grade 2 systolic murmur was heard at the apex and along the lower left sternal border. The edge of the liver extended 7 cm below the right costal margin, with a vertical span of 13 cm, and was non-tender; the splenic tip was barely palpable. Rectal examination was negative. The right femoral pulse was ++; the left femoral pulse and all distal pulses on both sides were absent; +++ edema of the left leg and ++ edema of the right leg were observed. Neurologic examination revealed moderate weakness of the legs; the tendon reflexes were ++ in the upper extremities and absent in the lower extremities; bilateral Babinski signs were found. There was diminished hearing in both ears.

The urine was normal. A stool specimen gave a negative test for occult blood. The hematocrit was 36.4 per cent; the white-cell count was 8400, with 57 per cent neutrophils. The urea nitrogen was 26 mg per 100 ml (9.3 mmol per liter), the creatinine 0.9 mg per 100 ml (75.6 μmol per liter), the glucose 99 mg per 100 ml (5.5 mmol per liter), the uric acid 11.2 mg per 100 ml (0.7 mmol per liter), the calcium 9.2 mg per 100 ml (2.3 mmol per liter), the phosphorus 2.7 mg per 100 ml (0.9 mmol per liter), the bilirubin 0.4 mg per 100 ml (6.8 μmol per liter), and the protein 7.6 g (the albumin 3.6 g, and the globulin 4.0 g) per 100 ml. The sodium was 132 mmol, the potassium 4.8 mmol. the chloride 97 mmol, and the carbon dioxide 26 mmol per liter. The serum aspartate aminotransferase (SGOT) was 29 U per milliliter (0.2 μmol $\cdot$ sec^{-1} per liter), the lactic dehydrogenase 137 U per milliliter (2.3 μmol $\cdot$ sec^{-1} per liter), the creatine phosphokinase 28 mU per milliliter (0.5 μmol $\cdot$ sec^{-1} per liter), the alkaline phosphatase 499 IU (8.3 μmol $\cdot$ sec^{-1}) per liter, and the acid phosphatase 0.4 Fishman-Lerner U. An electrocardiogram was normal. An x-ray film of the chest was unchanged. Films of the left knee revealed progression of Paget's disease, which involved the left femur and tibia; vascular calcification was evident. A venographic examination of the left leg showed a small clot in the superficial venous system distal to the knee, without other vascular abnormality. The vitamin B$_{12}$ level was normal.

Oxacillin was given by vein for one week, followed by dicloxacillin given by mouth. The dose of calcitonin was increased. The patient's intellectual function was intact, and the cranial nerves were normal aside from deafness. Motor function was normal in the upper extremities; muscle tone was diminished in the legs, with marked weakness, especially on the right side. Pain sensation was intact; position and vibratory sensations were absent at the toes and ankles and markedly decreased at the knees; bilateral Babinski

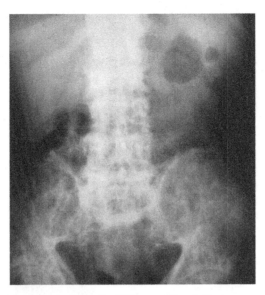

FIG 1 Radiograph of the Abdomen, Revealing Widespread Paget's Disease.

signs were present; no sensory level could be demonstrated on the trunk. X-ray films of the spine and pelvis demonstrated advanced pagetic changes throughout the axial skeleton (Fig. 1) and a mass adjacent to the 10th through the 12th thoracic vertebras, with smooth, elliptical lateral displacement of the left paravertebral stripe (Fig. 2). Films of the skull disclosed extensive pagetic change, with diffuse bony thickening, patchy sclerosis and osteolysis, and basilar impression. A lumbar and thoracic myelographic examination showed a questionable osteolytic lesion at the T10-T11 level; the procedure was technically difficult, and only a small amount of contrast material could be injected into the subarachnoid space; there was no evidence of a block in the lower thoracic or lumbar region. Tomographic examination of the lower thoracic spine (Fig. 3) revealed a large area of osteolysis that obliterated the vertebral end plates and rendered the vertebral bodies and intervertebral-disk spaces indistinguishable; the area did not appear invaded by or in communication with the paravertebral mass; residual contrast material showed no impingement on the vertebral canal at these levels. Nerve-conduction studies of the right extremities demonstrated diffuse and slightly abnormal motor-conduction velocity, slowed late responses, and electrophysiologic evidence of active denervation in all sampled muscles; there was evidence of right-carpal-tunnel compression.

During the first 10 days in the hospital the paraparesis progressed to almost complete flaccid paralysis of the lower extremities. A 10-day course of mithramycin (1.5 mg given intravenously over eight hours daily for 10 days) was substituted for calcitonin, with almost complete cessation of bone pain within four days and a marked increase in the strength of the legs over the ensuing six days; the patient gradually became able to walk with the aid of a stationary walker. The alkaline phosphatase fell to 176 IU (2.9μmol · sec^{-1}) per liter. A maintenance dose of mithramycin (1.0 mg given intravenously every two to four weeks) was continued for two years, with satisfactory ambulation and control of bone pain. Muscle cramps persisted, and quinine was substituted for phenytoin sodium. The patient was discharged to a nursing home.

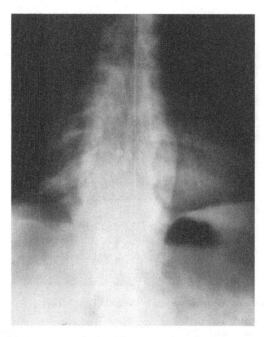

FIG 2   Radiograph of the Lower Dorsal Spine. Showing a Bilateral Soft-Tissue Paraspinal Mass.

Final admission (30 months later). Four months after discharge hematochezia occurred, and the patient returned to the hospital, where sigmoidoscopic examination disclosed internal hemorrhoids, without active bleeding; guaiac-positive liquid stool issued from a higher level. A barium-enema examination was negative. An upper gastrointestinal series revealed a large prepyloric gastric ulcer and deformity of the duodenal cap. A Pentagastrin stimulation test gave results normal for the patient's age. He returned to the nursing home, where he continued a barely ambulatory existence until the day of admission, when he fell and was unable to arise because of pain in the left leg.

The temperature was 37.1°C, the pulse 92, and the respirations 24. The blood pressure was 140/60 mm Hg.

On examination the patient was agitated, in pain, and very deaf. Extensive bony deformities were again noted. Rhonchi were audible throughout both lungs. The heart was enlarged, and a Grade 2 systolic ejection murmur was heard along the lower left sternal border. Abdominal examination was negative. There was no peripheral edema. No pulses were palpated distal to the femoral arteries; the toes were cool. Neurologic examination was inadequate because of the patient's disoriented and uncooperative state. There was spontaneous movement of the right leg and toes and of the left hip and thigh but none distal to the level of a left femoral fracture. Noxious stimuli resulted in grimacing and withdrawal of the right leg and left thigh.

The urine was normal. The hematocrit was 28.4 per cent, and the white-cell count 12,600. The platelet count was 270,000. The prothrombin time and the partial thromboplastin time were normal. The urea nitrogen was 42 mg per 100 ml (14.9 mmol per liter), the creatinine 2.1 mg per 100 ml (185.6 µmol per liter), the glucose 130 mg per

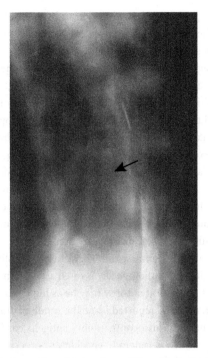

FIG 3 Polytomogram of the Lower Dorsal Spine, Lateral View, Disclosing Lytic Defects in the Ninth, 10th, and 11th Thoracic Vertebral Bodies (Arrows).

Retained myelographic contrast material discloses anterior displacement of the spinal cord by a posterior extradural mass.

100 ml (7.2 mmol per liter), and the bilirubin 0.3 mg per 100 ml (5.1 μmol per liter). The SGOT was 22 U per milliliter (0.18 μmol · sec^{-1} per liter), the amylase 26 U, and the alkaline phosphatase 773 IU (12.9 μmol · sec^{-1} per liter. An electrocardiogram and an x-ray film of the chest were unchanged. X-ray films of the left femur confirmed the presence of a fracture through an area of pagetic bone.

A cast was applied to the left lower extremity. The hospital course was complicated by a urinary-tract infection and by cholecystitis that required a cholecystectomy. Recurrent upper gastrointestinal bleeding led to a hemigastrectomy and vagotomy, which were succeeded by decubitus ulceration, pneumonia, pulmonary edema, renal failure, and sepsis. The patient died on the 76th hospital day.

DIFFERENTIAL DIAGNOSIS

Dr. Martin A. Samuels[*]: This case has multiple facets that are interwoven in a very interesting way. I shall discuss it in five parts: Paget's disease (PD) of bone;

[*] Chief, Neurology Section, Veterans Administration Medical Center. West Roxbury, Mass.; junior associate in medicine (neurology). Brigham and Women's Hospital; assistant professor of neurology, Harvard Medical School. Currently Chair, Department of Neurology, Brigham and Women's Hospital.

extramedullary hematopoiesis (EMH); the relation between PD and EMH; the neurologic picture; and the treatment of the patient with calcitonin and mithramycin, including the possible complications of such therapy.

In 1877 Sir James Paget[1] described an advanced case of a bone disease that he called "osteitis deformans" because of the gross thickening and elongation of the bones and the associated deformities. An excellent discussion of the history, clinical manifestations, and pathological findings of Paget's disease was written by Jaffe.[2] This disease is "a focal disorder of unknown etiology characterized initially by excessive resorption and subsequently by excessive formation of bone culminating in a 'mosaic' pattern of lamellar bone associated with extensive local vascularity and increased fibrous tissue in adjacent marrow."[3] Epidemiologic investigation has shown an extremely variable prevalence throughout the world and even within single countries. The disease is known worldwide, but most cases are seen in the United Kingdom, Australia, New Zealand, Germany, France, and the United States. It is very rare in India, China, Japan, the Middle East, Africa, and Scandinavia.[4] There may be a slight male preponderance.[5] The disorder as defined pathologically is often asymptomatic. The frequency in patients over the age of 40 years at autopsy may be as high as 3 per cent.[6] Some cases of familial clustering have been reported,[7] but the mode of transmission is unclear, and no specific distribution of histocompatibility antigens has been found.[8] The histopathologic evolution of PD is generally considered to occur in three phases. The initial osteolytic phase is believed to result from focal resorption of bone by bizarre osteoclasts, which may contain as many as 100 nuclei, more than are seen in any other known metabolic bone disease.[9] Rarely, the osteolytic phase is seen in pure form as osteoporosis circumscripta; which may be an incidental finding in x-ray studies done for other reasons. Even in these cases, however, biopsies usually show some evidence of osteoblastic response. Prominent bone formation characterizes the second, or mixed, phase of the disease, in which abnormal lamellar bone is found adjacent to areas of resorption. Replacement of the normal marrow by connective tissue and hypervascularity are also observed. Both trabecular and cortical bone participate in this phase. The third phase, the osteoblastic or sclerotic phase, is marked by decreased osteoclastic activity with an increase in the amount of bone per unit volume due to the continued deposition of lamellar bone in a typical mosaic pattern.

In the vast majority of cases there is a striking coupling of bone formation and resorption, so that the absolute concentrations of calcium and phosphate ions in the serum are normal despite greatly increased rates of release and reutilization of these ions.[10] In a few patients this coupling is disrupted slightly, perhaps because of fracture, resulting in hypercalciuria or, even more rarely, hypercalcemia. Another metabolic consequence of bone resorption reflects the resorption of bone matrix as well as mineral. The bone matrix consists mainly of a fibrillar protein-collagen. When this collagen is resorbed, amino acids are released into the serum, metabolized, and excreted in the urine. The amino acids hydroxyproline and hydroxylysine, however, are not reutilized for collagen biosynthesis and thus serve as markers for collagen degradation. The rates of hydroxyproline excretion in the urine reflect the amount of osteoclastic activity, whereas the serum alkaline phosphatase level indicates the degree of osteoblastic activity. These two indexes remain roughly proportional to one another and also to the erythrocyte sedimentation rate,[11] thus reflecting the activity of the disease. A considerable number of patients with PD have hyperuricemia, some with clinically evident gout, presumably due to accelerated rates of nucleic acid metabolism secondary to increased turnover of the active cells in pagetic bone. The patient under discussion had an elevated uric acid level of 11.2 mg per 100 ml (0.7 mmol per liter) but no clinical evidence of gout.

It is well known that the marked increase in blood flow in pagetic bone is sometimes enough to cause high-output congestive heart failure.[12] This patient had cardiomegaly of long duration, possibly as a result of this mechanism. It has been found that skeletal blood flow is increased up to threefold in patients with PD.[13] Some of the clinical manifestations may reflect vascular-steal mechanisms that result in ischemia of tissue in close proximity to pagetic bone. Ischemia may explain many of the neurologic syndromes seen in the course of PD, in which direct compression of neural tissue does not seem to account adequately for the clinical picture. The vascular-steal explanation may apply to the case at hand, as I shall mention later. However, the warmth of the skin overlying pagetic bone probably results from vasodilatation rather than increased blood flow through the bone itself since it can be suppressed by epinephrine iontophoresis, which is known to decrease blood flow to the skin but not to underlying tissues.[14]

The most feared complication of PD is the development of bone sarcoma, which fortunately occurs in less than 1 per cent of the cases.[15] The sarcoma may involve any site, and the histologic type varies from fibrosarcoma or osteosarcoma to an undifferentiated sarcoma.[16] The clinical picture associated with the appearance of sarcoma includes increased local pain, an unexplained explosive rise in the alkaline phosphatase level, and suggestive radiologic findings. There is no evidence in the case record that this patient had an osteosarcoma. Certainly, the dismal prognosis for these tumors in the setting of PD excludes the possibility that such a tumor was the cause of the paraparesis, which occurred 2½ years before his death.

Pain, fracture, and neurologic disturbances are the most frequent clinically important manifestations of PD. The neurologic changes are due to either pressure exerted by pagetic bone on the brain, cranial nerves, spinal cord, or nerve roots or to changes in the weight-bearing ability of the bone, with local invasion, compression, or vascular insufficiency of neural structures. The entire spectrum of the neurologic manifestations of PD has been reviewed recently.[17] Several points are relevant to this case. The patient's deafness undoubtedly reflected involvement of the middle-ear ossicles or compression of the cochlear nerve in the temporal bone, or both. X-ray films of the skull were said to show basilar impression, but the patient was never described as having a syndrome referable to the cervical medullary junction—namely, lower-cranial-nerve dysfunction, cerebellar ataxia, cervical myelopathy, hydrocephalus, hydromyelia, or hydrobulbia.

The patient did, however, have a syndrome that may have been construed as a myelopathy or radiculopathy. The spinal cord is most frequently compromised in the upper thoracic spine, presumably because that is the site of the narrowest width of the canal. It is tempting to postulate that the neurologic syndrome was due to simple compression of the spinal cord or roots by hypertrophic bone, collapsed vertebras, or extruded intervertebral disks. However, that explanation is probably too simple. Although there is impressive myelographic evidence of compression in some patients, others with severe myelopathy or radiculopathy have normal myelograms. A vascular steal in these cases has been postulated but not proved. Surgical decompression in the absence of myelographically demonstrated block has not been effective.

The nature of Paget's disease remains a mystery. It has been thought variously to be a neoplasm because of the bizarre morphologic pattern of the bone cells and the frequency of malignant bone tumors, a vascular disorder perhaps mediated by the autonomic nervous system, an endocrine disease, an inborn error of connective-tissue biosynthesis, an inflammatory process, and most recently, a latent viral infection. The basis for the last hypothesis has been the ultrastructural demonstration of characteristic nuclear inclusions in osteoclasts. No such inclusions have been detected in patients with metabolic bone diseases other than Paget's disease or in normal bone. These inclusions have been found in only one other known bone disease, osteosarcoma. They resemble most closely those discovered in neurons of patients with subacute sclerosing panencephalitis. However, proof that a viral agent is present is not yet available.[18] The possible relation between PD and a known neurologic disease therefore deserves comment but has no relevance to this case.

The second interesting aspect of this case is the occurrence of extramedullary hematopoiesis. There is no question that active bone marrow existed outside the intramedullary cavities in this patient. We are told that a large mass was removed from the pelvis and found on histologic examination to be a myelolipoma. Myelolipoma, originally described in the adrenal gland,[19] is a mass of ectopic bone marrow, which may be located in multiple sites. EMH usually occurs in the reticuloendothelial system, particularly in the liver, spleen, and lymph nodes, but has been seen in many other locations, including the thymus gland, appendix, lungs, kidneys, peripheral nerves, and the extradural space, both paraspinally and intracranially. Of pertinence to this case is the possibility that epidural hematopoietic tissue compressed neural structures or their blood supply. Intracranial EMH is very rare,[20] and that diagnosis is not pertinent to this case. Slightly more common is EMH in the spinal epidural space, resulting in myelopathy. There are 21 examples of this phenomenon in the world's literature.[21–23] In every case the mass was located in the midthoracic region posteriorly, usually extending over several spinal levels. Treatment with decompressive laminectomy and radiotherapy has often resulted in very prompt recovery, which is frequently maintained for the rest of the patient's life. This patient's presentation with a paravertebral mass in the thorax is consistent with EMH in that location.

Three explanations for the origin of extramedullary hematopoietic tissue have been advanced. The first is that it is a manifestation of a myeloproliferative disorder, in which heterotopic totipotential cells are transformed into hematopoietic cells. The second is that EMH is a compensatory phenomenon when the bone marrow fails or hemolytic anemia is present. The third explanation is that a connection exists between the marrow cavity and the masses of EMH. None of these theories explain all the findings in cases of EMH.

It is clear that EMH sometimes occurs as part of a myeloproliferative disorder, such as polycythemia vera, agnogenic myeloid metaplasia, acute and chronic myelocytic leukemia, essential thrombocythemia, and the DiGuglielmo syndrome. The platelet and white-cell counts and the hematocrit were not elevated in the case under discussion, and we have no evidence that it fits into any of those categories. A bone-marrow biopsy might have been informative in this regard.

Could this case be an example of compensatory EMH because of bone-marrow injury or replacement or hemolytic anemia? There is no history of exposure to any agents toxic to the bone marrow, such as benzene and radium. The peripheral blood did not contain nucleated red cells, the presence of which would have been compatible with premature release of normoblasts from a replaced bone marrow. A bone-marrow biopsy might have been helpful in this regard as well, but we have no reason to suspect infiltration of the marrow. The normal acid phosphatase value probably excludes widespread adenocarcinoma of the prostate gland, which is a common myelophthisic tumor and one that could be confused with PD on radiologic examination. Multiple myeloma can also replace the marrow and appear as a paraspinal mass. Serum immunoelectrophoresis or protein electrophoresis and a bone-marrow biopsy would have been useful in establishing that diagnosis. However, it is unlikely that the patient would have lived for 2½ years after a major myelophthisic tumor became manifest. We have no evidence of hemolytic anemia. Although the patient was mildly anemic, the serum bilirubin level remained normal. The serum haptoglobin level was not determined and a Coombs' test was not performed, but a major hemolytic anemia causing this degree of EMH is improbable in this case.

Could a primary disease of bone result in enough marrow destruction to produce EMH as a compensatory phenomenon? Aside from myelophthisis the only bone disease known to result regularly in EMH is osteopetrosis, which is characterized by defective osteoclastic activity resulting in abnormally thickened bone and fibrous obliteration of the bone marrow. This disorder probably includes a group of hereditary syndromes that present in childhood and is not a consideration in this case. Could Paget's disease cause enough fibrosis of marrow cavities to result in EMH as a compensatory phenomenon? Although conceptually feasible, it is highly unlikely that a multifocal disorder such as PD would be widespread enough to produce this devastating effect on the bone marrow.

Thus, we are left with the third theory of the pathogenesis of EMH in this case—namely, leakage of bone marrow outside the bone through a defective cortex. In several reported cases of EMH (none with Paget's disease) a connection between the hematopoietic tissue and the adjacent vertebra has been demonstrated. The underlying diseases in these cases were agnogenic myelofibrosis,[24] thalassemia,[25] and pernicious anemia.[26] This very rare mechanism could have been involved in the case under discussion, with Paget's disease disrupting the bony cortex and leading to EMH. My review of the world's literature revealed only four cases in which EMH was related specifically to Paget's disease (Table 1). The first case was that of a presacral myelolipoma in a 74-year-old woman who had an incidental radiologic diagnosis of Paget's disease.[27] The authors did not postulate leakage of marrow through pagetic

Table 1 Reported Cases of Paget's Disease with Extramedullary Hematopoiesis

Authors Year	Age yr	Sex	Location	Neurologic Status	Comment
Dodge and Evans/1956[27]	74	F	Retroperitoneal presacral	Normal	Attached to sacrum
Kadir, Kalisher, and Schiller/1977[29]	61	M	Paraspinal T3-T8	Normal	Attached to vertebras
	66	M	Paravertebral and pelvic	Normal	Attached to pubic bone
Devulder et al./1979[28]	77	M	Paravertebral	Normal	Nuclear study demonstrated connection to vertebra

bony cortex but considered the myelolipoma a true neoplasm. The most recent case report is that of a 77-year-old man who had a paravertebral mass in the lower thoracic region and Paget's disease but no myelopathy.[28] In that case nuclear scanning with Indium 111 ferritin showed a connection between a pagetic vertebra and the paravertebral mass. Such a study would have been of interest in this case. A thoracic computed tomographic (CT) scan may also be useful in this circumstance. The other two cases, which were reported from this institution by Kadir, Kalisher, and Schiller,[29] are the most instructive. One was that of a 61-year-old man with Paget's disease and a paraspinal mass extending from the third to the eighth thoracic vertebra; the mass was biopsied and proved to be EMH. No myelopathy was described. The second case clearly concerned the patient under discussion, but the case report ended with excision of the pelvic myelolipoma. After reviewing other case reports of Paget's disease with paraspinal masses[5] the authors concluded that the process was probably EMH rather than extraosseous PD in all of them. Despite that interpretation in this case as well, there is as yet no recorded case in which PD led to EMH with a resultant neurologic syndrome. None of the patients in the 21 published cases of myelopathy due to EMH had Paget's disease (10 had thalassemia, seven had myelofibrosis, two had polycythemia, one had sickle-cell anemia, and one had pyrurate-kinase deficiency). Nonetheless, a logical syllogism is difficult to avoid: PD can result in EMH; EMH can produce myelopathy; therefore, Paget's disease can cause a myelopathy via the mechanism of EMH. This leads us to an analysis of the neurologic syndrome in this patient in an effort to determine its cause.

The patient's first admission to this hospital was precipitated by his inability to walk. We cannot be certain of the pace of this problem from the case record. He became unable to walk three days before admission, but it is not clear whether the onset was sudden or gradual. That knowledge is important from the viewpoint of the differential diagnosis. When faced with the problem of a patient with a paraparesis the physician has to determine the location of the disease, which may be in muscle, nerve roots, the spinal cord, or the brain. Primary muscle disease cannot explain the sensory loss in this case. Neuropathic disease could account for some of the picture. The absent ankle jerks and the lower-extremity sensory loss noted two years before the first admission may have reflected a mild neuropathy, which could have progressed. The absent reflexes, the weakness and sensory loss, and the widespread lower-extremity denervation and slightly slowed nerve-conduction velocity all support the diagnosis of an axonal polyneuropathy. Diseases of nerve roots may also be associated with widespread denervation, absent reflexes, weakness, and sensory loss. An elevated spinal-fluid protein level might have been helpful in determining that a radiculopathy was present, but none was reported.

I believe that the patient had a myelopathy. The strongest evidence is the finding of bilateral extensor plantar responses that had not been present two years earlier. Extensor plantar responses per se are not of much diagnostic help in the setting of Paget's disease, since it can affect the spinal cord at multiple levels. The frequency of extensor plantar responses in asymptomatic patients with PD is very high, and it is difficult to attribute their presence to another lesion. In this case, however, it was a new finding, probably reflecting the appearance of upper-motor-neuron disease. Furthermore, the degree of loss of joint position and vibratory sense in the legs is probably not totally ascribable to the polyneuropathy. With loss of sensation at the level of the knees on the basis of an axonal neuropathy one would expect some loss in the fingers as well, and that was not described. Although the dissociated sensory loss (i.e., loss of joint-position sense with preserved pain sense) could be ascribed to a large-fiber neuropathy, it is more likely that it resulted from a myelopathy affecting the posterior columns of the spinal cord. Conspicuously absent among the findings on neurologic examination is a sensory level or sweat level on the trunk, either of which would have pointed unequivocally to a myelopathy. The absent deep tendon reflexes do not argue strongly against such a diagnosis since areflexia is seen with acute myelopathies because of "spinal shock." Also, a superimposed neuropathy or radiculopathy could ablate reflexes, even in the presence of a myelopathy. One other location in the nervous system in which disease could lead to a paraparesis is the most rostral portion of the frontal cortex near the falx cerebri. EMH can occur in this region. However, the presence of sensory loss and widespread denervation argues against a process in that location as the only lesion. We have no way of excluding an intracranial lesion since no CT scan of the brain was done.

In view of the available clinical information, it appears probable that the patient had a myelopathy, a radiculopathy, and a polyneuropathy. With respect to the polyneuropathy, most of the neuropathic disorders seen with Paget's disease have been entrapment mononeuropathies, thought to be due to either direct compression by pagetic bone or vascular-steal mechanisms. This patient did have one such problem—a right carpal-tunnel syndrome. However, there are no specific axonal polyneuropathies associated with PD. It is interesting that involvement of the peripheral nerves by EMH has been reported[30] and could be the explanation in this case.

Myeloradiculopathy is a relatively common manifestation of Paget's disease. The mechanisms of myelopathy in this disorder are obscure. In many cases the myelograms show a subarachnoid block with pagetic changes in the contiguous vertebras, which may be collapsed or hypertrophic, and clear encroachment on the vertebral canal. Whether the mechanism is direct compression or vascular compromise, it is clear in these cases that Paget's disease itself leads directly to the spinal-cord disorder. In a minority of cases, however, there is no such block or clear evidence of direct encroachment on the spinal canal. This is an appropriate time to review the relevant radiologic studies.

DR. KENNETH R. DAVIS: X-ray films obtained on the first admission show evidence of widespread Paget's disease (Fig. 1). These changes are visible also on the x-ray films taken 25 years before admission. A bilateral thoracic paraspinal mass is evident (Fig. 2).

During the myelographic study on the first admission an unsuccessful attempt was made to introduce contrast material in the lumbar area; with some difficulty the material was then injected into the cervical subarachnoid space. Subsequent polytomograms (Fig. 3) show enlargement of the posterior extradural space in the lower thoracic region. The ninth, 10th, and 11th thoracic vertebras have radiolucent areas, but their cortical margins are preserved. These abnormalities are also unchanged in appearance in comparison with the findings on x-ray films obtained 25 years previously. The radiolucent changes are not associated with an anterior extradural mass effect. The diameter of the thoracic spinal cord is widened on an anteroposterior view and narrowed on a lateral view because of compression of the cord by the posterior extradural mass.

DR. SAMUELS: These x-ray films demonstrate large osteolytic lesions in the ninth, 10th, and 11th vertebral bodies, but the contrast material flowed by this region. The area of greatest spinal-cord narrowing was above that level. Furthermore, the cord is clearly shown to be widened in the anteroposterior view and flattened in the lateral view, with an epidural soft-tissue mass posterior to it. The subarachnoid space was small, having been compressed but not obliterated by the mass. The difficulty encountered in introducing contrast material into the subarachnoid space probably reflected its small size because of compression by the mass, which explains the severity of the signs of posterior-column involvement. After the myelographic study the patient's condition worsened rapidly to complete paraplegia. This deterioration after the lumbar subarachnoid space was violated provides further evidence of the existence of an intraspinal mass.

The patient had a striking, almost unbelievable response to the change of medication from calcitonin to mithramycin, so that within 10 days a total flaccid paraplegia became a mild paraparesis, with ability to walk. What is the explanation for this type of response? All the systemic treatments for Paget's disease depend on the administration of agents that inhibit bone resorption. Salmon, porcine, and human calcitonin have been used the longest. There is no question that pain, the alkaline phosphatase level, and subjective and objective neurologic deficits may all improve with calcitonin treatment. Although pain may decrease within the first few weeks or even days, the neurologic deficit almost never improves in less than several weeks and usually months. Whether the mechanism is vascular compression or direct neural compression, the objective neurologic response to treatment with calcitonin is usually only slight and slow in its evolution.[31,32] This patient's condition worsened considerably while he was being treated with calcitonin. The diphosphonate compound sodium etidronate, which was not used in this patient, is also able to inhibit bone resorption, but its effectiveness for the neurologic complications of PD has not yet been well demonstrated. Because PD has some characteristics of a neoplasm, cytotoxic drugs have been used as a treatment. The first such drug in this category was actinomycin D, an inhibitor of DNA-dependent RNA synthesis. A slight transient response in terms of the alkaline phosphatase level has been observed, but most investigators believe that the toxicity of the drug outweighs its therapeutic efficacy.[33] Mithramycin is another oncolytic antibiotic once used in the treatment of testicular germ-cell tumors. It acts by inhibiting DNA-dependent RNA synthesis. In smaller doses than those used in oncolytic therapy, it has been shown to be effective in the treatment of hypercalcemia and Paget's disease, probably because it damages osteoclasts. The dose used is 15 to 25 μg per kilogram per day for 10 days, followed by a weekly maintenance dose of 15 μg per kilogram. The drug is potentially toxic to the liver, kidneys, platelets, and bone marrow, but in these small doses effects on those organs and tissues are minimized. Nonetheless, about 5 per cent of the patients will have a rise of the urea nitrogen and creatinine levels, and the hepatic enzymes typically increase, at least transiently.[34] The terminal rise in the urea nitrogen and creatinine levels in this case could have reflected mithramycin toxicity. Furthermore, therapy with this drug has been associated with a hemorrhagic diathesis, often in the absence of thrombocytopenia, which has occasionally been fatal.[35] This drug-dependent platelet dysfunction is associated with a prolonged bleeding time, decreased platelet aggregation to adenosine diphosphate (ADP), collagen, and epinephrine, and depleted platelet stores of ADP.[36] This patient had a normal platelet count, but no tests of platelet function were performed. Perhaps the several cryptic episodes of gastrointestinal hemorrhage were a consequence of platelet dysfunction.

The patient's unusually favorable response to mithramycin therapy is well outside the known effects of the drug on PD alone. Clearly, the precipitous fall in the alkaline phosphatase level was expected, but the neurologic response is difficult to understand, especially in the face of the lack of response to calcitonin, a drug with a similar mechanism of action as far as Paget's disease is concerned. Perhaps the mithramycin, even in the small doses used, acted as an antimetabolite suppressing the EMH. In the past, extramedullary hematopoiesis has been treated with radiation therapy, with a prompt and often permanent response. There is no experience with the exclusive use of an oncolytic agent to treat it in the absence of an underlying malignant tumor, but it is possible that this drug, even in a small dose, acted dually in this patient, affecting both possible causes of the myelopathy—namely, Paget's disease and extramedullary hematopoiesis. This double effect may account for the response to mithramycin therapy after calcitonin failed.

In summary, I believe that this patient had Paget's disease of bone complicated by extramedullary hematopoiesis due to leakage of marrow through a defective bony cortex. The extramedullary hematopoiesis was probably found in multiple locations, including the epidural space involving a long span of the spinal cord and roots and infiltrating peripheral nerves, accounting for the polyneuropathy. He responded dramatically and uniquely to the mithramycin therapy because of its combined anti-PD and antimetabolic effects, but a bleeding diathesis developed because of mithramycin-related thrombocytopathic phenomena. The renal toxicity is attributable to mithramycin. With fracture of the left femur and subsequent gastrointestinal hemorrhage, he fell prey to a series of medical and surgical complications and died as a result of overwhelming sepsis.

DR. EDWARD P. RICHARDSON, JR.: Dr. Richter and Dr. Campion, you followed this patient closely. Do you have any comments?

DR. JAMES M. RICHTER: When we decided to administer mithramycin we thought that most of the neurologic disorder was based on Paget's disease alone and not associated with extramedullary hematopoiesis.

DR. EDWARD W. CAMPION: When the mithramycin was given we were aware of the possibility of bone-marrow suppression. We used very small doses, no greater than 15 µg per kilogram. The mithramycin was discontinued long before the terminal complications occurred. We suspected that we were alleviating either direct nerve-root compression or a vascular-steal phenomenon.

DR. RICHARDSON: Dr. Bodnar, what was the diagnosis of the medical students?

DR. ANDREW G. BODNAR: Initially, they postulated a vascular steal as the source of an ischemic cord syndrome. After a review of the myelograms, when compression was evident, they considered the possibility of a tumor, such as a chondrosarcoma. They finally made a diagnosis of myelopathy due to pressure on the spinal cord by an area of extramedullary hematopoiesis.

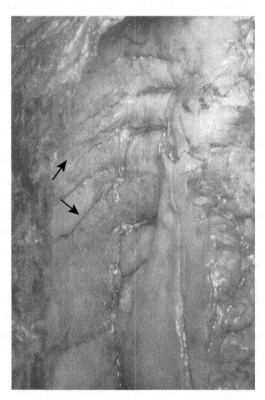

FIG 4 Fleshy Paraspinal and Paracostal Masses of Extramedullary Hematopoiesis. Partially Surrounded by a Thin Shell of Bone (Arrows).

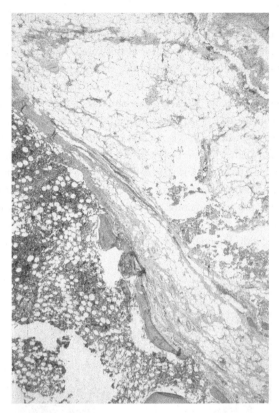

FIG 5 Extramedullary Hematopoiesis Adjacent to a Rib (Left) (×37).
Note the thin bony shell (middle), which was partially pagetic, and the peripheral normal fibrofatty tissue (right).

CLINICAL DIAGNOSES

Paget's disease of bone, with extramedullary hematopoiesis.
    Myelopathy, radiculopathy, and polyneuropathy due to compression.

DR. MARTIN A. SAMUELS' DIAGNOSES

Paget's disease of bone.
    Extramedullary hematopoiesis, extradural, causing polyneuropathy, myelopathy, and radiculopathy.
    Thrombocytopathia and renal toxicity due to mithramycin therapy.

PATHOLOGICAL DISCUSSION

Dr. Alan L. Schiller: The post-mortem examination revealed Paget's disease involving the spine, ribs, skull, clavicle, pelvis, and long bones and a right paraspinal mass. The mass was composed of fibrofatty tissue that contained fine, calcified spicules and extended from the fifth to the 10th thoracic vertebras. Similar tissue was seen along several ribs (Fig. 4). Microscopical examination revealed extramedullary hematopoiesis (Fig. 5). In contrast to the distribution of EMH in hematopoietic disorders, the liver, spleen, and lymph nodes were uninvolved in this case. The location of the hematopoietic tissue along bones involved by PD lends credence to the pathogenetic concept of mechanical weakening of the pagetic bone with extrusion of marrow into the soft tissues. Although pagetic bone appears coarser and thicker than normal on x-ray examination, it is actually weaker. The trabeculae tend to become organized along lines of stress, but they are intrinsically inferior because the lamellar bone units have a chaotic, purposeless arrangement. The interfaces between these units produce the characteristic mosaic pattern of pagetic bone.[3] Such a situation is akin to building a brick wall by placing the bricks in a helter-skelter pattern and creating an unstable structure. Therefore, it is not surprising that microfractures occur in foci of Paget's disease, with extrusion of hematopoietic tissue. A specimen x-ray film of the spine (Fig. 6A) revealed various stages of collapse, with potential defects in the cortex allowing extrusion of marrow.

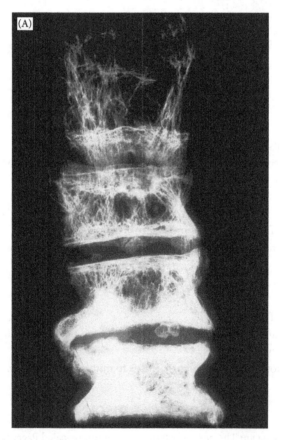

FIG 6 (*Continues*)

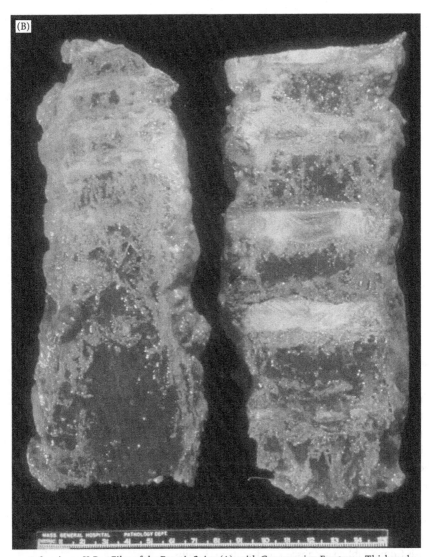

FIG 6 Specimen X-Ray Film of the Pagetic Spine (A), with Compression Fractures, Thickened and Coarsened Trabeculae, Thin Cortexes, and Large Marrow Spaces, and Sectioned Specimen of the Spine (B), with Large Marrow Spaces Filled with Red Marrow, Distortion of the Shape of Vertebras, and Loss of Intervertebral Disks.

The intervertebral disks had degenerated. In extreme cases a vertebral body may appear radiologically as a transverse compressed bar. Examination of the gross specimen of the spine (Fig. 6B) illustrated how hematopoietic marrow fills up the large empty spaces between the pagetic bone trabeculae and extends into the thin cortex.

A similar picture was seen in the left femur, with marked distortion of the normal bony architecture and exaggeration of the trabeculae. It is interesting that the callus of the fracture that the patient sustained before the last admission also had the features of pagetic bone. The marrow of the femur contained hematopoietic tissue, which is abnormal for an adult, and, more prominently, fibrovascular tissue in

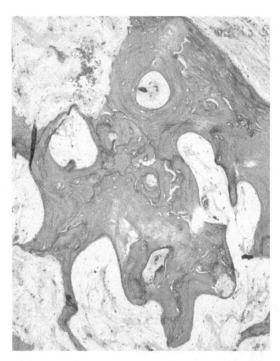

FIG 7   Pagetic Bone of the Femoral Cortex with a Mosaic Pattern (× 100).

which osteoclasts and osteoblasts were present. The femoral cortex was porous, with extension of marrow into the widened cortical spaces. Examination of the skull disclosed thickening and coarsening of the diploe trabeculae and outer and inner tables. Microscopical examination of the vertebral and femoral cortexes (Fig. 7) revealed the fibrovascular marrow and pagetic bone. Pagetic bone was even found in the areas of EMH.

The heart weighed 425 g, with marked biventricular dilatation and moderate hypertrophy. An interesting gross correlation with the neurologic manifestations was the finding of marked pallor and fatty infiltration of the psoas muscles. Death was due to sepsis from a subhepatic abscess and acute peritonitis.

DR. RICHARDSON: Dr. Samuels was correct in his interpretation of the neurologic disorder. Hematopoietic tissue was found in the spinal epidural space in the thoracic region, where it produced narrowing of the spinal canal. The cord was compressed in this region and appeared somewhat flattened, but on microscopical examination its structure was remarkably intact, with minimal loss of fibers in the posterior and lateral columns. This sparing of the nerve cells and fibers within the cord is compatible with some recovery of function, such as occurred with treatment.

The best explanation for the evidence of peripheral-nerve involvement is probably a lumbosacral radiculopathy due in part to encroachment on the nerve roots as they left the vertebral canal and in part to the deposition of fibrous tissue and bone in the lumbar subarachnoid space, which narrowed the space available for the cauda equina. We found an increase in endoneurial connective tissue and loss of fibers in some of the cauda equina roots, which typically occur with chronic compression. There was enough impingement on neural structures by extraneural tissues to account for the neurologic deficits. We found no evidence to suggest that a vascular-steal syndrome played any part in their pathogenesis.

ANATOMICAL DIAGNOSES

Paget's disease of bone, polyostotic.
  Extramedullary hematopoiesis, with compressive myelopathy.
  Radiculoneuropathy, lumbosacral, compressive.

REFERENCES

1. Paget J. On a form of chronic inflammation of bones (osteitis deformans). Trans R Med-Chir Soc (London). 1877; 60:37–63.
2. Jaffe HL. Paget's disease of bone. Arch Pathol. 1933; 15:83–131.
3. Singer FR, Schiller AL, Pyle EB, Krane SM. Paget's disease of bone. In: Avioli LV, Krane SM, eds. Metabolic bone disease. New York: Academic Press. 1978:489–575.
4. Krane SM. Paget's disease of bone. Clin Orthop Rel Res. 1977; 127:24–36.
5. Barry HC. Paget's disease of bone. Baltimore: Williams & Wilkins, 1969.
6. Schmorl G. Über Ostitis deformans Paget. Virchows Arch [Pathol Anat]. 1932; 283:694–751.
7. McKusick VA. Heritable disorders of connective tissue. St Louis: CV Mosby, 1972.
8. Simon L, Blotman F, Seignalet J, Claustre J. Étiologie de la maladie osseuse de Paget. Rev Rheum. 1975; 42:535–44.
9. Rasmussen H, Bordier P. The physiological and cellular basis of metabolic bone disease. Baltimore: Willimas & Wilkins, 1974.
10. Nagant de Deuxchaisnes C, Krane SM. Paget's disease of bone: clinical and metabolic observations. Medicine (Baltimore). 1964; 43:233–66.
11. Nagant de Deuxchaisnes C, Rombouts-Lindeman C. Exploration biologique de la maladie de Paget. J Belge Rheum Med Phys. 1974; 29:243–54.
12. Edholm OG, Howarth S, McMichael J. Heart failure and bone blood flow in osteitis deformans. Clin Sci. 1945; 5:249–60.
13. Wootton R, Reeve J, Veall N. The clinical measurement of skeletal blood flow. Clin Sci Mol Med. 1976; 50:261–8.
14. Heistad DD, Abboud FM, Schmid PG, Mark AL, Wilson WR. Regulation of blood flow in Paget's disease of bone. J Clin Invest. 1975; 55:69–74.
15. Collins DH. Pathology of bone. London: Butterworths, 1966.
16. McKenna RJ, Schwinn CP, Soonj KY. Higinbotham NL. Osteogenic sarcoma arising in Paget's disease. Cancer. 1964; 17:42–66.
17. Schmidek HH. Neurologic and neurosurgical sequelae of Paget's disease of bone. Clin Orthop Rel Res. 1977; 127:70–7.
18. Singer FR, Mills BG. The etiology of Paget's disease of bone. Clin Orthop Rel Res. 1977; 127:37–42.
19. Collins DC. Formation of bone marrow in the suprarenal gland. Am J Pathol. 1932; 8:97–106.
20. Polliack A, Rosenmann E. Extramedullary hematopoietic tumors of the cranial dura mater. Acta Haematol. 1969; 41:43–8.

21. Rutgers MJ, van der Lugt PJ, van Turnhout JM. Spinal cord compression by extramedullary hematopoietic tissue in pyruvate-kinase-deficiency-caused hemolytic anemia. Neurology (Minneap). 1979; 29:510–13.

22. Stahl SM, Ellinger G, Baringer JR. Progressive myelopathy due to extramedullary hematopoiesis: case report and review of the literature. Ann Neurol. 1979; 5:485–9.

23. Rice GPA, Assis LJP, Barr RM, Ebers GC. Extramedullary hematopoiesis and spinal cord compression complicating polycythemia rubra vera. Ann Neurol. 1980; 7:81–4.

24. Bree RL, Neiman HL, Hodak JA, Flynn RE. Extramedullary hematopoiesis in the spinal epidural space. J Can Assoc Radiol. 1974; 25:297–9.

25. Marinozzi V. Aspetti insoliti dell'iperplasia midollare nelle anemie emolitiche. Haematologica (Pavia). 1958; 43:737–59.

26. Lyall A. Massive extramedullary bone marrow formation in a case of pernicious anemia. J Pathol. 1935; 41:469–72.

27. Dodge OG, Evans DMD. Haemopoiesis in a presacral fatty tumour (myelolipoma). J Pathol Bacteriol. 1956; 72:313–17.

28. Devulder B, Remy J, Marchandise X, Plouvier B, Prin L, Rouget JP. Pseudo-tumeur hématopoïétique paravertébrale au cours d'une maladie de Paget. Ann Med Interne. 1979; 130:93–6.

29. Kadir S, Kalisher L, Schiller AL. Extramedullary hematopoiesis in Paget's disease of bone. AJR. 1977; 129:493–5.

30. Dieterich H. Studien über extramedulläre Blutbildung bei chirurgischen Erkrankungen. Arch Klin Chir. 1925; 134:166–75.

31. Chen J-R, Rhee RSC, Wallach S, Avramides A, Flores A. Neurologic disturbances in Paget's disease of bone: response to calcitonin. Neurology (Minneap). 1979; 29:448–57.

32. Walpin LA, Singer FR. Paget's disease: reversal of severe paraparesis using calcitonin. Spine. 1979; 4:213–19.

33. Ryan WG, Schwartz TB, Perlia CP. Effects of mithramycin on Paget's disease of bone. Ann Intern Med. 1969; 70:549–57.

34. Ryan WG. Treatment of Paget's disease of bone with mithramycin. Clin Orthop Rel Res. 1977; 127:106–10.

35. Kennedy BJ. Metabolic and toxic effects of mithramycin during tumor therapy. Am J Med. 1970; 49:494–503.

36. Ahr DJ, Scialla SJ, Kimball DB Jr. Acquired platelet dysfunction following mithramycin therapy. Cancer. 1978; 41:448–54.

Perspectives and Updates

This CPC, now 30 years ago, marks the beginning of my identification as a neurologist with a special interest in complications of general medical and surgical diseases. Having trained as an internist at the Boston City Hospital, I had always aspired to become expert in the borderlands between internal medicine and neurology. This remarkable case of a rare complication of Paget disease of bone gave me an opportunity to begin to investigate the fascinating world of neurological medicine.

Two issues arising from this case history are worthy of continued analysis: the usual neurological manifestations of Paget disease of bone, and the mechanisms and typical locations of extramedullary hematopoiesis (EMH)[1] when it affects the nervous system.

Most patients with Paget disease of bone are asymptomatic, having had the typical imaging features recognized as an incidental finding. Bone pain is by far the major symptom of the disorder, but a very small number of patients (perhaps fewer than 1 per cent) suffer the serious, but potentially very important complication, of the development of an osteosarcoma. The most important neurological complication of Paget disease of bone is that of platybasia and/or basilar impression. Modern MRI techniques have made these diagnoses much easier to make. Platybasia is a flattening of the skull base characterized by an abnormally obtuse basal angle. Many lines have been used over the years to make these measurements, but the basal angle, defined by Koenigsberg et al.[2] as the angle formed by a line from the nasion to the center of the pituitary fossa to a line from the center of the pituitary fossa to the anterior border of the foramen magnum, should be less than about 143 degrees. The term "basilar impression," often associated with platybasia, refers to an abnormal rostral encroachment of the upper cervical spine into the posterior fossa (i.e., above various lines such as Chamberlain's line, which runs from the dorsal soft palate to the dorsal foramen magnum). By producing softening of bone, Paget disease of bone may produce platybasia and/or basilar impression thereby producing a myelopathy or rarely a vascular syndrome due to interference with the course of the vertebral arteries. Deafness, caused by Paget involvement of the temporal bone, is another important neurological manifestation of Paget disease and one that may have led to Beethoven's premature deafness.

The cause of Paget disease remains a mystery, though several genes (sequestosome 1 on chromosome 5 and two tumor necrosis factor receptor superfamily members, TNFRS11A and TNFRS11B, both on chromosome 8) have been implicated in some familial cases. Most cases remain apparently sporadic and the question of an environmental factor, such as a virus, remains a consideration, though it is unproved. The peculiar multinucleated osteoclasts seen in the first phase of Paget disease resemble those seen in some osteosarcomas, raising a viral etiology as a possibility, though none has been definitely found.

We now know that EMH is much more common than previously recognized. Sensitive techniques, such as radionuclide scanning and PET scanning can detect EMH much more sensitively than in the past. Despite this impressive technical progress, it remains true that most EMH is due to failure of the bone marrow and/or to a hematologic malignancy. Leakage of bone marrow through defective bony cortex remains a very rare but conceptually important cause of EMH. As far as neurological EMH is concerned, I have learned in the intervening 30 years that it tends to occur in the epidural spinal space and the subdural intcracranial compartment. When it occurs in the latter space, it may imitate a traumatic subdural hematoma. I have seen, for example, a dramatic example of a patient with thalassemia who presented with bilateral abducens neuropathies and a mass in the subdural space on the surface of the clivus. Another patient with chronic myelogenous leukemia presented with bilateral asymmetric cerebral convexity masses. Both of these proved to be EMH. EMH, being bone marrow, is exquisitely sensitive to therapies aimed at cell multiplication (e.g., chemotherapy and radiation therapy).

One last amusing feature of this case relates to my finding the case, reported earlier in a radiology journal. In the modern era, with electronic search engines, this could have been an easier task, but when this CPC was discussed, I recall poring through the stacks of the Countway Library of Medicine, looking for information on the obscure topic of EMG in Paget disease of bone, when I was surprised and delighted to find what was clearly this very case, reported a few years earlier by the same bone pathology group who were to provide the pathology for my CPC discussion. I still recall the shocked expression on Dr. Schiller's face when, during my discussion, I produced a slide of this very patient, taken from his own case report. Please note that I did not hide this fact but rather included it in my table of cases already reported. Dr. Schiller, who fortunately had a sense of humor, stood for his part of the discussion, and simply said that he had nothing further to add; everything he had had to say was already published.

Martin A. Samuels

REFERENCES

1. Kadir S, Kalisher L, Schiller AL. Extramedullary hematopoiesis in Paget's disease of bone. AJR 1977; 129: 493–5.
2. Koenigsberg RA, Vakil N, Hong TA, Htaik T, Raerber E, Maiorano R, Dua M, Faro S, Gonzoles C. Evaluation of platybasia with MR imaging. AJNR 2005; 26:89–92.

A 16-Year-Old Boy with Confusion

PARAINFECTIOUS ENCEPHALOPATHY
FROM MYCOPLASMA
CPC 35-1981

PRESENTATION OF CASE

A 16-year-old boy was admitted to the hospital because of confusion.

He was well until the early hours of the day of entry, when he was observed in a parked car having a seizure. When the police arrived he was wandering on a nearby street. He was taken to another hospital, where he became combative, with occasional choreoathetoid movements. Naloxone hydrochloride, physostigmine, thiamine hydrochloride, and glucose were administered by vein, without response, and he was transferred to this hospital. On arrival in the Emergency Ward he responded only to painful stimuli. Decerebrate posturing developed, followed by a tonic-clonic seizure of 30 seconds' duration, with deviation of the eyes to the right side.

Earlier in the evening the boy had attended a party at which methaqualone, diazepam, alcohol, and other, unknown drugs were used. Two years earlier he was treated at another hospital for meningococcal meningitis. He had received poliomyelitis vaccine on schedule, with a booster dose one year before admission. A mild respiratory-tract infection with fever had occurred two weeks before entry. He was said to have frequent headaches. There was no history of head trauma, previous seizures, or prior drug abuse.

The temperature was 37.7°C, the pulse 96, and the respirations 30. The blood pressure was 130/60 mm Hg.

On examination the patient was stuporous, coughing or moaning periodically. General physical examination was negative. Neurologic examination showed that he lay immobile but responded to noxious stimuli by withdrawal. Tone was increased in the lower extremities. The pupils were 3 mm, equal, and reactive. The left eye did not abduct fully, but extraocular movements were otherwise normal, as were the optic fundi. The gag reflex was intact. No snout or grasp reflex could be elicited. When the arms were pinched he raised the left arm less than the right arm.

The urine gave a + test for protein and a + + + test for glucose but was otherwise normal. The hematocrit was 43 per cent; the white-cell count was 27,000, with 93 percent neutrophils. The erythrocyte sedimentation rate was 7 mm per hour. The urea nitrogen was 10 mg per 100 ml (3.6 mmol per liter), the glucose 268 mg per 100 ml (14.9 mmol per liter), the calcium 10.2 mg per 100 ml (2.5 mmol per liter), the phosphorus 2.9 mg per 100 ml (0.9 mmol per liter), the uric acid 8.2 mg per 100 ml (0.5 mmol per liter), and the protein 8.1 g (the albumin 5.2 g, and the globulin 2.9 g) per 100 ml. The alcohol level was 100 mg per liter. An electrocardiogram disclosed a normal rhythm at a rate of 100, with occasional premature ventricular contractions. An x-ray film of the chest was normal. A computed tomographic (CT) scan of the brain, performed without the injection of contrast material, revealed small ventricles; the basal cisterns were not identified; the findings were considered normal for the patient's age. A lumbar puncture yielded clear, colorless cerebrospinal fluid under an initial pressure of 260 mm; the fluid contained 5 red cells and 2 lymphocytes per cubic millimeter; the glucose was 132 mg per 100 ml (7.3 mmol per liter), and the protein 188 mg per 100 ml; a culture yielded no growth of microorganisms. An electroencephalogram showed continuous, diffuse high-voltage 1 to 2 Hz delta slowing with superimposed fast activity. An electrographic seizure was recorded, beginning in the left frontotemporal area, with subsequent generalization, and was accompanied by a generalized clinical seizure that began with turning of the head to the right side. A screening test for substances subject to abuse, including phencyclidine, was negative. Serum immunoelectrophoresis showed that IgG and IgA were normal; IgM was slightly increased. Agarose-gel electrophoresis gave a normal pattern. A test for cold agglutinins was positive in a titer of 1:16. An antistreptolysin-O test, a serologic test for syphilis, tests for rheumatoid factor and antinuclear antibodies, and a heterophil-antibody agglutination test were negative. Tests on urine for myoglobin and porphobilinogen were negative.

Specimens of blood, urine, and tracheal aspirate were obtained for culture; endotracheal and nasogastric tubes were inserted, ventilatory assistance was begun, and phenytoin sodium was administered by vein. The patient was admitted to the Pediatric Intensive Care Unit. Repeated grand-mal seizures occurred, and diazepam was administered by injection, with additional doses of phenytoin sodium; fluid intake was restricted. On the second hospital day no seizures occurred; the patient opened his eyes in response to noise. The temperature rose to 39.4°C. An x-ray film of the chest was normal. Penicillin was begun. All cultures failed to yield pathogenic micro-organisms. The white-cell count was 20,900, with 95 percent neutrophils, the platelet count was 176,000. The erythrocyte sedimentation rate was 49 mm per hour. Another lumbar puncture yielded clear, acellular cerebrospinal fluid under an initial pressure of 360 mm; the glucose was 85 mg per 100 ml (4.7 mmol per liter), and the protein 170 mg per 100 ml.

On the third hospital day the patient was more alert; he followed simple commands and nodded his head appropriately to queries; nystagmus was present on gaze to either side. Fever persisted. A repeated x-ray film of the chest was unchanged. Another lumbar puncture yielded clear, colorless cerebrospinal fluid that contained 86 red cells, 4 lymphocytes, and 2 neutrophils per cubic millimeter; the glucose was 87 mg per 100 ml (4.8 mmol per liter), and the protein 139 mg per 100 ml. On the next day the patient appeared fully alert and mouthed questions, although he did not phonate.

Weakness on abduction of the left eye persisted. The tendon reflexes were equal, but the ankle jerks were absent; the plantar responses were flexor. The serum aspartate aminotransferase (SGOT) was 111 U per milliliter (0.9 μmol · sec⁻¹ per liter), the lactic dehydrogenase (LDH) 247 U per milliliter (4.1 μmol · sec⁻¹ per liter), the creatine phosphokinase (CPK) 3060 mU (51 μmol · sec⁻¹ per liter), the aldolase 11 mU per milliliter (183.4 nmol · sec⁻¹ per liter), and the alkaline phosphatase 30 IU (0.5 μmol · sec⁻¹) per liter. The LDH isoenzyme 5 was greatly elevated; the CPK isoenzyme MB was less than 1 per cent. X-ray films of the skull disclosed prominence of the soft tissues of the nasopharynx, with slight opacification of the left maxillary sinus, both ethmoid sinuses, and the right mastoid sinus; the frontal sinuses were not well developed. Another electroencephalogram disclosed marked improvement, with intermittent runs of 3 to 5 Hz background slowing and no seizure activity. Detailed electrophysiologic studies, including conventional motor and sensory conduction and late responses (H reflex, F responses, and blink reflexes) excluded the diagnosis of a segmental demyelinating neuropathy. The endotracheal and nasogastric tubes were removed.

On the fifth hospital day the patient was alternately confused and lucid; he continued to mouth words but was unable to phonate. There was prominent swelling of the nose and left cheek. Neurologic examination showed no change; sensation was intact. The white-cell count was 11,100, with 61 per cent neutrophils; the erythrocyte sedimentation rate was 90 mm per hour. Pencillin was discontinued. On the following day the temperature rose to 38.9°C. Another lumbar puncture yielded clear, colorless cerebrospinal fluid under an initial pressure of 300 mm; the fluid contained 90 red cells and 1 lymphocyte per cubic millimeter; the glucose was 74 mg per 100 ml (4.1 mmol per liter), and the protein 90 mg per 100 ml; the gold-sol curve was 0122211000. Cerebrospinal-fluid immunoelectrophoresis revealed that IgG was 12 mg (normal, 0 to 8.6 mg), and the albumin 64.5 mg per 100 ml (normal, 11 to 48 mg); agarose-gel electrophoresis of the fluid disclosed no abnormal band in an 80-fold concentrated specimen. On the seventh hospital day another electromyographic examination showed that the motor-unit potentials were of normal size and shape, and there was no evidence of primary muscle disease or active denervation.

On the eighth hospital day the temperature rose to 39.1°C, and the patient coughed up thick, white, mucoid sputum; examination revealed no change. Additional samples of blood were obtained for culture. The white-cell count was 6700, with 57 per cent neutrophils; the erythrocyte sedimentation rate was 120 mm per hour. The SGOT was 76 U per milliliter (0.6 μmol · sec⁻¹ per liter), the aldolase 27.2 mU per milliliter (453.4 nmol · sec⁻¹ per liter), and the CPK 680 mU per milliliter (11.3 μmol · sec⁻¹ per liter). An x-ray film of the chest disclosed that the lungs remained clear. On the following day the patient was more confused and confabulated. Repeated cultures of blood, sputum, urine, and cerebrospinal fluid failed to yield pathogenic microorganisms. The CPK was 376 mU per milliliter (6.3 μmol · sec⁻¹ per liter). Phenytoin sodium was discontinued. The lead level was 9 μg per 100 ml (0.4 μmol per liter), and the free erythrocyte protoporphyrin 17 μg per 100 ml (normal, 50 μg or less). On the 10th hospital day the patient remained somnolent, inattentive, and variably confused. Neurologic examination showed no change except that he exhibited good strength in all extremities. A tuberculin skin test (PPD,

5 TU) and a skin test with candida antigen were negative. A CT scan with contrast material was normal. On the 11th hospital day the patient was able to walk unsteadily with assistance. He continued to speak mainly in whispers. An x-ray film of the chest disclosed that both lung volumes were low, and there was a band of subsegmental atelectasis at the right-lung base; the remaining portions of the lungs and the heart and mediastinum were normal. An electroencephalogram demonstrated deterioration since the previous study, with long runs of diffuse, 3 to 4 Hz moderate voltage slowing; no paroxysmal features were noted. The patient was transferred from the Intensive Care Unit.

During the next week the temperature fell to the range of 37.2 to 37.8°C. He complained of a sore throat, spoke in a hoarse voice, and was observed to choke on eating solid foods. His mentation improved progressively, although there was marked memory loss. On the 17th hospital day the white-cell count was 6200, with 52 per cent neutrophils; the erythrocyte sedimentation rate was 78 mm per hour. The SGOT was 26 U per milliliter (0.2 μmol $\cdot$ sec^{-1} per liter), the LDH 104 U per milliliter (1.7 μmol $\cdot$ sec^{-1} per liter), the CPK 39 mU per milliliter (0.7 μmol $\cdot$ sec^{-1} per liter), and the aldolase 3.7 mU per milliliter (61.7 nmol $\cdot$ sec^{-1} per liter). On the following day the voice was whispered, and the cough was weak. Laryngoscopic examination showed a moderate decrease in abduction of the vocal cords and a slight decrease in adduction, but an adequate airway was present; granulomas and pus were observed on the cords, and the visible portions of the trachea were erythematous. Ampicillin was prescribed. On the 19th hospital day lumbar puncture yielded clear, colorless cerebrospinal fluid under an initial pressure of 230 mm; the fluid contained 12 red cells per cubic millimeter; the glucose was 53 mg per 100 ml (2.9 mmol per liter), and the protein 23 mg per 100 ml. A CT scan of the brain appeared normal. On the 20th hospital day ataxia persisted, and there was slight nystagmus on lateral gaze. Another electroencephalogram showed improvement, with a decrease in the amount of background slowing. The erythrocyte sedimentation rate was 55 mm per hour.

On the 25th hospital day laryngologic examination revealed normal adduction but incomplete abduction of the vocal cords; the granulomas were less prominent, and the trachea was less injected; no pus was observed. A dexamethasone inhaler was prescribed. Slow but progressive improvement in mentation continued. On the 26th hospital day the hematocrit was 38.8 per cent; the white-cell count was 5400, with 57 per cent neutrophils. The erythrocyte sedimentation rate was 32 mm per hour. On the 27th hospital day the patient was discharged to his home.

After discharge the result of a diagnostic test was received.

DIFFERENTIAL DIAGNOSIS

DR. ALLAN H. ROPPER[*]: This young adult came to the emergency room suffering from an acute encephalopathy with seizures. Two important pieces of information in the medical history were a recent upper-respiratory-tract infection accompanied by fever

---

[*] Assistant in neurology, Massachusetts General Hospital; instructor in neurology, Harvard Medical School. Currently Vice-Chair, Department of Neurology, Brigham and Women's Hospital.

and his attendance at a party where drugs were used on the evening before admission. He had a sixth-nerve palsy and persistently high spinal-fluid pressures suggesting intracranial hypertension, but there were few or no cells in the cerebrospinal fluid (CSF). Two additional problems were elevation of serum enzyme levels, which persisted for at least eight days after the initial seizures, suggesting muscle destruction, and laryngeal dysfunction with inflammatory changes in the vocal cords. There was otherwise no evidence of disease outside the nervous system. Recovery was protracted and associated with a gait ataxia.

Many diseases cause encephalopathy and seizures; few are associated with increased spinal-fluid pressure, and none are common. This case provides the opportunity to discuss these diseases, including several not often considered in cases of adult nervous-system disorders.

Encephalopathies related to drug use are the first consideration. The possibility of drug ingestion should be entertained whenever a young patient is brought to the emergency room in coma. The drug that is most commonly involved is a barbiturate, which causes progressive loss of consciousness and, as the coma becomes profound, may result in extensor posturing, Babinski signs, and loss of reflex eye movements. There is a bewildering array of drugs subject to recreational use, and their neurologic manifestations are similar. However, very few are associated with seizures.

Alcohol is the most frequently used intoxicant, but the blood alcohol levels of this patient indicated only mild intoxication. It is also unlikely that a withdrawal syndrome was responsible for the seizures and encephalopathy, but a related disorder, pathological alcohol intoxication, should be mentioned. Persons who are severely intoxicated become delirious and drowsy and frequently have hallucinations when exposed to even small amounts of alcohol.[1] This unusual susceptibility may become evident when an adolescent consumes alcohol for the first time. Since seizures do not generally accompany this disorder and recovery occurs within several days, pathologic alcohol intoxication can be ruled out in this case. Methyl alcohol, in contrast, is infrequently abused and is associated with an asymptomatic latent period and a distinctive syndrome, including signs of intracranial hypertension.[2] The other typical features—optic-disk edema, poorly reactive pupils, gastrointestinal symptoms, and residual visual impairment—were not found in this case. Also, there was no acidosis, which is typical of methanol poisoning and poisoning due to other organic-acid-producing drugs.

Among the most commonly used drugs that produce both encephalopathy and seizures are tricyclic antidepressants, amphetamines, salicylates, and isoniazid. Since the administration of physostigmine had no clear effect on this patient's confusional state, tricyclic overdose is unlikely. Amphetamines are associated with a hypersympathetic state characterized by hypertension, dilated pupils, vomiting, and hyperpyrexia,[3] none of which occurred in this case. Seizures can follow aspirin overdose as a direct central-nervous-system effect or as a secondary manifestation of hypoglycemia or effective hypocalcemia. However, despite the suggestive presence of hyperventilation, glycosuria, mild hypokalemia, and a very low sedimentation rate, the absence of acid-base disturbances and several other chemical and hematologic abnormalities associated with aspirin overdose excludes that possibility.[4] Isoniazid can cause convulsions, even in the usually administered doses, and large doses are associated with refractory seizures, hyperglycemia, and severe metabolic acidosis, which apparently was not a factor in this case. Strychnine is often mixed with both marihuana and heroin, particularly on the East Coast. It causes seizures, but its manifestations do not match those in the remainder of this patient's clinical course. Strychnine produces atonic seizures with extensor posturing but with little clonic movement. In summary, drugs can be exonerated on clinical grounds on the basis of the negative toxicologic screening, the persistently elevated spinal-fluid pressure, and the prolonged encephalopathy. Commercial drug screens do not test for substances not specifically requested, but comprehensive drug screens, which generally use gas-liquid chromatography, thin-layer chromatography, multiple-enzyme immunoassay, and mass spectrometry, test for over 100 substances.

Chemicals such as ethylene glycol are occasionally abused and cause coma with intractable seizures.[5] In the absence of an anion-gap acidosis, nephropathy, or cells in the spinal fluid, however, we cannot implicate this substance in the case under discussion. Poisoning with industrial toxins, such as mercury, arsenic, and thallium, deserves mention in the differential diagnosis of a peculiar encephalopathy. Ingestion of these substances produces severe gastrointestinal symptoms and frequently shock in addition to neurologic manifestations. Lead toxicity, however, could explain this patient's clinical syndrome. Lead encephalopathy is characterized by somnolence and seizures, eventually leading to coma with an increased pressure and often a minimally elevated protein content in the cerebrospinal fluid.[6] The normal lead and free erythrocyte protoporphyrin levels seemingly eliminate lead toxicity in this case but do not exclude it. Although inorganic lead poisoning is a major health problem in children, most sporadic examples of poisoning result from exposure of adults to organic lead. The most commonly implicated organic lead compound is tetraethyl lead, which is used as a solvent and antiknock agent in gasoline. Gasoline sniffing, a common way to become "high" two decades ago, should be considered in this case. In contrast to the finding in cases of inorganic lead poisoning, the blood lead concentration after tetraethyl lead exposure is normal. Because the exposure is usually acute, there is no anemia or basophilic stippling, and the free erythrocyte protoporphyrin level is normal. These three findings are manifestations of the lead effect on reticulocytes and do not appear until two or three weeks after its ingestion.[7] Therefore, the chemical tests for lead intoxication in this case do not rule out inorganic or organic lead poisoning, but it is unlikely in view of the rarity of encephalopathy after a single exposure to gasoline sniffing, the lack of previous psychologic problems or known drug abuse, and the apparent absence of a similar syndrome in the other party-goers.

Endogenous metabolic encephalopathies, such as those due to uremia or hepatic failure, are eliminated by the laboratory data. This patient's illness, however, was compatible with one genetic metabolic disease, acute intermittent porphyria. A history of recent drug exposure, seizures, sinus tachycardia, and confusion are all consistent with porphyria and require analysis of the urine for porphobilinogen early in the course.[8] Testing was performed in this case and found to be negative. The absence of electrophysiologic evidence of a neuropathy and the presence of persistently high spinal-fluid pressure also argue against porphyria.

Among the toxic and metabolic encephalopathies associated with seizures carbon monoxide poisoning should be considered, especially since this patient was initially observed in a car. The findings compatible with carbon monoxide poisoning are brain swelling with increased spinal-fluid pressure and slightly elevated protein content, a protracted recovery, ataxia, and memory difficulty, as well as elevated muscle enzyme values.[9] The arterial partial pressure of oxygen, routinely measured in blood-gas determinations, is of no use in cases of carbon monoxide poisoning because the combination of carbon monoxide with hemoglobin does not affect oxygen tension. If the carboxyhemoglobin concentration in the blood is not measured within the first day after exposure (or in the first hour if oxygen has been administered) the diagnosis cannot be confirmed. In addition, seizures usually occur after the patient becomes comatose in cases of acute hypoxic brain injury. The fact that this patient was able to walk away from his car after the initial seizure excludes carbon monoxide poisoning.

A final metabolic consideration is brain hypoxia or ischemia secondary to the seizures. Transient respiratory failure and hypotension are very common sequelae of catastrophic brain lesions but are often overlooked. Four patients with these complications were recently admitted to our Neurological Intensive Care Unit. The inciting events were a small subdural hematoma, a traumatic contusion, cortical-vein thrombosis, and an old stroke. These patients were unresponsive for days to weeks. In retrospect, we concluded on the basis of the x-ray films of the chest, the initial blood-gas values, and the electroencephalograms that hypoxia had occurred early in their illnesses. Unlike the findings in the case under discussion, increased intracranial pressure did not occur immediately, and the CSF protein content was normal in all four patients. Furthermore, this patient would not have been able to walk away from the car if he had had anoxia profound enough to cause seizures. Although not all endogenous and exogenous metabolic derangements, the most common causes of acute encephalopathy, can be disregarded, the ones that deserve most serious consideration are lead toxicity, porphyria, carbon monoxide poisoning, and secondary hypoxia, and all can be eliminated on the basis of the laboratory tests or specific clinical objections.

Although this patient's illness had focal features, overall it reflected a multifocal or diffuse affliction of the cerebral hemispheres. The CT scans should be viewed now for specific evidence of multifocal or diffuse disease and for help in the interpretation of the increased spinal-fluid pressures.

DR. KENNETH R. DAVIS: The initial CT scan shows generalized brain swelling, as indicated by obliteration of the subarachnoid space and the small size of the ventricles. The subsequent CT scans show a gradual slight decrease in the swelling.

DR. ROPPER: The incomplete abduction of the patient's left eye is consistent with a sixth-nerve palsy related to increased intracranial pressure. The opening pressures on serial spinal taps were 260 mm of water on admission, 360 mm on the second day, 300 mm on the fifth day, and 230 mm on the 19th hospital day. Above an intracranial pressure of approximately 15 mm Hg, equivalent to 210 mm of water, spinal-fluid pressures do not reflect intracranial pressures except in a qualitative way.[10] A second point is that positive-pressure ventilation-causes increased intrapleural pressure, which is transmitted to thoracic structures, including the superior vena cava, the vertebral veins, and the thoracic intervertebral foramina, resulting in increased intracranial and spinal-fluid pressure.[11] It is generally helpful to know if and for how long the patient had been detached from the ventilator when the CSF pressure was measured. It may be necessary to remove the patient from the ventilator for several minutes before thoracic and CSF pressures equilibrate and reflect the raised intracranial pressure due directly to the cranial lesion. In this patient the intracranial pressure was persistently high, and on the basis of the first CT scan it appears that the increase was due to diffuse brain swelling.

In any patient with an acute neurologic syndrome vascular disease must be excluded. When seizures are associated with an increased intracranial pressure, lateral or superior sagittal venous sinus occlusion is a consideration. In the presence of fever and severe seizures septic phlebitis with extension into adjacent cortical veins is likely,[12] but more red cells or xanthochromia in the spinal fluid or some residual focal deficit would be expected if that type of lesion had produced an illness of this severity. The absence of extracranial bacterial infection, ear disease, a tumor, and a hypercoagulable state makes cerebral venous thrombosis unlikely, but an angiographic study would have been of value in this regard. Other vascular disorders, such as carotid arterial occlusion, cerebral embolism, and vasculitis, are very improbable. Similarly, traumatic, neoplastic, and degenerative diseases of the brain can be excluded on the basis of the clinical course and incompatible CT scans.

Still to be considered are infections and other types of inflammation of the nervous system. In view of the fever, the leukocytosis, the abnormal CSF, and the diffuse encephalopathy that characterize both encephalitides and parainfectious encephalopathies we should find the correct diagnosis within one of these two remaining categories of disease. We can dispense with bacterial meningitis and a brain abscess because of the spinal-fluid findings and CT scans.

The most commonly used classification of encephalitis, which was devised by the Centers for Disease Control, is as follows: arboviral and enteroviral forms; the type of encephalitis associated with childhood infections, respiratory-tract illness, and immunization; and a general category in which herpes simplex, the most common sporadically occurring form, belongs. Perhaps a more informative classification should be devised to divide encephalitis into four categories. The first is viral encephalitis, in which the inflammation is caused directly by viruses that can be cultured from the nervous system. For practical purposes, this includes mainly herpes simplex and arbovirus encephalitis.[13] The second category consists of the postinfectious and postvaccinial encephalomyelitides. These are multifocal, immunologic, inflammatory, and demyelinating diseases.[14] Parainfectious encephalitis and the ataxic syndromes that occur after measles, mumps, varicella, and rubella may fall into this category rather than that of neurotropic infections, but a recent report suggests that varicella-associated ataxia is due to direct viral invasion of the nervous system.[15] The third category, parainfectious inflammatory encephalitis, which is clinically indistinguishable from viral encephalitis but differs in that the agent has never been cultured from the brain, is suggested by a rise in antibody titers and the associated clinical phenomena in this case. This group of disorders is exemplified by meningoencephalitis as a complication of Epstein–Barr virus, influenza, and mycoplasma infections. Separating the Epstein–Barr and the mycoplasma group from typical postinfectious encephalitis may be somewhat artificial but is pathologically sound. Pathological examination in several cases of the former has shown lack of the typical demyelination, perivascular cuffing, and gliosis generally associated with postinfectious encephalitis.[16] These disorders are also placed in a separate category because the infectious agents have frequently been associated with other immune neurologic disorders, including the Guillain-Barré syndrome, transverse myelitis, and cranial-nerve neuropathies.[17] Parainfectious disorders may occur with or without and before or after clinically apparent viral or mycoplasma infection, and it is unlikely that the encephalitis depends on the presence of the infectious agent within the nervous system. The fourth category consists of the parainfectious but noninflammatory encephalopathies, which are characterized pathologically by brain swelling rather than inflammation and glial reaction.[18] Reye's syndrome is identified as a special example of this type of encephalopathy. Parainfectious brain swelling includes a heterogeneous group of disorders, which have been variously designated acute toxic encephalopathy,[19] acute nonsuppurative encephalitis, and acute brain swelling.[18] This disease, usually of children, is characterized by the acute onset of confusion, frequently leading to coma, and in a large proportion of patients by early status epilepticus. The core of the disease, and the feature that distinguishes it from both postinfectious encephalomyelitis and viral encephalitis, is a persistent increase in intracranial pressure with few or no cells in the CSF. If death ensues it is the result of severe intracranial hypertension. The patients who survive have a slow recovery and are often left with persistent intellectual and other deficits. Pathological examination reveals cerebral edema but no inflammation, necrosis, or demyelination.[19] The cause of the encephalopathy is unknown, and it presents in at least two forms. One form, occurring in toxic-appearing children, is associated with an obvious bacterial infection and has been designated "acute toxic encephalopathy." The other form, of which Reye's syndrome is the paradigm, follows a more banal febrile illness. Reye's syndrome is defined by characteristics other than brain swelling.[20]

Dr. J.-J. Putnam, one of the first physicians to use this case teaching method, is credited with the earliest report of acute toxic brain swelling.[21] In 1895 at this hospital he observed a group of children who had a respiratory-tract illness that he called influenza, followed by the later development of encephalopathy. From his observation that there was no inflammation of the brain he proposed that the cerebral symptoms were due to a toxin elaborated by the infectious agent. Lyon, Dodge, and Adams.[19] described 16 children and adolescents in whom an acute encephalopathy, generally accompanied by seizures, developed after bacterial or viral infection. Most of these patients died, and the autopsy revealed acute, severe brain swelling. Subsequently, there have been scattered reports of cases of increased intracranial pressure without evidence of cerebral inflammation after infection. Some of these cases appear on careful scrutiny to have been examples of anoxic encephalopathy, and others were probably examples of what we now call Reye's syndrome. However, many stand apart as cases of brain swelling without other visceral disease. The average age of patients with acute toxic encephalopathy is three to eight years, although there have been a few reports of adolescents and adults with the illness, including a case reported in *The Diagnosis of Stupor and Coma* by Plum and Posner.[22] That patient, a 46-year-old man, presented with an initial pressure of 260 mm, a protein content of 90 mg per 100 ml, and no cells in the CSF. The nature of the brain edema is unknown except that it seems to be a response to a nonneural infection and can exist independently of inflammation. Interesting cases of Reye's syndrome with unexpected cells in the CSF[23] and, conversely, cases of varicella-associated ataxia, which is usually on an inflammatory basis, with severe brain swelling have been reported.[24] These cases are hybrids between the better understood cases of parainfectious encephalomyelitis and acute brain swelling, and they raise the question whether immune phenomena are involved in both reactions to infection. There are many experimental models of toxic cerebral edema; the form related to pneumococcal and cryptococcal polysaccharide is the most pertinent in relation to parainfectious brain swelling.[25] In Reye's syndrome the basic insult is said to be mitochondrial, but its cause is unknown.

Viral encephalitis and parainfectious encephalitis are both capable of producing seizures and prolonged encephalopathy. However, the absence of white cells in the CSF in this case rules out those diagnoses since pleocytosis is the cardinal sign of inflammation in the nervous system. It is possible that in rare cases of viral encephalitis a CSF sample taken early in the course will not contain any white cells. In this case the CSF white-cell counts were 2, 0, 1, and 0 cells on hospital days one, two, five, and 19, respectively. The single determination of 6 cells on the third hospital day does not reflect the general trend. It has also been stated that viral encephalitis due to neurotropic agents such as herpes simplex and arbovirus can exist without CSF pleocytosis, although that occurrence must be very rare. According to Dr. Richard Whitley, three of 123 patients with biopsy-proved herpes infection in the current prospective herpes simplex encephalitis study had normal spinal fluid. Two patients who were restudied again had no white cells, but neither of them had elevation of the CSF pressure or protein content. The atypical absence of cells in the CSF coupled with the persistent evidence of intracranial hypertension and a fairly high initial CSF protein content make the diagnosis of viral encephalitis in this patient very unlikely.

Postinfectious encephalomyelitis and the parainfectious encephalitis of Epstein–Barr virus and mycoplasma infection may also have a rapid onset with convulsions, coma, and persistent neurologic deficits. The CSF pleocytosis is more variable in cases of parainfectious encephalitis. Several reviews, especially of cases of parainfectious encephalitis after the childhood exanthems, recorded a 20 to 60 per cent frequency of acellular CSF.[26–28] An investigation of the original published sources disclosed that in the majority of those cases only single spinal-fluid samples were taken, either within the first two days or very late in the course.[27,28] Cases with acellular CSF and pathologically verified inflammatory encephalitis are even rarer, if they exist at all. Most importantly, even the few patients reported to have postinfectious or para-infectious encephalitis with acellular CSF have had normal or minimally elevated spinal-fluid pressure and protein content.[26]

This patient had an encephalopathy rather than encephalitis. His illness was characterized by increased spinal-fluid and intracranial pressure and was probably related to a non-neurologic infection. The best neurologic diagnosis, in my opinion, is parainfectious encephalopathy with brain swelling. A disorder of this nature can occur in adults without liver disease and differs from Reye's syndrome. Its relation to the more commonly recognized parainfectious encephalitis remains unclear, and it appears that the two have often been confused in the literature. Many patients with the diagnosis of postinfectious encephalitis accompanied by an acellular CSF have had a high CSF pressure and probably had encephalopathy with brain swelling. The result of the test that was received after discharge in this case was probably a rise in antibody titers in response to an infectious agent. The fact that there was a recent infection is more important than the identity of the particular agent, since brain swelling represents one type of nervous-tissue response to infection, and the individual causative agents have few distinguishing features.

A few other points might refine this diagnosis further. The first is the finding of elevated serum enzyme levels. A rise in CPK does not distinguish between the occurrence of seizures and direct skeletal-muscle involvement related to a parainfectious process. This distinction is important, because if there is an acute myopathy certain agents might be implicated ahead of others. The second issue is determining whether there was liver damage, which would relate the disorder to Reye's syndrome. On admission the SGOT and ammonia levels were normal. For this reason alone the presence of Reye's syndrome is doubtful, although in some reported cases of that disorder the results of liver-function tests and ammonia levels obtained early in the course were normal.[29] The SGOT and LDH isoenzyme 5 elevations are not helpful in making this distinction, and the diagnosis of atypical Reye's syndrome remains a possibility. On the fourth hospital day the CPK was 3060 mU per milliliter (51 μmol · sec^{-1} per liter), and it decreased only slowly, still being elevated on the ninth hospital day. In most cases of enzyme elevation due to seizures as well as in experimentally induced epilepsy the serum CPK level returns to normal in several days, although in rare cases it has remained elevated for up to two weeks.[30] Parallel aldolase determinations showed an increase between the fourth and eighth hospital days. If one excludes the effect of intramuscular injection, this patient apparently had muscle damage continuing well after the initial seizures. A myopathy or myositis associated with the encephalopathy would explain this phenomenon. The status of viral myositis or myopathy is very unclear. A few investigators have reported the isolation of viral particles by electron microscopical examination, but there has been no consistent evidence of direct viral invasion of muscle. Elevation of muscle enzymes and noninflammatory morphologic abnormalities are very common in association with Reye's syndrome as part of the generalized mitochondrial defect.[31] The most common parainfectious myopathies are due to influenza, other respiratory-tract viruses, mycoplasma, and varicella. Varicella can be excluded in the absence of a rash. The only other hint is the patient's previous febrile laryngotracheitis. If this infection incited the encephalopathy the possibility of influenza, respiratory-tract viruses, or mycoplasma must be reconsidered. The vocal-cord granulomas associated with the laryngotracheitis were more suggestive of endotracheal-tube trauma, but the severe persistent difficulty with phonation probably indicated a superimposed infection. Diphtheritic laryngitis should be mentioned only to exclude it, because many of the early cases of acute toxic encephalopathy with brain swelling were associated with diphtheria.

The final item that tenuously suggests a specific infectious agent is the ataxia that appeared during convalescence. When seizures precede ataxia one always suspects anticonvulsants. However, nystagmus is usually prominent with phenytoin toxicity, whereas it was mild in this case. Many postinfectious encephalitis syndromes have been associated with ataxia, particularly those due to varicella,[24] influenza, and mycoplasma,[32–35] although other viruses have also been implicated. The ataxia is usually due to inflammation of the cerebellum, with cells in the spinal fluid.

In summary, in view of the patient's age, the probable myopathy, the laryngotracheitis, the absence of a rash, and possibly the residual ataxia influenza and mycoplasma are the leading contenders as agents responsible for the encephalopathy. The neurologic features associated with mycoplasma infection are so diverse and nonspecific that the diagnosis cannot be made solely on clinical grounds.[33] There are reports of post-mycoplasma-infection encephalopathy associated with elevated spinal-fluid pressure[32,34]; the diagnosis in those cases was postinfectious encephalomyelitis despite a lack of CSF inflammatory cells. The recent report of viable mycoplasma in CSF and blood during the acute phase of the Guillain–Barré syndrome[36] may, if confirmed, require us to reconsider the concept of postinfectious neurologic diseases, but at the moment they are best regarded as immunologic responses to extraneural infection. The best neurologic diagnosis in this case is parainfectious encephalopathy with brain swelling, although it is admittedly difficult to distinguish this entity from postinfectious encephalomyelitis. Influenza and mycoplasma are suspect as the inciting agents and are consistent with the patient's myopathy.

CLINICAL DIAGNOSES

Postinfectious encephalopathy, ? due to mycoplasma.
  Granulomatous laryngotracheitis.

DR. ALLAN H. ROPPER'S DIAGNOSES

Parainfectious encephalopathy with brain swelling, ? due to influenza or mycoplasma.
  Parainfectious acute myopathy.
  Laryngotracheitis.

PATHOLOGICAL DISCUSSION

DR. EDWARD P. RICHARDSON, JR.: The patient was under the care of Dr. Dooling, who has been following him subsequently.

DR. ELIZABETH C. DOOLING: This case was puzzling, and it was difficult to understand completely the nature of the patient's problem during the course in the hospital. After discharge a convalescent mycoplasma complement fixation titer was 1:256, consistent with the diagnosis of mycoplasma encephalopathy.

Lerer and Kalavsky[32] described five children with a similar course; four presented with seizures, and three presented with increased intracranial pressure, with a high protein content but only a slight pleocytosis in the CSF. Mycoplasma infections are most frequent in children between five and 16 years of age. About 50 cases of encephalopathy associated with mycoplasma infection have been reported; about a third of the patients have had a poor outcome, with incapacitating neurologic residua. A poor outcome has usually been associated with an extremely elevated CSF protein content, which has been attributed to polyradiculitis or an encephalopathy.

This patient has made a good recovery but gained about 35 kg in weight over a period of several months. Also, his mother stated that he became apathetic, withdrawn, and indifferent to his friends. In part, his difficulty could be related to his concern about his mother's health, since she has had hip, spine, and lung metastases during this time. However, we have observed a syndrome of postencephalopathic depression in other children and adolescents. As in this patient, there has been a good response to stimulants such as dextroamphetamine or methylphenidate.

DR. ROPPER: What was the anticomplement titer?

DR. DOOLING: It was 1.8.

DR. ROPPER: The anticomplement titers are helpful in interpreting single convalescent titers. After an acute infectious illness patients acquire a high anticomplement titer and avidly complement-fix many antigens. Was mycoplasma grown from the patient's sputum?

DR. DOOLING: Culture of specimens of sputum for mycoplasma was negative.

DR. ROPPER: That fact seems somewhat against the diagnosis, since mycoplasma will grow after the administration of almost any antibiotic unless treatment is given for a prolonged period.

DR. DOOLING: Dr. Keim, of the Infectious Disease Service, may want to comment on this patient's illness.

DR. DANIEL E. KEIM: I did not see this patient, but I have reviewed the serologic data. They are consistent with a *Mycoplasma pneumoniae* infection at about the time of the patient's illness.

DR. RICHARDSON: In conclusion, it seems probable that the patient did have a mycoplasma infection, but the diagnosis is not established with absolute firmness. In a case such as this one, however, determination of the identity of the infectious agent is not as important as reaching an understanding of the nature of the encephalopathy that may follow it.

ANATOMICAL DIAGNOSIS

Parainfectious encephalopathy, associated with Mycoplasma pneumoniae *infection.*

REFERENCES

1. Kolb LC. Alcoholism and alcoholic psychoses. In: Noyes' modern clinical psychiatry. 7th ed. Philadelphia: WB Saunders, 1968:193–210.

2. Reiner ER. The cerebrospinal fluid in methyl alcohol poisoning. Arch Neurol Psychiatr. 1950; 64:528–35.

3. Espelin DE, Done AK. Amphetamine poisoning: effectiveness of chlorpromazine: N Engl J Med. 1968; 278:1361–5.

4. Anderson RJ, Potts DE, Gabow PA, Rumack BH, Schrier RW. Unrecognized adult salicylate intoxication. Ann Intern Med. 1976; 85:745–8.

5. Case Records of the Massachusetts General Hospital (Case 38–1979). N Engl J Med. 1979; 301:650–7.

6. Ludwig G. Lead poisoning. In: Goldensohn E, Appel S, eds. Scientific approaches to clinical neurology. Philadelphia: Lea & Febiger, 1977:1347–79.

7. Kehoe R. Free protoporphyrin content of erythrocytes in chronic tetraethyl lead poisoning. Lancet. 1964; 2:594.

8. Waldenström J. Neurological symptoms caused by socalled acute porphyria. Acta. Psychiatr Neurol Scand. 1939; 14:375–9.

9. Garland H, Pearce J. Neurological complications of carbon monoxide poisoning. Q J Med. 1967; 36:445–55.

10. Lehman EP, Parker WH. The unsolved problems of brain injury: a critical review of the literature. Int Clin. 1935; 3:180–226.

11. Don H. Cardiopulmonary problems associated with neurologic and neurosurgical emergencies. In: Thompson R, Green J, eds. Critical care of neurological and neurosurgical emergencies. New York: Raven Press, 1979:175–82.

12. Infections of the nervous system (nonviral). In: Adams RD, Victor M. eds. Principles of neurology. New York. McGraw-Hill, 1977:618–53.

13. Ho M. Acute viral encephalitis. In: Vinken PJ, Bruyn GW, eds. Handbook of clinical neurology. Vol. 34. Amsterdam: Elsevier/North-Holland, 1978:63–82.

14. DeVries E. Post vaccinial perivenous encephalitis. Amsterdam: Elsevier, 1960.

15. Peters AC, Versteeg J, Lindeman J, Bots GT. Varicella and acute cerebellar ataxia. Arch Neurol. 1978; 35:769–71.

16. Miller HG, Stanton JB, Gibbons JL. Para-infectious encephalomyelitis and related syndromes: a critical review of the neurological complications of certain specific fevers. Q J Med. 1956; 25:427–505.

17. Grose C, Henle W, Henle G, Feorino PM. Primary Epstein–Barr-virus infections in acute neurologic diseases. N Engl J Med. 1975; 292:392–5.

18. Eiben R. Acute brain swelling (toxic encephalopathy). Med Clin North Am. 1967; 14:797–808.

19. Lyon G, Dodge PR, Adams RD. The acute encephalopathies of obscure origin in infants and children. Brain. 1961; 84:680–708.

20. Reye RD, Morgan G, Baral J. Encephalopathy and fatty degeneration of the viscera: a disease entity in childhood. Lancet. 1963; 2:749–52.

21. Putnam JJ. Relation of infectious processes to diseases of the nervous system: pathology and etiology. Am J Med Sci. 1895; 109:254–77.

22. Plum F, Posner JB. The diagnosis of stupor and coma. 3d ed. Philadelphia: FA Davis, 1980.

23. Glick TH, Likosky WH, Levitt LP, Mellin H, Reynolds DW. Reye's syndrome: an epidemiologic approach. Pediatrics. 1970; 46:371–7.

24. Goldston AS, Millichap JG, Miller RH. Cerebellar ataxia with preeruptive varicella. Am J Dis Child. 1963; 106:197–200.

25. Levine S, Zimmerman HM, Wenk EJ, Gonatas NK. Experimental leukoencephalopathies due to implantation of foreign substances. Am J Pathol. 1963; 42:97–117.

26. Scott TFM. Postinfectious and vaccinal encephalitis. Med Clin North Am. 1967; 51:701–17.

27. La Boccetta A, Tornay A. Measles encephalitis: report of 61 cases. Am J Dis Child: 1964; 107:247–55.

28. Boughton CB. Morbilli in Sydney. II. Neurological sequelae of morbilli. Med J Aust. 1964; 2:908–15.

29. Applebaum MM, Thaler MM. Reye syndrome without initial hepatic involvement. Am J Dis Child. 1977; 131:295–6.

30. Belton NR, Backus RE, Millichap JG. Serum creatine phosphokinase activity in epilepsy: clinical and experimental studies. Neurology (Minneap). 1967; 17:1073–6.

31. Roe CR, Schonberger LB, Gelbach SH, Wies LA, Sidbury JB Jr. Enzymatic alterations in Reye's syndrome: prognostic implications. Pediatrics. 1975; 55:119–26.

32. Lerer RJ, Kalavsky SM. Central nervous system disease associated with *Mycoplasma pneumoniae* infection: report of five cases and review of the literature. Pediatrics. 1973; 52:658–68.

33. Hodges GR, Fass RJ, Saslaw S. Central nervous system disease associated with *Mycoplasma pneumoniae* infection. Arch Intern Med. 1972; 130:277–82.

34. Taylor MJ, Burrow GN, Strauch B, Horstmann DM. Meningoencephalitis associated with pneumonitis due to *Mycoplasma pneumonlae*. JAMA. 1967; 199:813–16.

35. Murray HW, Masur H, Senterfit LB, Roberts RB. The protean manifestations of mycoplasma pneumoniae infections in adults. Am J Med. 1975; 58:229–42.

36. Bayer AS, Galpin JE, Theofilopoulos AN, Guze LB. Neurologic disease associated with *Mycoplasma pneumonlae* pneumonitis: demonstration of viable *Mycoplasma pneumoniae* in cerebrospinal fluid and blood by radioisotopic and immunofluorescent tissue culture techniques. Ann Intern Med. 1981; 94:15–20.

Continued preparation of these Case Records has been made possible by a generous grant to the Massachusetts General Hospital from Pfizer Pharmaceuticals.

Perspectives and Updates

This was an odd case of a teenager with a severe acute encephalopathy, seizures, and a hint of drug use. His initial white count was over 20,000 with 95 per cent neutrophils, but he was not febrile. The cerebrospinal fluid showed no inflammation but a protein of 188 mg/dl initially. Several subsequent lumbar punctures showed a few lymphocytes and persistent but declining elevated protein. About three weeks after the onset of illness the patient returned to normal clinically and the protein content of the CSF was likewise normal at 23 mg/dl. I commented in my discussion on the practice of mixing strychnine with recreational drugs as a cause of encephalopathy and seizures, a problem I have encountered in patients twice since. I also gave a very long discussion of the usual causes of encephalitis, but there was little point in going on about this since the CSF was a cellular.

I find value in this case if for no other reason then it occurred in the pre-MRI era. I therefore chose to focus on the elevated CSF pressure in the first two spinal fluid measurements. The initial pressure was reported as 260 mm H_2O, and a second one soon after, was 360 mm H_2O. This remains a fascinating case because of these findings. I invoked a process that had been termed in the subtitle of an article, "acute toxic encephalopathy" by Lyon, Dodge, and Adams (reference 19 in the CPC). They identified Reye syndrome before Reye did but gave it a broader clinical description that was not retained by the neurology readers of the time. I thought the case under discussion was essentially Reye syndrome, or an equivalent form of post- or parainfections brain swelling. Even with the interdiction of aspirin for children with febrile illnesses, Reye-like cases continue to be reported. Lead intoxication and sagittal sinus thrombosis are the main alternative considerations for global brain swelling in children. It is likely that some cases of brain swelling are due to fluid and electrolyte disturbances— that was one of the criticisms of the Lyon, Dodge, and Adams article that could not be easily leveled at the Reye paper. A final note: Johnson reported the same brain swelling illness in children the same year that Reye did,[1] and the entity is sometimes termed Reye-Johnson syndrome.

The trigger of *Mycoplasma* was a guess as the patient had no overt pneumonia.

Allan H. Ropper

REFERENCE

1. Johnson GM, Scurletis TD, Carroll NB. A study of sixteen fatal cases of encephalitis-like disease in North Carolina children. N C Med J 1963; 24:464.

A 63-Year-Old Woman with Agitation and an Extrapyramidal Syndrome

MULTISYSTEM ATROPHY

CPC 23-1983

PRESENTATION OF CASE

A 63-year-old woman was admitted to the hospital because of agitation and an extrapyramidal syndrome.

She was well until 10 years earlier, when the death of her husband was followed by agitation, which improved with the administration of perphenazine and amitriptyline hydrochloride. Four years before admission she fell and injured her back. She became increasingly nervous and retired from her position as a bookkeeper. She became unable to sit still and paced repeatedly; her handwriting deteriorated, and she occasionally drooled from either side. Diphenhydramine hydrochloride, oxazepam, and carbidopa–levodopa were prescribed, without improvement, and she noticed a tendency to stagger while taking medications. Thirty-two months before entry she was first seen at this hospital. Examination showed that she was anxious, repeatedly pacing the floor and wringing her hands. The cranial nerves were normal except that the left nasolabial fold was slightly smaller than the right. Motor function was normal in all extremities; the tone was slightly increased bilaterally, and a fine tremor of the hands was observed. Sensation and coordination were intact. The tendon reflexes were symmetric, and the plantar responses were flexor; no clonus was noted. On the Romberg test the patient tended to fall in any direction but was able to stand after reassurance and practice; the tandem gait was normal. The urea nitrogen was 14 mg per 100 ml (5.0 mmol per liter), and the thyroxine 6.4 μg per 100 ml (82 nmol per liter). Perphenazine–amitriptyline was resumed, with improvement in the symptoms.

Twenty-nine months before entry she fell down a flight of stairs and began to experience more unsteadiness of gait with a tendency to veer to the left. Three months later examination showed mild cogwheel rigidity in the upper extremities, and she fell to the right on the Romberg test. Her spontaneous gait was stable, but the tandem gait was unsteady. Doxepin was substituted for perphenazine and amitriptyline. At followup examination 14 months before admission she felt increasingly unstable. The blood pressure was 160/90 mm Hg on sitting and fell to 130 mm Hg systolic on standing.

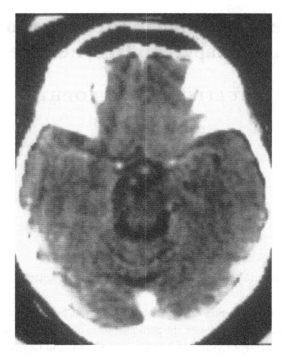

FIG 1 CT Scan Taken One Year before Entry, Showing Dilatation of the Cisterns around the Brainstem Consistent with Slight Atrophy.

Saccadic breakdown in pursuit eye movements was noted. Muscle tone was increased, more markedly on the right side. Her handwriting was small and cramped. The gait was slow and unsteady but with a normal base and arm swing; tandem gait was markedly unsteady. The vitamin B_{12} was 200 pg, and the folate 38.5 ng per milliliter. An electroencephalogram showed intermittent left anterior and midtemporal slowing and sharp waves. A computed tomographic (CT) scan of the brain (Fig. 1), performed after the injection of contrast material, revealed mild atrophic changes and was otherwise normal. The patient began to complain of dizziness when she turned her head; she continued to fall intermittently and had poor coordination of the right hand.

Ten months before entry she returned to the hospital, where examination disclosed slight stiffness on extension of the neck. There was mild dysarthria, but naming, comprehension, and repetitions were well performed. Decreased blink frequency was observed, the left palpebral fissure was widened and the left nasolabial fold flattened; the cranial nerves were otherwise normal. Strength was normal. Cogwheel rigidity was present and more prominent in the right extremities. Vibratory sensation was impaired in the toes and ankles. A mild terminal tremor and ataxia were observed in all extremities. Rapid alternating movements were slower on the right side. The gait was short-stepped, with no arm swing but with a relatively narrow base; tandem walk was poorly performed. On the Romberg test she fell backward without compensatory effort. The tendon reflexes were symmetric, with equivocal plantar responses bilaterally and brisk jaw jerks. X-ray films of the cervical spine showed no prevertebral soft-tissue swelling; the spine was straightened, and there was narrowing of the intervertebral spaces at C3-4 through C6-7, with anterior osteophyte formation predominantly at the level of C4-5; the sagittal diameter of the spinal canal was 17 mm at the level of C2, 14 mm from C3 to C6, and 16 mm at C7; there was slight encroachment on the left fourth through sixth neural foramina and the right fourth and fifth neural foramina. A lumbar puncture yielded clear, colorless, acellular cerebrospinal fluid; the glucose was 69 mg per 100 ml (3.8 mmol per liter), the protein 38 mg per 100 ml, and the gold-sol curve 0012100000; a serologic test for syphilis was negative; the cerebrospinal-fluid IgG was 3.2 mg, and the albumin 27.5 mg per 100 ml; an agarose-gel electrophoresis of the fluid disclosed no banding at an 80-fold concentration. Tests of visual, brainstem, and median somatosensory-evoked responses gave normal results. An electronystagmogram was abnormal because of saccadic breakdown of pursuit eye movements and large ocular deviations during caloric stimulation. Urinary urgency was noted; a urinary-tract infection due to *Escherichia coli* was treated with ampicillin. Doxepin hydrochloride and carbidopa–levodopa were administered, but the latter agent was discontinued five months later because of nausea and lack of improvement. The patient continued to complain of urinary urgency, frequency, and occasional incontinence; doxepin hydrochloride was also discontinued. An intravenous urographic examination showed marked degenerative changes of the lumbosacral spine, which predominantly involved the L4-5 and L5-S1 levels, accompanied by moderate narrowing of disk spaces; the sacroiliac joints were normal, and no soft-tissue calcifications were seen; after the injection of contrast material the kidneys, collecting systems, and ureters appeared normal; moderate trabeculation of the bladder was observed. Six days before entry cystoscopic examination disclosed urethral narrowing; a urethrotomy was performed, but urinary urgency persisted. The patient became more agitated and was light-headed, particularly after being upright for more than half an hour. She was admitted to the hospital.

There was a history of hypertension in previous years, which was treated briefly with an unknown agent. Her mother died at the age of 57 years of a stroke, and her father died at 70 years after a myocardial infarct. There was no history of loss of consciousness, head injury, diabetes mellitus, or amyloidosis. There was no family history of neurologic disease.

The temperature was 35.6°C, the pulse 88, and the respirations 16. The blood pressure was 150/85 mm Hg with the patient supine. With the patient standing the pulse was 100 and the blood pressure 130/90 mm Hg.

On examination the patient was an agitated woman with bradykinesia, a masklike facies, and a flexed posture on standing. The general physical examination was negative; no tenderness was noted over the spine. On neurologic examination she was alert and oriented, with an intact intellect. Mild dysarthria was present; the handwriting was small and barely legible. Lateral eye movements were slow, and upward gaze was impaired. There was cogwheel rigidity in all extremities, more marked on the right side. A fine action tremor was more marked in the right extremities than the left; occasional dystonic movements of the right toes were noted. The gait was shuffling, and tandem walk was impossible. Vibratory sensation was reduced in the lower extremities. The tendon reflexes were + + and symmetric, with equivocal plantar responses; a slight grasp reflex and right sucking response were observed.

The urine was normal. The hematocrit was 41.5 per cent; the white-cell count was 6300, with a normal differential count. The platelet count was 307,000, and the erythrocyte sedimentation rate was 11 mm per hour. The urea nitrogen was 16 mg per 100 ml (5.7 mmol per liter), the glucose 85 mg per 100 ml (4.7 mmol per liter), the uric acid 4.5 mg per 100 ml (0.27 mmol per liter), and the bilirubin 0.3 mg per 100 ml (5 μmol per liter). The sodium was 142 mmol, the potassium 4 mmol, the chloride 103 mmol, and the carbon dioxide 30 mmol per liter. The serum aspartate aminotransferase (SGOT) was 26 U per milliliter (0.21 μmol · sec⁻¹ per liter), the lactic dehydrogenase (LDH) 120 U per milliliter (2.0 μmol · sec¹ per liter), and the alkaline phosphatase 25 IU (0.42 μmol · sec⁻¹) per liter. An electrocardiogram and an x-ray film of the chest were normal. A CT scan of the brain, an electroencephalogram, and tests of visual, brainstem, and median somatosensory-evoked responses showed no change.

Doxepin was resumed, and the patient promptly became less agitated. On the third hospital day the blood pressure was 80/60 mm Hg while she was standing. After she sat for a few minutes the blood pressure was 110/80 mm Hg. Urinary retention recurred, orthostatic dizziness persisted, and desipramine was substituted for doxepin. An endocrinologic consultant noted no abnormal pigmentation or varicose veins. The fasting cortisol was 12.1 μg per 100 ml (0.33 μmol per liter); 30 minutes after the intravenous administration of synthetic adrenocorticotropic hormone (ACTH) the cortisol was 27.8 μg per 100 ml (0.77 μmol per liter), and 60 minutes after the injection it was 33.3 μg per 100 ml (0.92 μmol per liter). The luteinizing hormone was 92.1 mIU, the follicle-stimulating hormone 130 mIU, the prolactin 6.9 ng, and the human growth hormone 6 ng per milliliter. The plasma catecholamines from specimens drawn while the patient was supine, with a pulse of 108 and a blood pressure of 150/90 mm Hg, were 574 pg; when she assumed a dangling posture the blood pressure fell to 90/75 mm Hg, and she complained of persistent dizziness; the plasma catecholamines were 995 pg per milliliter. Desipramine was discontinued; fludrocortisone acetate, aphedrine, and protriptyline hydrochloride were begun, but the symptoms were not improved.

She was discharged to a nursing home, where her symptoms gradually worsened. She required the assistance of two persons to walk and complained of severe dizziness after sitting for 20 minutes. Difficulty with chewing and swallowing developed, and she became unable to eat without assistance and lost an undetermined amount of weight. Her speech volume diminished markedly, the lower extremities became rigid, and the upper extremities had prominent cogwheel rigidity. The patient died two years after discharge from the hospital.

DIFFERENTIAL DIAGNOSIS

DR. ALLAN H. ROPPER*: We are confronted with the problem of a progressive illness evolving over a few years in a middle-aged woman. The process was complex but

---

* Director, Neurological/Neurosurgical Intensive Care Unit, and assistant neurologist, Massachusetts General Hospital; assistant professor of neurology. Harvard Medical School. Currently Vice-Chair, Department of Neurology, Brigham and Women's Hospital.

mainly involved abnormalities of movement, with severe rigidity and difficulty with gait. In addition, two constellations of neurologic abnormalities appeared as the illness progressed. One was ataxia—specifically, a cerebellar-like tremor—and dysarthria. The second was orthostatic hypotension, dizziness, and urinary urgency. The patient also experienced anxiety, with pacing and unsteadiness or imbalance leading to falling. Throughout this period her intellect, cranial nerves, power, and reflexes remained for the most part normal.

In discussing complex neurologic cases of this type one should define the outstanding features of the illness and then search for similarities to those of common or more clearly defined diseases. The central theme in this case is parkinsonism. It is also useful to distinguish among regional diseases such as stroke, multifocal diseases such as multiple sclerosis or multiple emboli, and systemic disease in which groups of anatomically disparate neurons involved in one functional activity are all affected simultaneously. Both diagnostic approaches are used implicitly by neurologists, and the distinction outlined is unique to neurologic diagnosis.

Three of the four cardinal manifestations of the core neurologic syndrome, parkinsonism, were prominent in this patient. The four are tremor at rest, rigidity, bradykinesia, and impaired postural reflexes. There was early deterioration of handwriting, which later became micrographic. The patient had cogwheel rigidity, bradykinesia, flexed and shuffling gait, drooling, mask-like facies, or hypomimia, decreased blink frequency, and eventually increasing rigidity. All these findings are typical of parkinsonism, and preservation of intellect, mild distal dystonic movements, a fine tremor, and impaired upward gaze commonly accompany this disorder. These manifestations do not necessarily indicate the presence of idiopathic Parkinson's disease, since several diseases simulate it or have parkinsonism as one component. This patient's illness exceeded the bounds of typical parkinsonism because of the presence of other features, but the similarities to Parkinson's disease attract the attention of the clinician, even early in the illness. Since parkinsonism is of diverse causes and not a distinct disease a differential diagnosis with an eye toward diseases with additional neurologic manifestations is warranted.

The parkinsonian syndrome may follow infection, such as encephalitis lethargica or syphilis. It may be toxic, may be related to drugs, may follow trauma, or may result from metabolic diseases. Postencephalitic parkinsonism deserves consideration in this case because it is associated with additional neurologic features. About 12 per cent of 802 patients with parkinsonism seen from 1949 to 1964 in a large neurology clinic were thought to have postencephalitic disease,[1] and in four of 119 pathologically studied cases from this hospital typical pathological features of postencephalitic parkinsonism were found.[2] Epidemics of encephalitis lethargica have not occurred for over 50 years, but postencephalitic parkinsonism was at one time the second most common type after the idiopathic form. All the clinical features of idiopathic parkinsonism may be present in the postencephalitic variety, with notable additions that make it a distant consideration in this patient. Dystonia, chorea, myoclonus, or tics, each generally a residuum of the acute encephalitis, are engrafted upon the movements of typical parkinsonism. Residual ocular palsies, mental changes, and sleep or autonomic disturbances also suggest postencephalitic parkinsonism. However, most characteristic of the disease are severe abnormalities of posture and oculogyric crises. In view of the absence of a clear episode of encephalitis or any of the typical features of the disease I do not believe that this patient had postencephalitic parkinsonism. Rarely, other types of encephalitis are associated with parkinsonism, generally as a transient state, and they can be excluded for similar reasons.

Toxins, particularly manganese compounds, should be considered as possible causes of unusual parkinsonian syndromes, but the absence of evidence of exposure excludes them in this case. Similarly, other rare toxic extrapyramidal syndromes due to carbon monoxide, cyanide, methanol, and carbon disulfide can be eliminated, particularly in the absence of an episode of coma or toxic psychosis. Other unusual causes of parkinsonism that can be ruled out for obvious reasons and are mentioned only for completeness are head trauma, a syrinx extending to the substantia nigra (of which there is a single report), deep brain tumors, which would not be compatible with the clinical course or CT findings, hypoparathyroidism with basal-ganglion calcification, acquired hepatocerebral degeneration, and Wilson's disease. Wilson's disease causes an extrapyramidal syndrome with dystonia and psychiatric disturbances and includes some features of cerebellar involvement, but it is distinguished from the disorder in this case by the presence of prominent and early pseudobulbar signs, with a pained-looking facies, severe dysarthria, and disturbed intellect; and by the absence of orthostatic hypotension or prominent falling. Finally, vascular or arteriosclerotic parkinsonism deserves brief comment. The unwarranted popularity of this diagnosis results in part from an article in 1929 by Critchley,[3] in which he suggested that vascular disease was the cause of parkinsonism when tremor was absent and there were accompanying signs of cerebral infarction. He noted in particular the occurrence of dementia, incontinence, pyramidal signs, and pseudobulbar palsy. Unfortunately, he presented no pathological findings. He later tempered his view, presumably because so many patients with parkinsonism have unrelated strokes. Although a few clinical features associated with bilateral deep strokes are similar to those of parkinsonism, there are rarely enough similarities to cause serious confusion between the two. In one study of 114 patients with lacunar infarction none had evidence of parkinsonism.[4] Most cases of "arteriosclerotic parkinsonism" in the literature are probably examples of normal-pressure hydrocephalus.[5]

Drug-induced parkinsonism should also be mentioned, but in this case it would not explain the inexorable progression of the illness or the other associated findings. The possibility that the patient's extra-pyramidal syndrome was exaggerated by neuroleptics, antidepressants, or minor tranquilizers cannot be excluded, but associated limb movements such as arm swinging while walking are prominently suppressed by neuroleptics, whereas they were spared early in this patient's illness.

Having excluded the major known causes of parkinsonism I am left with the problem whether this patient had the idiopathic form. In Parkinson's disease tremor is typically the first symptom; in one large series that was true of 70 per cent of the patients,[1] and only 10 per cent had no tremor even late in the course. Rather than the typical 4-Hz tremor present with the limb at rest and disappearing on initiation of movement, some patients have instead or in addition a faster, so-called action tremor. Action tremor, implying movement of 8 to 12 Hz elicited by maintaining a posture, was present in this patient, but it was neither prominent nor early. That fact and the absence of the slower parkinsonian tremor at rest are the first atypical features for idiopathic Parkinson's disease in this case. The absence of minimal evidence of the typical tremor in a patient with an extrapyramidal disorder raises the suspicion that the illness is not idiopathic Parkinson's disease. Also unusual in this case was the absence of response to carbidopa–levodopa. The major reason, however, for excluding idiopathic Parkinson's disease is the presence of neurologic symptoms indicating disease that extended beyond the substantia nigra, the only consistently affected structure in idiopathic Parkinson's disease.

This patient's disorder, in addition to producing parkinsonism, affected other fairly restricted groups of neurons, allowing some systems, such as those subserving intellect, power, cranial-nerve function, and for the most part sensation, to remain unaffected while functions of the basal ganglions, cerebellar system, and autonomic nervous system deteriorated progressively. The disease was therefore not regional or multifocal but involved neurons in several different functional systems. Systemic abnormalities of this nature always implicate degenerative processes. In this case one is led to consideration of a heterogeneous group of degenerative diseases of the basal ganglions characterized not only by parkinsonism but also by one or more nonextrapyramidal manifestations, such as ataxia, orthostatic hypotension, and amyotrophy. It is probable that the diagnosis is to be found within this group of degenerative diseases. In the large series of cases of parkinsonism to which I alluded these "parkinsonism-plus" constellations accounted for about 3 per cent of all the cases,[1] and in the series of pathologically studied cases of parkinsonism at this hospital 2 per cent of the patients did not have typical idiopathic Parkinson's disease or postencephalitic disease.

These degenerative diseases are striatonigral degeneration, olivopontocerebellar atrophy in cases with cell loss in the basal ganglions, idiopathic orthostatic hypotension or the related Shy–Drager syndrome, spinocerebellar-nigral degeneration, parkinsonism combined with motor-neuron disease, and two diseases that are less clearly tied to the others but nevertheless cause a parkinsonian syndrome—progressive supranuclear palsy and corticodentatonigral degeneration with neuronal achromasia. I shall not discuss the last disease, which is rare, because the movement disorder associated with it only superficially resembles parkinsonism[6] and because of its unclear classification.

For the purposes of classifying this case I have devised a scheme for organizing the diseases that I have mentioned on both a clinical and a pathological basis (Fig. 2). The process that occupies a central position among these degenerative diseases is striatonigral degeneration, characterized by loss of nigral and striatal cells.[7,8] Lewy bodies are not found, and their absence in addition to the presence of striatal atrophy distinguishes this disorder from idiopathic Parkinson's disease, although the two are identical clinically in most respects. In virtually all patients with striatonigral degeneration the diagnosis of Parkinson's disease is made during life. The original descriptions of the disease included rigidity and slowness, to which were later added

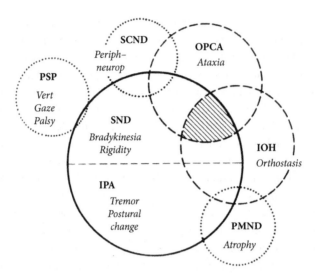

FIG 2 Interrelation among the System Atrophies with Parkinsonism as a Major Clinical Feature.
IPA denotes idiopathic Parkinson's disease, SND striatonigral degeneration, PSP progressive supranuclear palsy, IOH idiopathic orthostatic hypotension, OPCA olivopontocerebellar atrophy, PMND parkinsonism with motor-neuron disease, and SCND spinocerebellar-nigral degeneration.
The major clinical manifestations of each disease are italicized.
The central solid circle represents the parkinsonian syndrome, and the shaded area encompasses cases with features of SND, IOH, and OPCA, as in this case.

hypophonic, hesitant speech, slowness of chewing and swallowing, hypomimia, and slow, flexed walking; two of the four originally described patients had a 4-Hz rest tremor. Reports of subsequent cases, however, suggest that a tremor is not as frequent or prominent as it is in patients with idiopathic Parkinson's disease. The clinical features in the case under discussion were similar to but exceeded those of striatonigral degeneration because of the presence of additional findings, particularly orthostatic hypotension.

Progressive supranuclear palsy resembles parkinsonism but in addition includes axial and nuchal rigidity, a tendency to fall, and a distinctive feature, supranuclear ophthalmoplegia.[9] A rest tremor is rarely observed. The typical appearance of these patients, stiff-necked and sitting straight up, is usually identifiable.[9] Instead, this patient had a flexed, parkinsonian posture. The absence of early and progressive vertical ophthalmoplegia is enough to exclude the diagnosis of progressive supranuclear palsy in this case, but it is of interest that patients with idiopathic Parkinson's disease in whom sepsis developed have been reported to have reversible supranuclear ophthalmoplegia.[10] Progressive supranuclear palsy is not associated with orthostatic hypotension or ataxia and is not a satisfactory diagnosis in this case. The pathological features of progressive supranuclear palsy differ from those of striatonigral degeneration and the other degenerative system atrophies because of the presence of neurofibrillary tangles and widespread cell loss in many nuclear structures. This disorder is therefore only tangentially related to striatonigral degeneration (Fig. 2), mainly because of the presence of some parkinsonian clinical features. However, anxiety and an early tendency for unsteadiness and falling such as the patient under discussion experienced are common in that disorder and require explanation.

The second syndrome to consider in this case is the triad of orthostatic hypotension, urinary urgency, and later urinary retention, characteristic features of idiopathic orthostatic hypotension. These features may occur in isolation but more frequently are combined with a movement disorder, usually parkinsonism, to constitute the Shy–Drager syndrome (Fig. 2). In addition to orthostatic hypotension and sphincteric disturbances the syndrome may include other dysautonomic features such as anhydrosis, which may be patchy, atrophy of the iris, and impotence.[11-15] The substrate for the orthostatic hypotension is thought to be cell loss in the intermediolateral cell columns of the spinal cord, which is the pathological hallmark of the disorder. The cause of the impotence, urinary urgency, and later retention is probably loss of autonomic neurons of the sacral cord.[12] I strongly suspect that there was a central autonomic disturbance in this patient despite the somewhat inconsistent results of plasma catecholamine measurements, which demonstrated an elevated base-line catecholamine concentration with the patient supine and a doubling in concentration with sitting. Patients with idiopathic orthostatic hypotension typically have a low or normal basal catecholamine value and only a slight elevation with upright posture.[16] In the absence of another satisfactory explanation I shall discount the aberrant laboratory results in favor of the clinical data linking the orthostatic hypotension to sphincter disturbances and a movement disorder.

In the majority of the cases of the Shy–Drager syndrome pathological examination reveals cell loss and replacement gliosis in the striatum, nigra, and other pigmented nuclei, thereby relating the disease to striatonigral degeneration. In a few cases there have been cytoplasmic inclusion bodies in pigmented neurons indistinguishable from Lewy bodies and minimal loss of striatal cells, both of which have related the disease to idiopathic Parkinson's disease (Fig. 2).[14] The most striking pathological feature of the Shy–Drager syndrome, which suggests that it is the diagnosis in this case, is the frequently found cell loss in systems other than the basal ganglions and autonomic columns. In some cases the pontine nuclei, cerebellar cortex, and inferior olives are affected.[15] The disease in these cases overlaps with olivopontocerebellar atrophy (shaded area in Fig. 2). For this reason the associated movement disorder in the Shy–Drager syndrome may include, as in this patient, varying degrees of cerebellar ataxia and dysarthria, presumably as a result of pontine and cerebellar cell loss. In a recent analysis of 21 cases of this impure form of the Shy–Drager syndrome combining parkinsonism and dysautonomia[12] there were five with a predominance of nigral changes with Lewy bodies, indicating a relation to Parkinson's disease, six with striatonigral degeneration, and 10 with features of both striatonigral and olivopontocerebellar atrophy. This would be an appropriate time to review the CT scan for evidence of brainstem or cerebellar tissue loss.

DR. KENNETH R. DAVIS: The CT scans before admission (Fig. 1) and on admission are similar. Both demonstrate brainstem, cerebellar, cortical, and central atrophy.

DR. ROPPER: The patient's third major neurologic syndrome was limb ataxia with a terminal trajectory tremor and dysarthria. In most series of cases of olivopontocerebellar atrophy one finds a number of cases with rigidity and the pathological features of striatonigral degeneration.[17-19] Just as in the Shy–Drager syndrome, there frequently are cases of olivopontocerebellar atrophy in which the disease is more widespread than the clinical symptoms would lead one to believe. These crossover cases among the cases of idiopathic orthostatic hypotension, striatonigral degeneration, and olivopontocerebellar atrophy have the same pathoanatomical features but not necessarily the same causes. The manner in which an individual case is reported has often depended on the earliest or most prominent manifestation, whether it was rigidity, ataxia, or orthostatic dizziness. In summary, there are cases with mixtures of clinical manifestations among the system atrophies that simulate those in the case under discussion, and they include parkinsonism, cerebellar ataxia, and dysautonomia. It is worth noting that these cases point up a hierarchy of movement disorders, in that rigidity obscures cerebellar ataxia even if the cerebellar abnormality is more profound than the striatonigral degeneration. That phenomenon probably happened as the illness progressed in this case.

The best clinical diagnosis in this case, therefore, is multiple-system atrophy, a term coined by Graham and Oppenheimer[20] for cases with pathological features of more than one of the following—striatonigral degeneration, idiopathic orthostatic hypotension, and olivopontocerebellar atrophy. To this designation I would add "parkinsonian multiple-system atrophy" because the term is otherwise too vague and sounds somewhat like combined-system disease. The term "parkinsonian multiple-system atrophy" probably should be reserved for crossover cases such as this one, since the other system atrophy designations transmit information about the most prominent symptoms and many cases run true to form pathologically. In this case I suspect that prominent cell loss was found at least in the substantia nigra and putamen (the striatonigral-degeneration component) to explain the parkinsonian syndrome, in the cerebellar hemispheres and basal pons (the olivopontocerebellar-atrophy component) to explain the ataxia and dysarthria, and in the lateral columns of the spinal cord and sacral autonomic nuclei (the idiopathic-orthostatic-hypotension component) to explain the dysautonomia.

There undoubtedly were abnormalities in several other areas, as there typically are in parkinsonian multiple-system atrophy. I do not have enough data to determine if the diminished vibration sense was related to loss of fibers in posterior roots or columns or peripheral nerves. The late preservation of deep tendon reflexes, if indeed it included the Achilles tendon reflexes, is against appreciable neuropathy. Although spinocerebellar-nigral degeneration is inherited and has features of both Friedreich's ataxia and parkinsonism (Fig. 2), which differ from the findings in this case, there has been a large-fiber peripheral neuropathy in several cases of multiple-system atrophy.[21] I shall not be surprised to learn that there was loss of corticospinal-system fibers to explain the increased limb tone. Since the details of this patient's rigidity are not given, the abnormality of tone could have been exclusively extrapyramidal. Finally, in 8 of 10 patients with striatonigral degeneration and olivopontocerebellar atrophy careful pathological study also revealed loss of ventral horn cells despite the absence of amyotrophy during life,[12] and therefore this finding would not be unexpected in the case under discussion. The presence of upper and lower motor-neuron disease would tie the process to amyotrophic lateral sclerosis (Fig. 2).

Finally, severe anxiety, which heralded the onset of this patient's illness, has been an early symptom in a few cases of multiple-system atrophy, as have frequent falling and axial dystonia characteristic of progressive supranuclear palsy.[8,12] Although little insight is gained by this observation because the pathologic changes responsible for these signs are unclear, it at least makes the early history in this case consistent with multiple-system atrophy. Any pathoanatomical crossover between the disorder in this case and progressive supranuclear palsy might be an indicator of areas of the brain involved in producing anxiety. It would also be interesting to know if the patient continued to experience anxiety even after the sympathetic nervous system became severely affected, since much of the subjective and objective nature of anxiety is tied to a hypersympathetic state.

In summary, the disorder in the case under discussion combined features of three diseases, striatonigral degeneration, olivopontocerebellar atrophy, and idiopathic orthostatic hypotension, and is best termed parkinsonian multiple-system atrophy.

DR. STEPHEN W. PARKER: You raised the question of whether the patient had anxiety after the sympathetic nervous system was involved. That was one of the problems faced by the attending clinicians. Every time we stopped the antidepressant medication she experienced severe anxiety, and in fact it precipitated one of the admissions to the hospital. She was treated for the urinary retention with urologic procedures and discontinuance of the antidepressant medication. She then became markedly anxious within a week after admission. We tried to taper and stop the antidepressant medication because we thought that it might be contributing to the postural hypotension. That issue was never settled because she was never off medication for more than a week and a half. She preferred the symptoms of postural hypotension to the marked anxiety experienced when antidepressants were stopped.

CLINICAL DIAGNOSIS

Striatonigral degeneration.

DR. ALLAN H. ROPPER'S DIAGNOSIS

Parkinsonian multiple-system atrophy (combined features of striatonigral degeneration, idiopathic orthostatic hypotension, and olivopontocerebellar atrophy).

PATHOLOGICAL DISCUSSION

DR. E. TESSA HEDLEY-WHYTE: At the time of autopsy the patient was cachectic and dehydrated, with a weight of approximately 30 kg. The immediate cause of death was extensive bronchopneumonia.

The weight of the brain, 1240 g, was approximately normal, as it is in many cases of multisystem disease with parkinsonism. External examination revealed slight atrophy of the frontal lobes, but the most striking findings were the small size of the cerebellum and absence of bulging of the basis pontis. Coronal sectioning of the cerebrum revealed bilateral marked discoloration and shrinkage of the putamen, particularly its posterior portion. The cortex was slightly atrophic, but the ventricles were not unusually dilated for the age of the patient. The thalamus appeared normal. Microscopical examination disclosed almost complete disappearance of small nerve cells in the posterior and lateral portions of the putamen, with loss of their associated myelinated tracts. Occasional large neurons remained, however, even in the most gliotic areas (Fig. 3). The residual neurons and astrocytes contained large amounts of lipofuscin pigment. There was no noticeable loss of neurons in the anterior or medial portion of the globus pallidus, and gliosis was present only in its posterolateral portion. The cerebral cortex appeared normal.

Sectioning of the brainstem revealed bilateral depigmentation of the substantia nigra, particularly in its lateral portion (Fig. 4). Pigmented neurons were markedly decreased in number, and large amounts of melanin pigment were present within macrophages. The pars reticulata was very gliotic. There were no Lewy bodies or neurofibrillary tangles in the substantia nigra or the locus ceruleus.

The pons was markedly affected (Fig. 5). Usually the basis pontis makes up two thirds of the pons, but in this case the distance from the floor of the fourth ventricle to the medial lemniscus accounted for half its width. The middle cerebellar peduncles

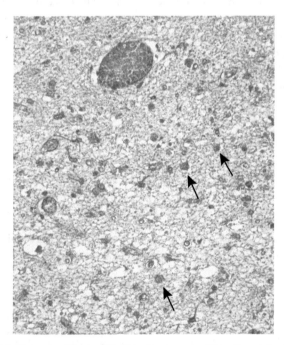

FIG 3 Section of the Putamen, Showing Fibrillary Astrocytes and Rare Remaining Large Neurons (Arrows) (Phosphotungstic-Acid Hematoxylin Stain, ×256).

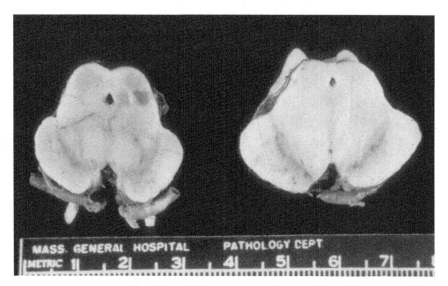

FIG 4 Loss of Pigment in the Shrunken Substantia Nigra (Left) as Compared with the Normal Content (Right).

were markedly discolored and shrunken, but the superior cerebellar peduncles, the dentate nucleus, the medial lemniscus, and the pyramidal tracts appeared normal. Microscopical examination revealed almost total disappearance of the crossing myelinated fibers of the basis pontis (Fig. 6), with a marked loss of neurons. Sectioning of the medulla disclosed a striking decrease in the size of the inferior olive (Fig. 7), and microscopical examination revealed a patchy depletion of its neurons accompanied

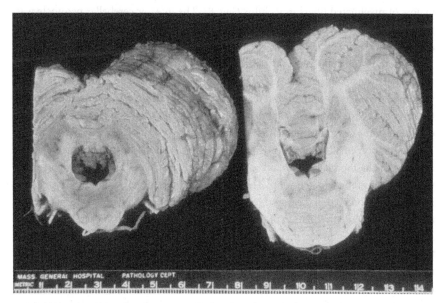

FIG 5 Marked Shrinkage of the Pons, Middle Cerebellar Peduncle, and Derebellar Folia (Left) as Compared with the Normal Appearance (Right).

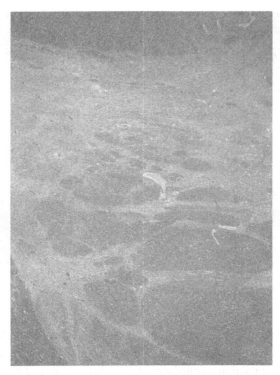

FIG 6 Basis Pontis with the Tegmentum and Medial Lemniscus (Top) and Descending Corticospinal Tracts (Bottom) (Luxol Fast Blue, Hematoxylin and Eosin Stains, ×11)
Note the loss of the normally dark-staining crossing pontine fibers in the center.

by loss of myelinated fibers in its hilus (Fig. 8). The inferior cerebellar peduncle was preserved (Fig. 7) but appeared vacuolated on microscopical examination, suggesting a loss of fibers.

The cerebellum (Fig. 5) was atrophic, with striking involvement of the folia, which were small, principally because of loss of central white matter. The dentate nucleus was well preserved. The myelin around its capsule and in its hilus and the myelin beneath the cerebellar cortex were almost normal in amount, but there was a very striking loss of myelin in the central white matter.

Examination of the spinal cord revealed loss of neurons in the intermediolateral columns in the thoracic region, accompanied by slight gliosis. This finding correlates with the orthostatic hypotension.[22] There were important negative findings as well. No changes were observed in the dorsal roots, their ganglions, or the sympathetic ganglions, and there was no demyelination of the corticospinal or ascending spinocerebellar tracts.

This case as an example, therefore, of multisystem degeneration.[23,24] The overlap of disorders in this category raises the question of the common denominator among the neurons in the putamen, substantia nigra, basis pontis, and lateral columns of the spinal cord. Connections between the putamen and the substantia nigra are well known, but I am not aware of any between the putamen and the basis pontis. It is tempting to speculate that there is a common metabolic denominator among these groups of

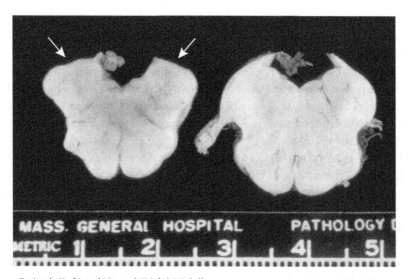

FIG 7 Patient's (Left) and Normal (Right) Medulla.
Note the small size of the inferior olivary nuclei and the preservation of the inferior cerebellar peduncles (arrows)

neurons. In conclusion, this is an example of striatonigral degeneration or perhaps better described as a multisystem degeneration, since this case, as well as some of the others reported in the literature, has features of the Shy–Drager syndrome and olivopontocerebellar degeneration.

DR. WALTER KOROSHETZ: In the reported cases of the Shy–Drager syndrome weren't the changes in the intermediolateral columns much more obvious than they were in this case?

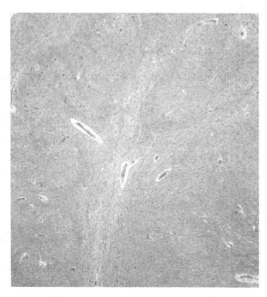

FIG 8 Inferior Olivary Nucleus with Partial Loss of Neurons and Loss of Normally Dark-Staining Myelin in the Hilus (Luxol Fast Blue, Hematoxylin and Eosin Stains, ×31).

DR. HEDLEY-WHYTE: They were more obvious in one of them,[20] in which examination of comparative levels of the thoracic cord showed an obvious gliosis in the intermediolateral columns.

DR. MICHAEL A. MOSKOWITZ: Other types of pathological examination can be performed in patients such as this one. Neurotransmitters can be measured by determining the levels and activities of enzymes involved in their synthesis and degradation. The changes that are observed are even more striking than those detected by the more traditional histologic approaches.

DR. HEDLEY-WHYTE: That is a very good point. When a disease with a probable metabolic background is being investigated at the time of autopsy tissue should be frozen not only for biochemical study but also for fluorescence and immunocytochemistry. One can also look for indexes of metabolic activity such as cytochrome oxidase[25] as well as for degenerating nerve endings.[26]

DR. KENNETH L. TYLER: In one of the original four cases of striatonigral degeneration studied by Dr. Raymond D. Adams pathological examination revealed cerebellar changes consistent with olivopontocerebellar atrophy. Have other cases with that combination been seen at this hospital?

DR. LAWRENCE R. WECHESLER: Case 4 in the paper by Adams et al.[8] was similar to this one, with the pathological findings of both striatonigral degeneration and olivopontocerebellar atrophy. Subsequently, there have been several similar reported cases.[12,15,23]

ANATOMICAL DIAGNOSES

Multiple-system atrophy with parkinsonism (striatonigral degeneration, olivopontocerebellar atrophy, and degeneration of intermediolateral spinal columns).
Bronchopneumonia.

REFERENCES

1. Hoehn MM, Yahr MD. Parkinsonism: onset, progression, and mortality Neurology (Minneap) 1967; 17:427–42.
2. Richardson EP Jr. Remarks on the pathology of Parkinson's disease. In: Barbeau A, Doshay LJ, Spiegel EA, eds. Parkinson's disease: trends in research and treatment. Monographs in biology and medicine. Vol. 4. New York: Grune and Stratton, 1965:63–8.
3. Critchley M. Arteriosclerotic Parkinsonism. Brain 1929; 52:23–83.
4. Fisher CM. Lacunes: small, deep cerebral infarcts. Neurology (Minneap) 1965; 15:774–84.
5. Earnest MP, Fahn S, Karp JH, Rowland LP. Normal pressure hydrocephalus and hypertensive cerebrovascular disease. Arch Neurol 1974; 31:262–6.
6. Rebeiz JJ, Kolodny EH, Richardson EP Jr. Corticodentatonigral degeneration with neuronal achromasia. Arch Neurol 1968; 18:20–33.
7. Adams R, van Bogaert L, Van der Eccken H. Dégénérescences nigro-striées et cerebello-nigro-striées. Psychiatr Neurol (Basel) 1961; 142:219–59.
8. Adams RD, van Bogaert L, Vander Eecken H. Striato-nigral degeneration. J Neuropathol Exp Neurol 1964; 23:584–608.

9. Steele JC, Richardson JC, Olszewski J. Progressive supranuclear palsy: a heterogeneous degeneration involving the brain stem, basal ganglia and cerebellum with vertical gaze and pseudobulbar palsy, nuchal dystonia and dementia. Arch Neurol 1964; 10:333–59.

10. Guiloff R, George R, Marsden CD. Reversible supranuclear ophthalmoplegia associated with Parkinsonism. J Neurol Neurosurg Psychiatry 1980; 43:552–4.

11. Shy GM, Drager GA. A neurological syndrome associated with orthostatic hypotension: a clinical-pathologic study. Arch Neurol 1960; 2:511–27.

12. Sung JH, Mastri DR, Segal E. Pathology of Shy–Drager syndrome. J Neuropathol Exp Neurol 1979; 38:353–68.

13. Roessmann U, van den Noort S, McFarland DE. Idiopathic orthostatic hypotension. Arch Neurol 1971; 24:503–10.

14. Vanderhaeghen J, Périer O, Sternon JE. Pathological findings in idiopathic orthostatic hypotension: its relationship with Parkinson's disease. Arch Neurol 1970; 22:207–14.

15. Bannister R, Oppenheimer DR. Degenerative diseases of the nervous system associated with autonomic failure. Brain 1972; 95:457–74.

16. Bannister R, Sever P, Gross M. Cardiovascular reflexes and biochemical responses in progressive autonomic failure. Brain 1977; 100:327–44.

17. Klawans HL, Zeitlin E. L-Dopa in Parkinsonism associated with cerebellar dysfunction (probable olivopontocerebellar degeneration). J Neurol Neurosurg Psychiatry 1971; 34:14–9.

18. Critchley M, Greenfield JG. Olivo-ponto-cerebellar atrophy. Brain 1948; 71:343–64.

19. Jellinger K, Degenerations and exogenous lesions of the pallidum and striatum. In: Vinken PJ, Bruyn GW, eds. Handbook of clinical neurology. Vol. 6. Amsterdam: Elsevier/North-Holland, 1968; 632–93.

20. Graham JG, Oppenheimer DR. Orthostatic hypotension and nicotine sensitivity in a case of multiple system atrophy. J Neurol Neurosurg Psychiatry 1969; 32:28–34.

21. Galassi G, Nemni R, Baraldi A, Gibertoni M, Colombo A. Peripheral neuropathy in multiple system atrophy with autonomic failure. Neurology (NY) 1982; 32:1116–21.

22. Johnson RH, Lee G de J, Oppenheimer DR, Spalding JMK. Autonomic failure with orthostatic hypotension due to intermediolateral column degeneration: a report of two cases with autopsies. Q J Med 1966; 35:276–92.

23. Tekei Y, Mirra SS. Striatonigral degeneration: a form of multiple system atrophy with clinical parkinsonism. In: Zimmerman HM, ed. Progress in neuropathology. Vol. 2. New York: Grune & Stratton, 1973;217–51.

24. Adams RD. The striatonigral degenerations. In: Vinken PJ, Bruyn GW, eds. Handbook of clinical neurology. Vol. 6. Amsterdam: Elsevier/North-Holland, 1968:694–702.

25. Horton JC, Hubel DH. Regular patchy distribution of cytochrome oxidase staining in primary visual cortex macaque monkey. Nature 1981; 292:762–4.

26. Mesulam M-M. Tracing neural connections of human brain with selective silver impregnation: observations on geniculocalcarine, spinothalamic, and entorhinal pathways. Arch Neurol 1979; 36:814–8.

Continued preparation of these Case Records has been made possible by a generous grant to the Massachusetts General Hospital from Pfizer Pharmaceuticals

Perspectives and Updates

This CPC of multiple system atrophy (MSA) was discussed at a time when the concept of these variant types of parkinsonism were just being articulated. They were previously included in the clinical grouping of "Parkinson plus syndromes," which contained progressive supranuclear palsy, striatonigral degeneration with autonomic failure, and Machado-Joseph disease among other disparate movement disorders. Lewy-body disease was known at the time of this discussion (1983) but had yet to be fully described and incorporated into thinking about multiple system degenerations. Corticobasal degeneration was still called corticodentatonigral degeneration with neuronal achromasia, after the characteristic pathologic change in parietal cortical neurons.

It is still not clear to me if there is truly a unifying theme that should bind cerebellar degeneration, autonomic failure, and parkinsonian types of MSA and the old designations of olivopontocereballar atrophy (which would now be called MSA-C, for cerebellar), Shy-Drager syndrome (MSA-A, for autonomic) and striatonigral degeneration (MSA-P, for parkinsonism); the older designations certainly transmit more clinically useful information than the new ones. I do not make this statement just to be iconoclastic. It is infrequent to find the cerebellar syndromes crossing over with the other two syndromes, and the adjective "multiple" fails to capture much beyond those cases of parkinsonism with orthostatic hypotension, a combination that is seen as often with idiopathic Parkinson disease. Machado-Joseph disease is its own entity and is more of a true multiple-system atrophy than are cases given the MSA denotation. However, this CPC is exemplary of MSA because the patient had rigidity, ataxia, and orthostatic hypotension, one of the few instances that make a case for MSA as a clinical, and perhaps pathologic, category of disease.

Again, this is not just polemical. Most textbooks of neuropathology adhere to the idea that all the forms MSA (the term coined by Graham and Oppenheimer) uniquely share the property of an oligodenroglial intranuclear inclusion.[1] The theme of synucleinopathy, not known at the time of this CPC discussion, has unfortunately failed to assist clinicians because of the phenotypic heterogeneity of diseases that it defines; but in MSA, the inclusion material is present in oligodendrocytes rather than in neurons, as it is in Lewy-body and Parkinson diseases. It is still not clear if MSA should therefore be considered to be a synucleinopathy and also unclear how the deposition of the protein creates vastly multiple phenotypes.

This CPC led to many requests for me to send a slide or permission to copy the Venn diagram of my conceptualization of the shared features between various parkinsonian disorders (Fig. 2). That diagram reflected a clinical perspective that was meant to capture the overlap of neurological signs between the various movement disorders.

It turned out to be a valuable way to teach about these diseases and to show how to approach them in an office practice, but it is now clear that this model offers limited biological insight.

The definitive articles on MSA are currently, in my opinion, the ones from Wenning's group[2,3] which were published after the appearance of this case report.

Allan H. Ropper

REFERENCES

1. Lantos P. The definition of multiple system atrophy: a review of recent developments. J Neuropathol Exp Neurol 1998; 57:1099.
2. Wenning GK, Ben-Shlomo Y, Magalhaes M, et al. Clinical features and natural history of multiple system atrophy: an analysis of 100 cases. Brain 1994; 117:835.
3. Wenning GK, Ben-Shlomo Y, Magalhaes M, et al. Clinicopathologic study of 35 cases of multiple system atrophy. J Neurol Neurosurg Psychiatry 1995; 58:160

A 29-Year-Old Woman with Myalgia and Muscle Weakness

PORPHYRIA

CPC 39-1984

PRESENTATION OF CASE

A 29-year-old woman was admitted to the hospital because of myalgia and muscle weakness.

She was well until three weeks earlier, when she awoke with pain in the lumbar region and abdomen that increased during the day. On the following day the pain extended into the proximal portions of the thighs. She entered another hospital, where she was treated for a urinary-tract infection with ampicillin. Shortly after admission two generalized grand mal seizures were observed. The sodium was 107 mmol per liter. An electroencephalogram was reported to be mildly abnormal, without focal or seizure activity. Phenytoin sodium was begun, and hypertonic saline was administered by vein. The patient improved and was discharged on the ninth hospital day. The pain persisted, and during the next few days it spread to involve the upper portions of the arms and occasionally the shoulders. Six days before admission, on attempting to lift a cup of coffee, she first noticed muscle weakness. On the next day weakness was observed in both arms, and during the next few days it affected her legs. She was admitted to this hospital.

The patient was a divorced mother of four children and worked at an electronics assembly plant. There was a history of several syncopal episodes 10 or more years before admission. A tubal ligation was performed in the past, and a urinary-tract infection was treated at another hospital three years before entry. She had noted occasional palpitation, arthralgia of the knees and elbows, constipation, and a nasal voice during the several weeks preceding admission. She smoked nearly one pack of cigarettes daily, consumed 6 to 12 bottles of beer and uncertain amounts of vodka daily, and used diazepam on a chronic basis but had discontinued use of alcohol and diazepam at the time of entry to the other hospital. Her mother was an alcoholic. There was no history of previous similar illness, fever, chills, diarrhea, previous seizures, difficulty in swallowing, sphincter disturbances, headache, diplopia, ptosis, dyspnea, dryness of the eyes or mouth, rash, Raynaud's phenomenon, periorbital edema, recent respiratory-tract infection or diarrhea, use of vaccines, increased weakness with sustained activity, or use of drugs other than diazepam. There was no family history of muscle weakness.

The temperature was 36.1°C, the pulse was 90, and the respirations were 18. The blood pressure was 140/85 mm Hg.

On examination the patient was a quiet woman who appeared mildly depressed and older than her stated age. No rash or lymphadenopathy was found, and the joints were normal. The lungs, heart, and breasts were normal. The abdomen and extremities were normal, and pelvic and rectal examinations were negative.

Neurologic examination revealed that the patient was alert and oriented but was irritable and had difficulty giving a coherent history and cooperating for a detailed neurologic examination. There was no aphasia or apraxia. The right pupil was 0.5 mm larger than the left, and both were reactive; no ptosis or diplopia was found. The remaining cranial nerves were normal. There was considerable muscle tenderness, particularly in the thighs. Strength in the upper extremities was graded 2 on a scale of 5 in the right arm and 2–3 in the left arm; in the lower extremities the hip flexors and extensors were graded 3 on the right side and 4 on the left; the knee flexors and extensors were 4 on the right side and 5 on the left. The more distal muscles were graded 3–4 in the right upper extremity, 4–5 in the left upper extremity, and 5 in the lower extremities. The neck flexors and extensors were 5 bilaterally. Sensation and coordination were normal. The tendon reflexes were + + and equal except that the triceps was + bilaterally; the plantar responses were flexor.

The urine was amber and had a specific gravity of 1.022 and a pH of 5.0; the sediment contained 15 white cells, rare granular casts, and a few bacteria per high-power field. A stool specimen gave a negative test for occult blood. The hematocrit was 38.9 per cent; the white-cell count was 6300, with 58 per cent neutrophils, 40 per cent lymphocytes, and 2 per cent monocytes. The platelet count was 291,000, and the erythrocyte sedimentation rate 8 mm per hour. The prothrombin time was 9.1 seconds, with a control of 10.7 seconds; the partial thromboplastin time was 27.5 seconds. The urea nitrogen was 23 mg per 100 ml (8.2 mmol per liter), the glucose 123 mg per 100 ml (6.83 mmol per liter), the calcium 9.3 mg per 100 ml (2.3 mmol per liter), the phosphorus 3.7 mg per 100 ml (1.2 mmol per liter), the uric acid 3.0 mg per 100 ml (0.2 mmol per liter), the bilirubin 0.3 mg per 100 ml (5.1 μmol per liter), and the protein 6.4 g (the albumin 3.7 g and the globulin 2.7 g) per 100 ml. The phenytoin level was 18.6 μg per milliliter. The sodium was 138 mmol, the potassium 4.1 mmol, the chloride 92 mmol, and the carbon dioxide 28 mmol per liter. The serum aspartate aminotransferase (SGOT) was 31 U per milliliter (0.25 μmol · sec^{-1} per liter), the lactic dehydrogenase (LDH) 78 U per milliliter (1.3 μmol · sec^{-1} per liter), the creatine kinase (CK) 13 mU per milliliter (0.22 μmol · sec^{-1} per liter), the amylase 10 U, and the alkaline phosphatase 54 IU (0.90 μmol · sec^{-1}) per liter. An electrocardiogram revealed sinus tachycardia at a rate of 126 and was within normal limits. X-ray films of the chest were normal. A lumbar puncture yielded clear, colorless cerebrospinal fluid that contained 2 red cells, 1 lymphocyte, and 1 mononuclear cell per cubic millimeter; the glucose was 80 mg per 100 ml (4 mmol per liter), and the protein 21 mg per 100 ml; a gold-sol test was 2222110000; a culture was negative. Serum immunoelectrophoresis showed a mild increase in IgG and a mild decrease in IgA, with a normal IgM precipitin arc; agarose-gel electrophoresis demonstrated a normal pattern with a mild, diffuse increase in gamma globulins. A serologic test for syphilis and tests for rheumatoid factor and antinuclear antibodies were negative. A culture of urine yielded a few colonies of *Torulopsis glabrata*. Vaginal cytologic examination disclosed no tumor cells.

The patient was continued on phenytoin sodium and was given prednisone, diphenhydramine hydrochloride, acetaminophen, codeine, folic acid, thiamine, multiple vitamins, chlordiazepoxide, and amoxicillin. She remained afebrile; the heart rate ranged from 100 to 120. On the second hospital day she continued to complain of pain and weakness in the extremities and experienced some difficulty with swallowing, although she ate well and ambulated and showered with minimal assistance. The urine was orange; the sediment contained 8 white cells and a few bacteria per high-power field. The urea nitrogen was 13 mg per 100 ml (4.6 mmol per liter). The sodium was 125 mmol, the potassium 3.5 mmol, the chloride 86 mmol, and the carbon dioxide 29 mmol per liter. Prednisone was discontinued. Indomethacin and hydroxyzine pamoate were administered; the dose of phenytoin sodium was tapered, and phenobarbital was substituted.

On the third hospital day weakness and myalgia continued. Physical examination revealed no change. The administration of edrophonium chloride by vein resulted in no increase in strength. On the following day the patient still complained of myalgia and weakness. Examination showed no change. The results of electrophysiologic studies, including conventional motor-nerve and sensory-nerve conduction and minimal latencies for late responses, were within normal limits. Needle electromyographic examination (EMG) revealed no evidence of active denervation (fibrillations and positive sharp waves), fasciculations, or primary muscle disease; the recruitment pattern in the biceps and mid-deltoid was "low mixed."

A diagnostic procedure was performed.

DIFFERENTIAL DIAGNOSIS

DR. MARTIN A. SAMUELS[*]: This patient clearly had acute hepatic porphyria. To dwell on a lengthy differential diagnosis would be artificial and misleading. As is often true in cases of porphyria, the attending physicians required some time in arriving at the proper diagnosis. This patient dwindled for nine days in another hospital and later for three days in this hospital before the proper diagnostic test was ordered. What could the doctors have been thinking? When she was admitted to the other hospital it is clear that the working diagnosis was a urinary-tract infection. This diagnosis was apparently based principally on the abdominal and back pain. We have no information about whether the urinalysis supported this interpretation. When seizures developed and she was found to be severely hyponatremic the diagnosis of a simple urinary-tract

* Chief, Neurology Service. Veterans Administration Medical Center. Brockton-West Roxbury: physician. Brigham and Women's Hospital; assistant professor of neurology. Harvard Medical School. Currently Chair, Department of Neurology, Brigham and Women's Hospital.

infection should have come into question. Perhaps it did, but nonetheless the attending physicians treated her with hypertonic saline and phenytoin, and the latter proved to a serious error in retrospect.

When the patient came to this hospital she had a six-day history of progressive weakness, several weeks of a nasal voice, and severe pain in the back, abdomen, and upper arms. She was an alcoholic. In addition to proximal muscle weakness the examination revealed considerable muscle tenderness. At that point and on the basis of the clinical history and examination alone one might have concluded that the illness was acute rhabdomyolysis associated with alcoholism. After all, the proximal muscle weakness suggested the possibility of a myopathy, and very few myopathies are associated with exquisite muscle tenderness. Acute rhabdomyolysis with myoglobinuria produces the most painful myopathy. The urine was later said to be orange, possibly supporting this interpretation. However, the creatine kinase level was only 13 mU per milliliter. No acute myopathy producing this degree of muscle weakness and pain could be associated with a normal CK level. This point was subsequently supported by the neurophysiologic studies, which failed to show any myopathic changes. At that juncture any consideration of an acute myopathy should have been dropped. There are no other reasonable differential diagnostic possibilities. The performance of an edrophonium test to exclude myasthenia gravis in this patient with severe pain, proximal weakness, hyponatremia, seizures, and orange urine was admirable for completeness but predictably was of no avail. The switching of the anticonvulsant from phenytoin to phenobarbital shows that the attending physicians still had not thought of porphyria.

A few points of historical interest have bearing on this disorder. George William Frederick was the third hanoverian king of England.[1] George III was born in 1738 and ruled from 1760 to 1811, when a regent was appointed because of a series of episodes of "madness" associated with abdominal pain, constipation, weakness of the limbs, hoarseness, a fast pulse, and darkening of the urine. On one occasion in 1788 he had seizures and nearly died. It is believed by some that an episode of illness in 1765, when the king was 26 years old, resulted in his allowing the enactment of the ill-advised Stamp Act, which led in part to the American Revolution. Although there is little evidence that the king was insane in 1765, it is clear that the serious illness in 1788 resulted in the "Regency Crisis," in which the Whigs tried to wrest power from members of the king's cabinet, including the prime minister, William Pitt. An analysis of the king's family history reveals that the illness may have originated from Mary, Queen of Scots,[1] a Stuart, and spread through her descendants to the hanoverian line and Prussian royal family. As such, the illness may well have had major implications, both politically and in the history of medicine, in particular in the development of modern psychiatry.[2] These insights regarding George III were, of course, made in retrospect, since the first case of porphyria was published in 1890.[3] The term "porphyria" was introduced by Hans Fischer and popularized by Waldenström.[4] The history of the elucidation of the biochemical defects in the porphyrias is fascinating but too complex to review in this context. It is summarized beautifully by Tschudy[5] in his role as the moderator of a conference at the National Institutes of Health in 1975 on the subject of acute intermittent porphyria. I shall limit my discussion to the clinicopathological correlations, since they are the major goal of this exercise.

The porphyrias are a group of disorders involving inherited abnormalities in heme biosynthesis, with clinical effects primarily on the nervous system, skin, and liver. To understand them we must review the heme biosynthetic pathways (Fig. 1).[6] Glycine, an amino acid, and succinyl CoA, a compound generated by the Krebs cycle, are combined in the mitochondrion to beta-delta-aminolevulinic acid (ALA) by pyridoxal phosphate and the enzyme ALA synthetase, which is the rate-limiting enzyme in the heme biosynthetic pathway. This ALA leaves the mitochondrion, and two molecules of it are condensed to form porphobilinogen (PBG), a monopyrrol, by ALA dehydrase. Four PBG molecules are combined to form a tetrapyrrol by the enzyme uroporphyrin-l-synthetase, also known as PBG deaminase. The tetrapyrrols uroporphyrinogen I and uroporphyrinogen III are produced from a postulated intermediate compound by cosynthetase enzymes. Uroporphyrinogen III has side chains of acetate and propionic acid. Decarboxylation of the acetate side chain leads

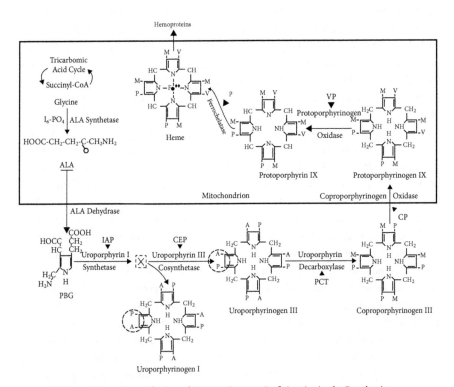

FIG 1. Outline of Heme Biosynthesis and Known Enzyme Deficiencies in the Porphyrias. (Copyright 1982, American Medical Association, Reproduced with Permission.[6])

ALA denotes delta-aminolevulinic acid, PBG porphobilinogen, X postulated intermediate, A acetic acid, P propionic acid, M methyl, and V vinyl.

Arrows show the location of enzyme deficiency for each of the porphyrias. IAP denotes intermittent acute porphyria, CEP congenital erythropoietic porphyria, PCT porphyria cutanea tarda, CP coproporphyria, VP variegate porphyria, and P protoporphyria.

to coproporphyrinogen III, which returns to the mitochondrion for the final steps in heme biosynthesis. These final steps consist of oxidation of coproporphyrinogen III to protoporphyrinogen IX by coproporphyrinogen oxidase, followed by further oxidation to protoporphyrin IX by protoporphyrinogen oxidase. Iron is then added by the enzyme ferrochelatase to form heme.

It is estimated that 250 mg of heme is synthesized per day; four fifths of the heme appears in hemoglobin. The synthesis occurs with only 4 mg of excess ALA, 1.5 mg of excess PBG, 0.1 mg of excess uroporphyrinogen, 0.3 mg of excess coproporphyrinogen, and 0.1 mg of excess protoporphyrinogen. Excess porphyrins are not converted to bilirubin but are excreted. The mode of excretion is determined by water solubility. Thus, ALA, PBG, and porphyrinogen are almost exclusively excreted in the urine owing to their high water solubility, whereas protoporphyrin, being water insoluble, is excreted in the feces. Coproporphyrin, which is of intermediate solubility, is excreted in both the urine and the feces.[6]

The porphyrias are characterized by excessive excretion of porphyrins or their precursors. Each porphyria is a distinct genetic entity, with specific biochemical features and a well-defined enzyme defect.[7] Intermittent acute porphyria is due to a deficiency of porphobilinogen deaminase, formerly known as uroporphyrinogen I synthetase. Congenital erythropoietic porphyria is due to a deficiency in the enzyme uroporphyrinogen III cosynthetase. Porphyria cutanea tarda (symptomatic porphyria) is caused by a deficiency of the enzyme uroporphyrinogen decarboxylase. Coproporphyria is due to a deficiency of the enzyme coproporphyrinogen oxidase. Variegate porphyria (South African porphyria) is due to a deficiency in the enzyme protoporphyrinogen oxidase. Protoporphyria is due to a deficiency in the enzyme ferrochelatase (Fig. 1).

With knowledge of the enzyme deficiencies, the normal heme biosynthetic pathway, and the excretion patterns it is easy to work out the expected pattern of precursor excretion for each of the porphyrias. For example, in intermittent acute porphyria PBG deaminase is deficient. Thus, ALA and PBG will be the accumulated precursors. Since these are both water soluble they should appear in the urine in elevated amounts, whereas the stool should be normal. In variegate porphyria the enzyme block is well down the biosynthetic pathway, leading to excessive levels of ALA, PBG, uroporphyrinogen, corproporphyrinogen, and protoporphyrinogen. Since protoporphyrinogen is not water soluble, patients with variegate porphyria have an elevated level of protoporphyrin in the stool as well as elevated levels of ALA and PBG in the urine. In coproporphyria the enzyme deficiency of coproporphyrinogen oxidase leads to a very elevated level of coproporphyrinogen, which can be found in the stool.

One last biochemical point is important. Heme acts through a negative feedback mechanism in the mitochondrion to inhibit ALA synthetase. If heme biosynthesis is defective, then ALA synthetase is induced. Despite these partial blocks in the heme synthesis mechanism none of the porphyrias ever cause enough heme deficiency to result in anemia.

The porphyrias have traditionally been divided into three categories on the basis of the locus of the associated enzyme deficiency—erythropoietic, erythrohepatic, and hepatic. Congenital erythropoietic porphyria (Gunther's disease) is characterized by photosensitivity of the skin with bullous lesions appearing early after birth. It is the only porphyria inherited as an autosomal recessive trait. It is not characterized by acute attacks and is clearly not a consideration in this case. There is also an erythropoietic coproporphyria in which the red-cell coproporphyrin level is elevated in association with photosensitivity.[8] Erythrohepatic protoporphyria is inherited as an autosomal dominant trait and is characterized by skin sensitivity to light and by hepatic disease, which can lead to severe cirrhosis and hepatic failure. Acute attacks do not occur, and it is also clearly excluded in this case.

The hepatic porphyrias are divided into two types—acute and chronic—based on their clinical features. The only chronic hepatic porphyria is porphyria cutanea tarda (PCT), or symptomatic porphyria. PCT is known to have two forms: one is inherited as an autosomal dominant disorder, and the other is sporadic. The clinical characteristics of the two forms are identical, consisting of blistering, friability, hyperpigmentation, and scarring of the light-exposed skin. There are no acute attacks.[9] Clearly, this patient did not have porphyria cutanea tarda.

The remaining hepatic porphyrias are designated acute because of their tendency to produce attacks. They are intermittent acute porphyria (IAP), variegate porphyria (VP), and coproporphyria (CP). These entities are clearly distinct on the basis of their biochemical analyses, but they may be difficult or impossible to separate on clinical grounds. The combination of acute attacks plus skin lesions suggests either VP or CP. However, patients with the biochemical disorders of variegate porphyria and coproporphyria may present with only acute attacks. Thus, in the absence of skin lesions there is no definite clinical method for distinguishing IAP from VP and CP. This patient presented with nearly all the typical clinical features of acute hepatic porphyria, but since no skin lesions are described we cannot be certain which of the three acute hepatic porphyrias she had. This distinction requires the clinical pathologist's analysis of urine for ALA and PBG, of stool for protoporphyrin and coproporphyrin, and of red cells or white cells for the specific enzyme deficiency—PBG deaminase for IAP, protoporphyrinogen oxidase for VP, and coproporphyrinogen oxidase for CP.

Since this is a clinicopathological conference it might be interesting to speculate for a few moments on the proposed pathogenesis of the various clinical features of the illness, so nicely demonstrated by the case history today.

This patient presented with pain, which began in the abdomen and lower back and spread to involve the limbs. It was confused with urinary-tract pain, and in fact three years previously she had been treated for another alleged urinary-tract infection that may also have been an attack of porphyria. Pain of this type occurs in the vast majority of patients during an acute attack of porphyria. It has been postulated that the pain is due to an autonomic neuropathy, although hard evidence for that concept is difficult to find and the rationale for pain in such a circumstance is not clear. Bowel spasm has been observed at laparotomy,[10] autonomic neuropathy has been found at autopsy,[11] and ganglionic blocking agents may relieve the pain.[12] It may be the ganglionic blocking effects of phenothiazines that render them effective in treating some patients in this setting.

Tachycardia is a common manifestation of the acute attack, and the patient under discussion had pulse rates that ranged from 100 to 120. Tachycardia may also be a manifestation of an autonomic neuropathy affecting the vagus nerve. The same explanation of vagal neuropathy has been used to understand the constipation that is often present, as it was in this patient.

This patient also had hyponatremia, another common manifestation of acute porphyric attacks. In some cases gastrointestinal loss of sodium partially explains this finding, whereas in others a subtle renal lesion may be present. However, in most cases all the physiologic indexes of the syndrome of inappropriate secretion of antidiuretic hormone (SIADH) are found. Vacuolation has been observed in neurons in the supraoptic nucleus of the hypothalamus in patients who have died of acute porphyria with hyponatremia. It is believed by some that this change is pathognomonic of SIADH of any cause and results in this circumstance from a toxic stimulus to the supraoptic nucleus.[5]

Weakness is another characteristic manifestation of the illness and is well documented in this case. It is frequently greater proximally, thus leading one to consider myopathy. However, no evidence of a myopathy in acute porphyria has ever been convincingly documented on either physiologic or pathological grounds. Most observers believe that the weakness is due to a short-fiber peripheral neuropathy.

Sensory loss may also be present, and it, too, is greater proximally than distally, thus producing the typical "bathing-trunk" sensory-loss pattern. The results of most physiologic studies in patients with porphyria are normal. Some studies have shown findings consistent with an axonal neuropathy. In only one case have the findings been consistent with a demyelinating type of neuropathy.[13] The few pathological studies that have been done have shown mainly axonal loss, with some degree of probably secondary demyelination. The question of why neuropathy should affect short fibers more than long fibers is an interesting one in itself. Most polyneuropathies, of course, affect long fibers predominantly, presumably because the primary lesion is a neuronopathy, which results in failure of the most distal parts of the axon first, receding as the disease worsens (the so-called dying-back phenomenon). Dr. Thomas Sabin, chief of neurology at the Boston City Hospital, has speculated that short-fiber neuropathies such as porphyria may be due to retrograde axonal flow of a toxic material picked up by axonal terminals in the periphery. When the toxin reaches the nerve-cell body it disables the cell. Thus, the short fibers would be intoxicated first.

Seizures occur in about 10 per cent of patients during an acute attack of porphyria. Most of these seizures are probably related to hyponatremia, but some clearly occur when there are normal electrolytes. The mechanism is unknown. Mental symptoms, including confusion, delirium, mania, psychosis, abnormal behavior, and depression, develop in at least a third of patients with porphyria. These features can dominate the clinical picture. This patient's irritability and inability to give a coherent history were probably due to the porphyria.

The orange urine in this case undoubtedly reflected the presence of porphyrin precursors. It should have been possible to make the diagnosis of acute porphyria quickly, using the so-called Watson–Schwartz test.[14] It involves the condensation of dimethylparaminobenzaldehyde (Ehrlich's reagent) with PBG, which instantly forms a cherry-red color. The color remains in the aqueous phase after organic solvent extraction. In fact, Willis, the doctor of George III, said that he passed port-wine–colored urine. The color can often be obtained by leaving the urine exposed to sunlight for several hours so that the precursors can be converted to the visible porphyrins.

The mechanism of the effects of porphyria on the nervous system is not known, but several theories have been proposed. The first is the concept of a toxic effect of the porphyrin precursors. Porphyrin precursors have been shown in vitro to inhibit ATPase in the brain,[15] to interfere with presynaptic neuromuscular transmission,[16] and to decrease monosynaptic impulses from the spinal cord.[17] However, the administration of ALA or PBG to human beings and animals has not resulted in a neurologic dysfunction characteristic of acute porphyria.[18,19] A second theory is that there may be a deficiency of pyridoxine caused by overproduction of ALA and PBG,[20] but the administration of pyridoxine (vitamin B_6) has had no consistent clinical benefits in patients with acute attacks of porphyria.[21] Impaired NADH oxidation has been postulated as a mechanism on the basis of experiments on animals,[22] and there is some evidence of abnormalities in steroid-hormone biotransformation that could be related to the pathogenesis of the disease.[23] The last major theory is that heme deficiency results in the neurologic impairment. Defective heme biosynthesis could lead to a deficiency of hemoproteins within nerve cells, such as the microsomal cytochromes required for the mono-oxygenase system or the mitochondrial cytochromes necessary for oxidative phosphorylation.[24] It is of interest that partial blockade of the heme biosynthetic pathway has been shown experimentally to cause an impairment of drug-mediated induction of the heme-containing liver-enzyme cytochrome P-450 system.[25]

All three acute hepatic porphyrias are inherited in an autosomal dominant manner. However, there is considerable variability in expressivity, probably largely because of the pharmacogenetic nature of the disease. Probably less than half the persons with the gene express it clinically. In those carrying the gene an acute attack may be precipitated by four major factors. The first and most important is the use of drugs. Drugs that induce the enzyme ALA synthetase should always be avoided in persons in whom porphyria is suspected. Unfortunately, since lists of such drugs are compiled largely from anecdotal reports they are incomplete and unreliable. Patients at risk should therefore avoid all drugs unless absolutely needed. In general, drugs are placed in four categories: those that have been implicated in precipitating an acute attack (e.g., barbiturates, sulfonamides, griseofulvin, some benzodiazepines, meprobamate, phenytoin, alcohol, methsuximide, glutethimide, and ergot preparations); those that produce porphyria in experimental systems (e.g., mephenytoin, phensuximide, and chloramphenicol); those that are safe or probably safe (e.g., opiates, penicillin, streptomycin, tetracycline, corticosteroids, antihistamines, phenothiazines, digoxin, vitamin C, atropine, prostigmine, and propoxyphene); and those about which nothing is known. The second precipitating factor is the level of hormones and related steroids. The disease has been known to be exacerbated in puberty, with menses, and during pregnancy, as well as during treatment with steroids. The third precipitating factor is infection, either bacterial or viral, and the fourth is starvation or dieting.

The best treatment for porphyria is prophylaxis by avoidance of the four precipitating factors by persons known to be at risk for the disease. Treatment of the acute attacks consists of removal of the precipitating agents, a high-carbohydrate diet of at least 300 g per day, which inhibits ALA-synthetase activity, and management of pain with opiates and phenothiazines. Propranolol is sometimes useful to control the tachycardia if that becomes necessary. Anticonvulsant therapy is difficult, since most seizure medications are known to induce ALA synthetase. The electrolyte levels should be corrected first, since that will terminate many seizures related to hyponatremia. If that fails, use of clonazepam or valproate is probably the safest therapy. Treatment with intravenously administered hematin (ferriheme hydroxide) will inhibit ALA synthetase.[26] Dr. Peter V. Tishler, at our institution, has shown that the use of solid-phase sorbents to remove porphyrin precursors is technically possible and practical.[27] However, this approach could cause further induction of ALA synthetase by removing the agents that tend to inhibit it. Dr. Tishler believes that the ideal therapy may require both hematin to suppress ALA synthetase and methods to remove the potentially toxic precursors.

In conclusion, it is possible that this patient had acute hepatic porphyria. Whether it was intermittent acute porphyria, variegate porphyria, or coproporphyria is impossible to decide on purely clinical grounds in the absence of skin lesions. Dr. Tishler and members of the dermatology staff of this hospital[28] have emphasized the various features of the hepatic porphyrias and contrasted them with porphyria cutanea tarda. In the absence of skin lesions the clinical pictures of the three forms of acute hepatic porphyria are identical. Only an analysis of the porphyrin precursors in the urine and the stool and the demonstration of the specific enzyme deficiency can separate them. Statistically, it is most likely that this patient had intermittent acute porphyria since it is the most common form of acute hepatic porphyria in North America. Coproporphyria is rare throughout the world. Variegate porphyria is common in South Africa, where its prevalence is estimated to be 3 per 1000 in the white population. Formerly, it was thought that variegate porphyria was very rare in the United States, but it has been found in several families in New England.[28] Therefore, it remains a possibility in this case. I believe that it is now time to turn to the clinical physiologist and pathologist to hear about the electrophysiologic studies, the results of the urine and stool analysis for porphyrin precursors, and the specific enzyme deficiency found in this patient.

In summary, my final diagnosis is acute hepatic porphyria, probably the intermittent acute form, although variegate porphyria and coproporphyria cannot be excluded vigorously on clinical grounds.

DR. ARTHUR S. PIER, JR.: Does this disease cause damage to the liver, such as cirrhosis?

DR. SAMUELS: There is associated liver disease in some forms of porphyria, but in the three acute porphyrias clinically important liver disease is not common. It was not a problem in the patient under discussion.

DR. EDWARD P. RICHARDSON, JR.: Dr. O'Gara, will you tell us the impression of the medical students?

DR. PATRICK T. O'GARA: The students also thought that the patient had acute hepatic porphyria and agreed on statistical grounds that acute intermittent porphyria was most likely. They suggested that the next diagnostic steps were analyses of the urine and stool for porphyrin precursors.

CLINICAL DIAGNOSIS

Acute hepatic porphyria.

DR. MARTIN A. SAMUELS' DIAGNOSIS

Acute hepatic porphyria, probably intermittent acute porphyria.

PATHOLOGICAL DISCUSSION

DR. RICHARDSON: The first diagnostic procedure was an electrophysiologic study, and Dr. Shahani will describe the findings.

DR. BHAGWAN T. SHAHANI: Detailed electrophysiologic studies, including conventional motor and sensory conduction, needle electromyography, late responses, sympathetic skin responses (SSR), estimation of conduction in alpha motor axons of different diameters, and measurements of beat-to-beat variation of the heart rate (R-R interval), were performed. When the patient was first seen in our laboratory she had weakness that was most prominent in the proximal muscles. The values for maximum motor-conduction velocity in the right median, ulnar, and tibial nerves were within normal limits (Table 1). Minimal latencies of F responses, which provide information regarding conduction in the entire length of alpha motor axons from the motor neuron to terminal axons, were also normal (Table 1). There was, however, a slight increase in the minimal–maximal latency difference (normal, less than 2 msec in ulnar and median nerves and less than 4 msec in peroneal and tibial nerves when 10 F responses are recorded), suggesting a mild peripheral neuropathy. Orthodromic sensory-nerve action potentials, which evaluate the function of sensory-nerve fibers of large diameter, recorded from the median and sural nerves, had normal latency, duration, and amplitude (Table 2). Electromyographic studies performed with concentric needle electrodes showed normal duration, amplitude, and shape of motor-unit potentials

Table 1. Motor Conduction Studies.

Nerve	Distal Latency	Muscle Action-Potential Amplitude	Conduction Velocity	F-Response Latency (Minimum-Maximum)
	msec	μV	meters-sec	msec
Right median	3.8	10.500	56	28–32
Right ulnar	2.8	5.000	50	27–30
Right tibial	3.5	15.000	41	51–54

Table 2. Sensory Conduction Studies.

Nerve	Duration	Latency	Amplitude
	Cm	msec	μV
Right median	15	2.8	15
Right sural	16	3.5	8

(MUPs) recorded from proximal muscles; however, with maximal voluntary effort only a few MUPs could be recruited (low-mixed recruitment pattern). Needle electromyographic and late responses were compatible with a neurogenic lesion rather than primary muscle disease as the underlying pathologic process.

We then performed serial electrophysiologic studies to monitor the course of the illness. A motor-nerve conduction study performed approximately two weeks after the first study showed a reduction in the amplitude of compound muscle-action potentials evoked by stimulation of median and peroneal nerves, whereas maximum motor-conduction velocity values remained normal. Similarly, orthodromic median sensory-nerve action potentials showed a reduction of more than 50 per cent in the amplitude, whereas sensory-conduction velocity and minimal latency values remained almost unchanged. With the exception of the first study, needle electromyographic examination showed spontaneous activity in the form of fibrillations and positive sharp deflections. Reduction in the amplitude of compound nerve and muscle-action potentials with relatively normal conduction velocity and the presence of spontaneous activity at rest (fibrillations and sharp waves) are characteristic findings in patients with "axonal" neuropathies—neuropathies in which the primary disease affects the axon rather than the myelin sheath.

Other interesting features became apparent when the patient was seen for the second time in our laboratory. For example, signs and symptoms of ulnar-nerve compression at the elbow had developed. At that time and during subsequent examinations we studied the function of alpha motor axons of different diameter of the ulnar nerve and recorded minimum–maximum motor-conduction velocity using "collision" techniques. During the second study, when the patient had clinical evidence of ulnar compression, the minimum–maximum conduction-velocity difference was 6 m per second, whereas in the third study, when there was no more evidence of ulnar compression, the difference was 18 m per second (normal, 15 to 20 meters per second difference in conduction velocity of alpha motor axons of different diameter of the ulnar nerve). A narrower range of conduction-velocity values with the use of collision techniques is seen in compression neuropathies and is due to involvement of alpha motor axons of larger diameter. The improvement of values of minimum–maximum conduction shown on subsequent studies suggests that the compression of the ulnar nerve had produced a reversible "conduction block" (during the second study) rather than axonal degeneration.

In some patients with porphyric neuropathy and proximal muscle weakness needle electromyographic studies demonstrate brief-duration MUPs and a normal recruitment pattern with maximal voluntary activity, characteristic electromyographic findings of primary muscle disease. If these patients are followed, however, subsequent studies show electromyographic findings typical of the axonal type of neuropathy—spontaneous activity (fibrillations and positive sharp deflections), a reduced recruitment pattern with maximal voluntary effort, and prolonged duration of highamplitude MUPs. Why does one find "myopathic" electromyographic changes during the acute stage of the illness? There are two possible mechanisms. One is predominant involvement of terminal axons (terminal axonopathy), resulting in a conduction failure at branching points during the acute stage of porphyric neuropathy. The second possible explanation is that toxins released in porphyria may behave like a botulin toxin and act presynaptically by interfering with the release of acetylcholine from synaptic vesicles. Both these pathophysiologic mechanisms can explain "myopathic" electromyographic findings. In this patient, however, we did not find any other electrophysiologic evidence typical of botulism or the Eaton–Lambert syndrome.

In addition to performing serial physiologic studies with electromyography and nerve-conduction examinations we investigated several functions related to the autonomic nervous system, which is also affected in some of these patients. We first recorded sympathetic skin responses (SSR), which give information regarding the function of postganglionic sympathetic unmyelinated C fibers innervating sweat glands.[29] SSRs evoked by single electric stimuli delivered to the median nerve at the level of the wrist were recorded from the hands and feet, indicating preservation of the function of unmyelinated nerve fibers of small diameter. We also recorded R-R interval variation, which presumably depends on intact parasympathetic innervation of the heart, to assess autonomic dysfunction. In normal persons there is a variation of the R-R interval, which increases noticeably during deep inspiration. In this patient the variation was reduced, and there was no substantial increase in this variation with deep breathing, providing objective evidence of autonomic neuropathy.

One of the interesting features of porphyric neuropathy is that although examination of proximal muscles shows weakness and appropriate electrophysiologic changes in the acute stages of the disease, studies performed months or years later may show evidence of chronic denervation–reinnervation in distal muscles more than in proximal muscles, characteristic features of neuropathies of the dying-back axonal type. It is possible that proximal muscle weakness seen during the acute illness is produced by reversible changes such as failure of conduction at branching points of distal axons or at neuromuscular junctions. In a few patients seen in our laboratory we have not found electrophysiologic evidence suggesting presynaptic involvement at the neuromuscular junction similar to that of botulism. It is therefore more likely that some of these changes during early stages of the illness are due to a terminal axonopathy rather than a disorder of neuromuscular transmission.

DR. RICHARDSON: The other diagnostic procedure was a positive Watson–Schwartz test for porphyrin excretion. The patient has been followed very closely by Dr. Sealfon and Dr. Robert R. Young. Dr. Sealfon, will you comment about the clinical course, and do you have a follow-up report on the patient?

DR. STUART C. SEALFON: As soon as the diagnosis of porphyria was suspected all offending medications were stopped. After the confirmatory Watson–Schwartz test was obtained carbohydrate was administered orally and glucose was given intravenously.

Despite a carbohydrate intake of 600 g per day the patient became weaker, and the tendon reflexes became unobtainable in the upper extremities. The extensor muscles in the upper extremities became profoundly weak, and she was unable to walk. We followed the measurements of the daily urinary porphobilinogen excretion, which were performed in Dr. Tishler's laboratory. They remained elevated at about 100 times normal. Hematin was obtained from Dr. C. A. Pierach (Abbott–Northwestern Hospital, Minneapolis) and was begun on the 11th hospital day. Her clinical condition then became stable, and the porphobilinogen and delta-aminolevulinic acid excretion fell. She was subsequently transferred to a rehabilitation facility and after three months was able to return home. I have seen her recently. She is able to walk well and has minimal iliopsoas weakness. The deltoid and triceps muscles and the extensors of the fist and fingers have improved considerably and are about grade 3 of 5. The tendon reflexes have all returned to normal.

The results of the initial laboratory studies were most consistent with coproporphyria. The erythrocyte uroporphyrinogen I synthetase activity was normal. The fecal coproporphyrin was elevated, and the protoporphyrin excretion was normal.

DR. RICHARDSON: Dr. Pathak has done some excellent work on the porphyrias. Are there any points that you wish to make, Dr. Pathak?

DR. MADHUKAR A. PATHAK: In the dermatology clinic we use a simple test for the diagnosis of porphyria. A freshly voided specimen or a 24-hour specimen of urine is subjected to ultraviolet examination before being sent to the laboratory for determination of porphobilinogen or delta-aminolevulinic acid. An orange-red fluorescence indicates the presence of one of two types of porphyria, either porphyria cutanea tarda or variegate porphyria. When there is a problem in differentiating acute intermittent porphyria and variegate porphyria two specimens must be sent to the laboratory. Neither coproporphyrin nor protoporphyrin is elevated in patients with acute intermittent porphyria, whereas variegate porphyria is consistently associated with increased levels of protoporphyrin.

ANATOMICAL DIAGNOSIS

Coproporphyria with polyneuropathy.

REFERENCES

1. Macalpine I, Hunter R. Porphyria and King George III. Sci Am 1969: 221:38–46.
2. *Idem.* A clinical reassessment of the "insanity" of George III and some of its historical implications. Bull Inst Hist Res 1967; 40:166–85.
3. Ranking JE. Pardington GL. Two cases of haemato-porphyrin in the urine. Lancet 1890: 2:607–9.
4. Waldenström J. Neurological symptoms caused by socalled acute porphyria. Acta Psychiatr Neurol 1939: 14:375–9.
5. Tschudy DP, Valsamis M, Magnussen CR. Acute intermittent porphyria: clinical and selected research aspects. Ann Intern Med 1975: 83:851–64.
6. Vavra JD, Avioli LV. Intermittent acute porphyria. Arch Inten Med 1982: 142:1527–9.
7. Tishler PV. The porphyrias. In: Conn HF, ed. Current therapy. Philadelphia: WB Saunders. 1982:329–33.

8. Heilmeyer L, Clotten R. Die kongenitale erythropoetische Coproporphyrie: Eine dritte erythropoetische Porphyrieform. Dtsch Med Wochenschr 1964; 89:649–54.

9. Day RS, Eales L, Meissner D. Coexistent variegate porphyria and porphyria cutanea tarda. N Engl J Med 1982; 307:36–41.

10. Mason VR, Courville C, Ziskind E. The porphyrins in human disease. Medicine (Baltimore) 1933; 12:355–439.

11. Gibson JB, Goldberg A. The neuropathology of acute porphyria. J Pathol Bacteriol 1956; 71:495–509.

12. Wehrmacher WH. New symptomatic treatment for acute intermittent porphyria. Arch Inten Med 1952; 89:111–4.

13. Stein JA, Tschudy DP. Acute intermittent porphyria: a clinical and biochemical study of 46 patients. Medicine (Baltimore) 1970: 49:1–16.

14. Watson CJ, Schwartz S. A simple test for urinary porphobilinopen. Proc Soc Exp Biol Med 1941: 47:393–4.

15. Becker D, Viljoen D, Kramer S. The inhibition of red cell and brain ATPasc by δ-aminolevulinic acid. Biochim Biophys Acta 1971; 225:26–34.

16. Feldman DS, Levere RD, Lieberman JS, Cardinal RA. Watson CJ. Presynaptic neuromuscular inhibition by porphobilinogin and porphobilin. Proc Natl Acad Sci USA 1971: 68:383–6.

17. Loots H, Goldstuck N, Carter RJM, Becker D, Viljoen D, Kramer S. Delta-aminolaevulinic acid in acute porphyria. S Afr Med J 1972: 46:524.

18. Goldberg A. Rimington C. Fate of porphobilinogen in the rat: relation to acute porphyria in man. Lancet 1954: 2:172–3.

19. Jarrett A, Rimington C, Willoughby DA. δ-Aminolacvulinic and porphyria. Lancet 1956: 1:125–7.

20. Cavanagh JB, Ridley AR. The nature of the neuropathy complicating acute intermittent porphyria. Lancet 1967: 2:1023–4.

21. Kosower NS. Rock RA. Seizures in experimental porphyria. Nature 1968: 217:565–7.

22. Tschudy DP, Bonkowsky HL. Experimental porphyria. Fed Proc 1972; 31:147–59.

23. Kappas A, Bradlow HL, Gillette PN, Gallagher TF. Studies in porphyria. I. A defect in the reductive transformation of natural steroid hormones in the hereditary liver disease, acute intermittent porphyria. J Exp Med 1972: 136:1043–53.

24. Laiwah ACY, Goldberg A. Moore MR. Pathogenesis and treatment of acute intermittent porphyria: discussion paper. J R Soc Med 1983: 76:386–92.

25. Smith AC, De Matteis F. Drugs and the hepatic porphyrias. Clin Haematol 1980; 9:399–425.

26. Watson CJ, Pierach CA, Bossenmaier I, Cardinal R. Use of hematin in the acute attack of the "inducible" hepatic porphyrias. Adv Inten Med 1978; 23:265–86.

27. Tishler PV, Gordon BJ. Sorbent therapy of the porphyrias, II. Experimental plasma or hemoperfusion with a commercial charcoal cartridge. Methods Find Exp Clin Pharmacol 1983: 5:185–91.

28. Muhlbauer JE, Pathak MA, Tishler PV, Fitzpatrick TB. Variegate porphyria in New England. JAMA 1982: 247:3095–102.

29. Shahani BT, Halperin JJ, Boulu P, Cohen C. Sympathetic skin response—a method of assessing unmyelinated axon dysfunction in peripheral neuropathies. J Neurol Neurosurg Psychiatry 1984: 47:536–42.

Continued preparation of these Case Records has been made possible by a generous grant to the Massachusetts General Hospital from Pfizer Pharmaceuticals

Perspectives and Updates

This case marks the first time that I stated that a differential diagnosis was not appropriate. An apocryphal story goes that a senior professor was asked to give a differential diagnosis for a particular syndrome. He allegedly responded: "I can't give you a differential diagnosis. If you wish, I can give you a list of wrong diagnoses followed by the right diagnosis." The exercise of listing many obviously impossible diagnoses is possibly one of the more serious allegations against the CPC method of learning medicine. I have attempted in many of my cases to avert this criticism by focusing in on the correct diagnosis and then explaining why this must be the case. The patient with porphyria was the first of my efforts in this regard.

One of the remaining interesting features of this case is the use of genetic testing for neurological diseases. At present genetic tests are available for seven of the porphyrias: acute intermittent porphyria, coproporphyria, variegate porphyria, porphyria cutanea tarda, hepatoerythropoietic porphyria, erythroporphyria, and congenital erythropoietic porphyria.[1,2] Each genetic test now costs about $850, so a complete screen would cost about $6,000. Thus it remains important to use clinical criteria as well as less expensive urine and stool studies to select patients who would most benefit by genetic testing. In this case, it was possible to determine that the patient had a form of acute hepatic porphyria, but because of the absence of a history of skin lesions, it was impossible to carry the analysis any further. The final diagnosis could have been acute intermittent porphyria, variegate porphyria, or coproporphyria. As mentioned in the CPC discussion, this could have been resolved using an analysis of the porphyrin precursors in the urine and the stool and/or a demonstration of the specific enzyme deficiency. Today, genetic testing would be done. One would start with the most likely and then proceed to the others if necessary. The total cost for an absolutely certain diagnosis in this case would now range from about $850 to about $2,500. Family members at risk could then be tested in a focused manner for about $150 each. Similar principles apply to the use of genetic testing for a large array of neurological disorders, including the spinocerebellar atrophies, peripheral neuropathies, muscular dystrophies and many more on the near horizon. In other words, genetic testing should be considered an extension of the clinician's arm, very much as we consider the use of neuromuscular testing.

Also important in this case's discussion is the role of the porphyrias in world history. Had George III not had this disease, his judgment might have been better and the American revolution might never have occurred. Many of my CPCs include a reflection on the history of the disorder and/or the physicians who recognized it. It is surprising to realize how few truly new ideas are created by each new generation.

Martin A. Samuels

REFERENCES

1. www.porphyriafoundation.com
2. Thadani H, Deacon A, Peters T. Diagnosis and management of porphyria. BMJ 2000; 320:1647–58.

A 62-Year-Old Man with Progressive Polyneuropathy

AMYLOIDOSIS

CPC 26-1986

PRESENTATION OF CASE

A 62-year-old man was admitted to the hospital because of progressive polyneuropathy.

The patient was well until two or three years earlier, when he began to experience burning sensations in the soles of his feet, with numbness of the feet and ankles. Several months later a feeling of pins and needles developed in all his fingers. Electromyographic studies, performed elsewhere, were reported to show abnormalities. Twenty-three months before entry surgical release of the right carpal tunnel was performed, without improvement; four months later the region of the right elbow was explored, again without benefit. By this time the patient's feet were so sensitive that he found the touch of bedsheets intolerable. His hands were weak, especially the right, after the second operation. "Shooting pains" appeared and radiated up from the hands, and he was disturbed by painful throbbing as well as burning in the hands and feet, particularly when his limbs were warm. He noticed occasional twitching of the right hand and the muscles of either leg, and during the six months before admission he experienced severe nocturnal cramps in the feet and lower legs. His gait became unsteady, and he had several episodes of dizziness or imbalance when he stood up quickly. He was admitted to the hospital.

The patient was born in this country. There was a history of hypertension for five years, for which he took hydrochlorothiazide and spironolactone, but he used no other medications. Operations were performed because of a small-bowel obstruction and cholelithiasis 25 years earlier, and an incisional hernia was repaired on three occasions during the succeeding 6 years. He had worked as a shop foreman in a plumbing firm in the past, with intensive exposure to lead and tin, and for the 10 years before entry he had a clerical position. He smoked cigars infrequently and rarely drank alcohol. A tentative diagnosis of diabetes mellitus was made elsewhere but was not confirmed on further testing. The patient noted no nocturnal penile tumescence during the year or two before admission and was totally impotent for the past year. His father and an uncle with diabetes had difficulty with walking in their 60s, but both resided in Italy and further details were unavailable; there was no other family history of neuromuscular disease. There was no history of bladder or bowel dysfunction, arthritis, rash, cough, dyspnea, diarrhea, weight loss, allergy, visual symptoms, diplopia, dysarthria, dysphagia, change in mentation, loss of consciousness, postural syncope or dizziness, headache, or recent exposure to toxic chemicals.

The temperature was 36.7°C, and the respirations were 18. The blood pressure was 120/55 mm Hg and the pulse 72 supine; the blood pressure was 100/60 mm Hg and the pulse 80 standing.

The patient was alert and sat with his arms flexed and with the tops of his shoes cut off to reduce contact with his toes. No rash was found. The head and neck were normal, and the lungs were clear. A Grade 2 systolic ejection murmur was heard along the left sternal border. Abdominal examination was negative; the liver and spleen were not felt. Hair was absent over the lower legs; there was no peripheral edema, and the pulses were intact. No enlargement of the ulnar nerves was palpated. Rectal examination disclosed ++ prostatic enlargement, without nodules; a stool specimen gave a negative test for occult blood.

Neurologic examination showed that mentation was intact and speech was fluent. The right pupil was slightly larger than the left, but both reacted normally; there was a slight decrease in lateral gaze bilaterally; the optic fundi and the remaining cranial nerves were normal. Atrophy of the intrinsic muscles of the hands was observed and was more prominent in the right hand; occasional fasciculations were seen in the right first dorsal interosseous muscle. Tone was normal throughout, and strength was normal except for mild weakness of the grips, finger and wrist flexors and extensors, and biceps bilaterally. There was a slight decrease in vibratory and proprioceptive sensation in the distal portions of the lower extremities. There was marked loss of pinprick and temperature sense in all the extremities, to the midportion of the forearms and in the feet and legs to above the knees. There was a mild decrease in pinprick sensation over the anterior aspect of the chest. Graphesthesia was intact, but stereognosis was poor in the upper extremities. There was no extinction to double simultaneous stimulation. There was a fine action tremor of the extremities, without dysmetria. The gait was slightly wide-based, and Romberg's test was mildly positive. The biceps and triceps reflexes were barely obtainable, and the responses were flexor, and no palmomental or grasp reflex was elicited. Lack of sweating was noted in the lower extremities.

The urine was normal. The hematocrit was 47.6 per cent; the white-cell count was 6500, with 73 per cent neutrophils, 22 per cent lymphocytes, 4 per cent monocytes, and 1 per cent eosinophils. The platelet count was 212,000, and the erythrocyte sedimentation rate 4 mm per hour. The urea nitrogen was 16 mg per 100 ml (5.7 mmol per liter), the glucose 146 mg per 100 ml (8.10 mmol per liter), the bilirubin 0.6 mg per 100 ml (10 μmol per liter), the thyroxine 6.9 μg per 100 ml (89 nmol per liter), and the protein 7.0 g per 100 ml. A protein electrophoresis revealed that the albumin was 54 per cent, the alpha$_1$ globulin 3 per cent, the alpha$_2$ globulin 14 per cent, the beta globulin 13 per cent, and the gamma globulin 16 per cent. The sodium was 138 mmol, the potassium 4.3 mmol, the chloride 102 mmol, and the carbon dioxide 29 mmol per liter. The serum aspartate aminotransferase (SGOT) was 18 U, the creatine kinase (CK)

37 U (new normal for men, 17 to 148), and the alkaline phosphatase 37 U per liter. An electrocardiogram disclosed a normal rhythm at a rate of 88, with a PR interval of 0.18 second and a QRS interval of 0.12 second; there was a pattern of complete right bundle-branch block, with left-axis deviation; Q waves were present in Leads 2, 3, and a VF, suggestive of an old inferior myocardial infarct. X-ray films of the chest revealed that the heart was enlarged and the lungs were clear; the bony thorax appeared normal except for degenerative changes in the thoracic spine. A serum immunoelectrophoresis showed normal precipitin arcs for IgG, IgA, and IgM; an agarose-gel electrophoresis gave a normal pattern. A serologic test for syphilis, tests for rheumatoid factor, antinuclear antibodies, and cryoprotein, and an LE-cell test were negative; a 50-fold concentrated specimen of urine gave a negative test for Bence Jones protein. The vitamin B_{12} was 478 pg per 100 ml (353 pmol per liter) (new normal, 205 to 876 pg per 100 ml [151 to 646 pmol per liter]), and the folic acid was 5.2 ng per milliliter (12 nmol per liter) (new normal, greater than 3.3 ng per 100 ml [7.5 nmol per liter]). A lumbar puncture, performed with difficulty, yielded slightly pink, hazy fluid, with xanthochromia graded 3 on a scale of 0 to 10; the fluid contained 814 red cells and 4 white cells per cubic millimeter, of which 12 per cent were neutrophils, 68 per cent lymphocytes, and 20 per cent monocytes; the glucose was 91 mg per 100 ml (5.1 mmol per liter), and the protein 74 mg, the IgG 4.9 mg (normal, 0 to 8.6), and the albumin 43.3 mg per 100 ml (normal, 11 to 48); cytologic examination revealed no malignant-tumor cells, and a culture was negative. Electrophysiologic studies showed slowing of maximal motor conduction velocity, abnormalities of late responses (H reflex and F responses), and absence of sensory-nerve action potentials and sympathetic skin responses. Needle electromyographic examination revealed evidence of spontaneous activity (fibrillations and positive sharp deflections) and reduced recruitment patterns with maximal voluntary effort. The findings were believed consistent with a sensorimotor peripheral neuropathy. An echocardiogram revealed concentric left ventricular hypertrophy: there was thickening of the aortic-valve cusps, without valvular stenosis. Examination of a 24-hour specimen of urine disclosed no mercury, lead, arsenic, or thallium.

Codeine, acetaminophen, carbamazepine, propoxyphene, clonazepam, doxepin, and imipramine were administered, without satisfactory relief of symptoms.

A diagnostic procedure was performed.

DIFFERENTIAL DIAGNOSIS

DR. MARTIN A. SAMUELS[*]: In the mid-19th century the renowned pathologist Karl von Rokitansky described a curious chronic disease characterized by a waxy, enlarged liver and sometimes an enlarged spleen.[1] Rudolph Virchow[2] noted that these enlarged organs were stained with iodine and sulfuric acid. He believed that the substance was a polysaccharide similar to cellulose and referred to it as amyloid, from the Latin *amylum*, meaning starch. The term "amyloid" had been coined by Schleiden in 1838 to

---

* Chief, Neurology Service. Brockton-West Roubury Veterans Administration Medical Center, associate professor of neurology. Harvard Medical School. Currently Chair, Department of Neurology, Brigham and Women's Hospital.

describe a normal starch-like constituent of plants. Wilks[3] reported the first case of primary amyloidosis in 1856. In 1872 Adams[4] described a 61-year-old woman who had pathologic fractures as a result of bone marrow infiltration by small spherical and oval cells with one or two nuclei and prominent nucleoli, and she also had a lardaceous change in the liver and spleen. It probably was the first report of multiple myeloma with amyloidosis. Peripheral neuropathy associated with systemic amyloidosis was first reported by Koenigstein,[5] who observed a patient with weakness and atrophy of hand muscles as a result of amyloid in the epineurium and vessels of the nerves. Familial amyloid polyneuropathy was initially described by Corino de Andrade[6] in 1939. He found a lower-limb neuropathy in a 37-year-old woman from Póvoa de Varzim, a fishing village near Oporto, Portugal. She suffered from a familial illness known in that area as *mal dos pèsinhos* (foot disease), which was characterized by severe, progressive impairment of thermal and pain sensation in the legs, with associated autonomic dysfunction.

You may ask why I leap unabashed to the diagnosis of amyloid neuropathy. After all, nothing is more bewildering than the differential diagnosis of a peripheral neuropathy. In fact, nothing is more useless in neurology than a long differential diagnosis of a generic syndrome, such as a neuropathy. One must instead depend on the particular flavor of the individual case, allowing it to leave an impression from which one can have only a handful of real possibilities.

Reduced to its essentials, this is the story of a late-middle-aged man who had a painful, symmetric pseudosyringomyelic sensorimotor polyneuropathy with some autonomic dysfunction, having presented with what at least some physicians thought was a carpal- tunnel syndrome. He was not diabetic, had no overt signs of cancer, and had a questionable family history of neurologic disease. By pseudosyringomyelic it is meant that the neuropathy predominantly affected small fibers, thus producing a deficit that was greater for pain and thermal sensation than for vibration and proprioception. The dissassociated sensory loss was sufficiently prominent in this patient to produce loss of pinprick sensation over the anterior portion of the chest while sparing the biceps and triceps tendon reflexes. This carapace pattern of sensory loss implies that very short sensory nerves were affected. At the same time motor nerves of larger diameter in the upper extremity were apparently at least partial spared, allowing for intact tendon reflexes.

Only amyloidosis really explains this unique picture. Diabetic polyneuropathy might rarely produce vaguely similar syndrome, but usually large fibers are affected at least as much as small fibers. Moreover this patient did not have diabetes. Tangier disease is a rare autosomally inherited disorder marked by deficiency of alpha-lipoprotein, a low cholesterol level low levels of phospholipids, and high triglyceride levels in the serum. It can produce a pseudosyringomyelic neuropathy but usually presents in childhood. In addition to the wrong age at the onset of the illness this patient had none of the abnormal laboratory findings characteristic of this disorder. Fabry's disease, due to an accumulation of ceramide trihexoside, is an uncommon sex-linked, recessively inherited disorder that may produce a very painful neuropathy but is associated with a characteristic skin lesion known as angiokeratoma corporis diffusum and progressive renal failure. The various hereditary sensory neuropathies may produce a dissociated sensory loss but do not cause severe pain, and the patients usually present much earlier in life than this patient presented. The familial dysautonomic neuropathies (the Riley–Day syndrome and related disorders) result in much more prominent autonomic failure than that produced in this patient. Although there may be a dissociated sensory loss pain is not a prominent feature, and most of the patients are symptomatic in childhood or infancy.

This patient had a remote exposure to metals, but his syndrome does not fit that seen in metal neuropathies. In such cases there is generally a direct temporal relation to the metal exposure, and the disease is subacute and is primarily motor and asymmetric. Autonomic abnormalities are uncommon. Much the same can be said about the neuropathies caused by various industrial toxins. He had no known exposure to any of the well-described substances that cause neuropathy, and most of them produce a subacute sensorimotor neuropathy without autonomic involvement. The toxic clinical syndrome that is most similar to this patient's disorder is the one caused by dimethylaminopionitrile (DMAPN), which is used as a catalyst in a grouting mixture that is called A-9 and as a catalyst in the manufacture of polyurethane foam.[7] This substance is known to produce a small-fiber neuropathy with prominent bladder symptoms, numbness and tingling of the feet, and loss of pain and thermal sensation distally, with relative preservation of tendon reflexes. The patient under discussion had no known continuing exposure to this substance. Furthermore, this intoxication would not account for the carpal-tunnel syndrome, the cardiac enlargement, and the electrocardiographic abnormalities. He also did not complain of bladder difficulty, a finding that is very prominent in DMAPN toxicity. It is very unlikely that this patient's disorder was any form of toxic or metal neuropathy.

Leprosy can produce a small-fiber neuropathy, but it characteristically affects cooler areas of the body, such as the ears, the dorsal surfaces of the hands, the forearms, and the feet. That distribution was not noted in this patient. Although it is perhaps the most common neuropathy in the world, the type related to leprosy is relatively rare in the United States except for regions around the Gulf of Mexico. We do not know this man's geographic background, but he had none of the characteristic skin lesions and no systemic illness. It is very unlikely that this disorder was any form of lepromatous neuropathy.

Amyloidosis is the only disorder that fits the case history. Before I discuss amyloidosis, however, three points regarding the clinical and laboratory findings should be made.

Pain was one of the major hallmarks of this man's illness. What determines whether a small-fiber neuropathy produces pain? There is no clear answer to this question, but I shall speculate. If a patient has a neuronopathy affecting the cells in the dorsal-root ganglia, which give rise to the small fibers, one might expect analgesia but not pain. The process should lead to an imbalance of impulses reaching the substantia gelatinosa of the spinal cord from large and small fibers in favor of relatively more input from large fibers. To the extent that the gate theory of pain has any truth, this should result in analgesia but no spontaneous pain, unlike the situation in this patient. On the other hand, if the process is an axonopathy caused by compression, ischemia, or some immune-mediated destruction of axons it might be expected to cause pain and analgesia. The pain would be due to the damage to the axons before their death, whereas the analgesia would be due to the failure of conduction and finally death of small fibers. In such a circumstance pain would lead the way, followed by analgesia, as observed in the patient under discussion. Thus, a system degeneration, such as the hereditary sensory neuropathy of Denny-Brown, would produce analgesia without pain, whereas infiltration of amyloid or a related immune attack on axons would probably cause pain followed by analgesia.

The second point is in regard to the lumbar puncture because it is difficult to explain the xanthochromia on the basis of the findings. The lumbar puncture may have been traumatic since it was difficult to perform.

DR. E. TESSA HEDLEY-WHYTE: The lumbar puncture was considered traumatic.

DR. SAMUELS: The third clinical point concerns the cardiac findings, which could have been the result amyloid infiltration but could also have been simple manifestations of hypertension and coronary atherosclerosis. The echocardiogram in patients with amyloid cardiomyopathy may be very helpful, almost pathognomonic, if it shows the characteristic speckle pattern in the heart muscle. However, that finding was not mentioned in the case record, and therefore the aspect of the illness does not clarify the diagnosis. It is important clinically, however, since amyloid heart disease is the major cause of death of patients with primary amyloidosis.

The diagnosis of amyloid polyneuropathy is straightforward in this case, but it is very difficult to say precisely what kind of amyloid neuropathy it was. The challenge is to decide whether this is a case of familial amyloid polyneuropathy, an example of amyloid polyneuropathy as part of the syndrome of primary amyloidosis, or amyloid neuropathy associated with a chronic disease. By exploring this challenge perhaps we can learn something about the nature and pathogenesis of amyloidosis and even suggest further evaluation and therapy for the patient under discussion. To accomplish this goal we shall have to review a few basic issues about amyloid and amyloidosis. It is not appropriate in this context to review the voluminous literature on this subject, and I shall merely outline the nature of the issues. The interested reader should be referred to several excellent reviews of the subject.[8–10]

Amyloidosis is defined as a "group of disorders characterized by the extracellular deposition of a fibrillar protein, amyloid, in one or more sites of the body."[9] It has been possible in recent years to characterize the amyloid molecules in great detail. As a result of this work it has become obvious that there is a great deal of heterogeneity among the various amyloids. Despite these differences all forms of amyloid demonstrate green birefringence under the polarizing microscope after Congo-red staining, a feature that is due to their organization as fibrils arranged in a twisted, beta-pleated sheet. Studies to date indicate that amyloid fibrils are composed of normal serum proteins, which are different for each form of amyloidosis. This understanding has led to the modern classification of the so-called beta fibrilloses. Fibrils isolated from primary or myeloma-associated amyloid consist of all or part of an immunoglobulin light chain ranging from 5,000 to 23,000 daltons and are designated as AL. The serum proteins associated with primary or myeloma-associated amyloid are Bence Jones proteins and are designated A kappa or A lambda. It should be borne in mind, however, that not all Bence Jones proteins are amyloidogenic. Amyloid fibrils isolated from patients with secondary amyloidosis—i.e., those associated with chronic diseases (e.g., rheumatoid arthritis, systemic lupus erythematosus, seleroderma, polymyositis, rheumatic fever, some tumors, including Hodgkin's disease, renal-cell carcinoma, and medullary carcinoma of the thyroid gland, tuberculosis, chronic osteomyelitis, leprosy, and familial Mediterranean fever) are designated as AA amyloid protein. Amyloid fibrils derived from patients with heredofamilial amyloidosis are composed of monometric units of prealbumin, otherwise known as transthyretin because it is a transport molecule for thyroxine and retinol. This form of amyloid is known as AF. Amyloid in various localized regions of the body has not yet been characterized fully. This category of amyloid includes that frequently found in the pancreas and the heart of aging persons. Of particular interest is the amyloid found in the brain as amyloid angiopathy, as cores of senile plaques, and as the paired helical filaments within neurofibrillary tangles. The exact role of this amyloid in the pathogenesis of neuronal degeneration is not yet known, and a debate rages about whether the amyloid is instrumental in initiating the process of cell death in the brain or is merely the result of cell death, perhaps produced by the action of microglial cells.[11] A unified hypothesis for the major lesions of Alzheimer's disease has been proposed in which amyloid has a major role.[12] This hypothesis, however, is yet to be substantiated.

For the sake of understanding the disorder in the patient under discussion it would be fruitful to review the three major categories of amyloidosis—AA, AL, and AF—making special reference to the issues of polyneuropathy.

AA, or secondary amyloidosis, is the easiest to exclude in this case. It is seen in the context of chronic inflammatory illnesses, some tumors, and the syndrome of familial Mediterranean fever. It is also present in animals with amyloidosis produced by injections of casein. The AA protein weighs about 8500 daltons, contains about 76 amino acids, and is probably derived from proteolysis as an amino terminal fragment of the associated serum protein SAA (serum amyloid-associated protein). Serum amyloid-associated protein weighs about 100,000 daltons and is an alpha$_2$ globulin acute-phase reactant present in normal persons in small amounts. Patients with AA amyloidosis may have a neuropathy, but the neuropathy is greatly overshadowed by the primary disease. This diagnosis is clearly not a consideration in this case, since the patient had none of the diseases that underlie this form of amyloidosis.

AL amyloidosis is probably always the result of a plasma-cell dyscrasia in the sense that the amyloid consists of the amino acid terminal region of the variable fragment of an immunoglobulin light chain, kappa or lambda. AL amyloid is presumably made by a clone of plasma cells located within the bone marrow or elsewhere in the body. Considerable information about the clinical and laboratory features of AL amyloidosis has been provided by Kyle and Greipp[10] from their experience with 229 patients at the Mayo Clinic. Approximately 20 per cent of patients with AL amyloidosis have multiple myeloma, defined by the authors as a disorder with more than 15 per cent plasma cells in the bone marrow or with an M component in the serum of a patient with lytic bone lesions, and 80 per cent do not. About 90 per cent of patients with AL amyloidosis have a monoclonal protein (M component) in the serum or urine. The patients with M components in the serum or urine in whom the findings do not fulfill the criteria for the diagnosis of myeloma are said to have a benign gammopathy. This leaves about 10 per cent of patients with AL amyloidosis who are found to have a normal bone marrow on examination, no lytic lesions on a bone survey or bone scan, and no M component in the serum or Bence Jones protein in urine. Presumably, there is a small clone of plasma cells producing this AL amyloid somewhere in the body beyond the sensitivity of the laboratory tests.

In this case an adequate search for a serum M component was carried out, to no avail. No Bence Jones protein was found in urine, even after 50-fold concentration of the specimen, which is the proper method for seeking its presence. However, the patient did not undergo a bone marrow examination, a bone survey, or a bone scan. I am unable to exclude AL amyloidosis with confidence without these studies. In view of the abnormal spinal fluid findings a complete spinal fluid immunoelectrophoresis would have been of interest, since M components can sometimes be found in the spinal fluid.[13–15] Rarely, a plasma-cell tumor develops in the central nervous system, and an M component may be demonstrable in the cerebrospinal fluid and absent in the serum.[16–19] If this patient had had some of the other features of AL amyloidosis, such as the nephrotic syndrome, congestive heart failure, gastro-intestinal involvement, or particularly macroglossia, we might have been able to make the diagnosis without further studies. However, in the absence of clinical evidence of other organ involvement there is nothing about the neuropathy in or by itself that distinguishes this form of amyloidosis from the other forms. The carpal-tunnel syndrome and the painful, progressive small-fiber neuropathy with autonomic difficulties are consistent with but not diagnostic of AL amyloidosis.[20]

It is interesting that there are many polyneuropathy syndromes related to myeloma and other plasma-cell dyscrasias in which no amyloid can be demonstrated in nerves or elsewhere. Among patients with multiple myeloma two major forms of peripheral neuropathy exist.[21] One is a primary motor subacute illness that resembles the Guillain–Barré syndrome, with a high cerebrospinal fluid protein level. This form is most often associated with osteosclerotic myeloma. Most but not all of the patients with this disorder have an M component in the serum.[22] Although I cannot exclude osteosclerotic myeloma in this patient since a bone survey was not done, it is unlikely as judged by the characteristics of the neuropathy. The second form of myeloma-associated neuropathy is the type related to typical myeloma. The associated neuropathy can take many forms, including mild sensorimotor, pure sensory, or subacute remitting and relapsing, and in this respect resembles carcinomatous neuropathy. Major autonomic dysfunction is rare unless the myeloma is complicated by AL amyloidosis.[23]

One point is clear. Most myeloma neuropathies are not associated with amyloidosis. What then is the mechanism of these plasma-cell–dyscrasia neuropathies? It may be that clues to their pathogenesis will yield ideas about the mechanism of amyloid neuropathy as well. In the past several years a sizable literature has appeared, largely generated at the laboratory of Dr. Norman Latov and his colleagues at Columbia University's

Neurology Department. They have demonstrated the binding of IgM M proteins in patients with plasma-cell dyscrasias and neuropathy to myelin-associated glycoprotein (MAG), a minor constituent of myelin from central or peripheral nerves.[21,24–26] Most patients with a gammopathy and a neuropathy have a demyelinating type of neuropathy; in some patients axonal neuropathies develop, and in these patients IgM M proteins have been found to be reactive with endoneurium rather than MAG.[27] Hafler and his associates[28] found that only patients with IgM monoclonal gammopathies had anti-MAG reactivity and that these patients had a characteristic slowly progressive, mild sensory neuropathy with no autonomic change. Patients with osteosclerotic myeloma and IgG paraproteinemia, on the other hand, do not show anti-MAG reactivity and differ clinically from the anti-MAG group in that they have a more severe and progressive sensorimotor neuropathy.[28] It is possible, therefore, that anti-MAG activity is the mechanism for the neuropathic disease in some patients with an IgM gammopathy, but it does not seem to be the mechanism in patients with other gammopathies.

The mechanism of nerve damage in amyloid neuropathies has never been settled. Various hypotheses have been proposed, including ischemia caused by amyloid infiltration of vessels, compression caused by amyloid deposits around and within the nerves, an inflammatory response elicited by the amyloid, an amyloid ganglionopathy, and a toxic metabolic process. None of these hypotheses can explain all the findings in cases of amyloidosis and related illnesses. One concept is that the plasma-cell clone responsible for the neuropathy produces a so-called "assassinating" molecule that may or may not be amyloidogenic.[29] Recall that all light chains are not amyloidogenic. Thus, some patients with plasma-cell dyscrasias may have amyloid and others may not. The amyloid would in a sense be a co-produced marker for the abnormal clone of plasma cells but would not in itself be neurotoxic. There is to my knowledge no direct evidence to support or refute this unifying hypothesis.

The last type of amyloid neuropathy to be discussed is familial amyloid polyneuropathy (FAP), in which the fibril designated AF is related to prealbumin in the serum. There is no good theory of pathogenesis of this form of the disease, although the gene for retinol-binding protein has been successfully cloned and sequenced.[30] Several major kindred are known but new families are being described regularly. There are four types of familial amyloid polyneuropathy. The prototype, Type I, is the Portuguese (Andrade) type, which is known to affect over 300 families and has now been seen in persons of Portuguese descent around the world. It is an autosomal-dominant trait, with the usual age at onset about 25 to 35 years, although cases with later onset are well known to occur.[31] The neuropathy itself is exactly as described in the patient under discussion. The carpal-tunnel syndrome may be part of the illness, and cardiac involvement with enlargement of all the chambers and conduction abnormalities is common. The findings in this patient are all consistent with this form of the disease except that the age at onset was a little late and he was of Italian ancestry. No cases have yet been reported from Italy. Affected Japanese and Swedish families were soon discovered, with an essentially identical picture. The Swedish families have some members with a later onset, averaging about 53 years. Many other families from numerous other ethnic groups have been reported to have the disorder. Recently, Cohen and Skinner[32] described a family of German–English ancestry residing in Texas in which the age at onset was in the seventh decade in all the family members affected by the disease. Aside from the late onset, all the other features are typical of the Type I familial amyloid polyneuropathy, including the fact that the fibril protein contains prealbumin.[33] The patient under discussion may well have Type I familial amyloid polyneuropathy, but it is impossible to substantiate that diagnosis on clinical grounds. The family history of a father and uncle with gait difficulties late in life is too vague. These relatives could, of course, have had the disease, with a pattern of inheritance consistent with the known autosomal-dominant pattern. Some patients with Type I familial amyloid polyneuropathy have a characteristically scalloped pupil, which some observers believe is pathognomonic of the disorder.[34] It is present in only about a third of the cases, however, and can easily be overlooked if not specifically sought. Some patients with familial amyloid polyneuropathy have a decreased level of serum prealbumin, which was not determined in this case. It is thus impossible to make a firm diagnosis of familial amyloid polyneuropathy in this case without the demonstration of prealbumin as the building block of the amyloid fibril obtained by biopsy.

The other three types of familial amyloid polyneuropathy do not fit this case very well. Type II, the Indiana or Rukavina type, is characterized by a peripheral neuropathy that affects the upper limbs more than the lower limbs and by the presence of vitreous opacities. The carpal-tunnel syndrome is also common in Type II FAP, and the age at onset is in the fourth or fifth decade, with an autosomal-dominant inheritance pattern. Type III familial amyloid polyneuropathy, the so-called Iowa or the Van Allen type, is characterized by a severe upper and lower limb sensorimotor polyneuropathy and severe progressive renal amyloid deposition, leading to death from uremia. Type IV, the Meretoja type, is marked by lattice dystrophy of the cornea and cranial-nerve palsies. Two other rare forms of familial amyloidosis that are not associated with neuropathies are known as familial oculoleptomeningeal amyloidosis and hereditary cerebrovascular amyloidosis. None of these disorders apply to the case under discussion.

It seems, therefore, that this patient had amyloid neuropathy of either the AL or the AF (Type I) variety. It is impossible on the basis of the available information to resolve this issue further. This is an important distinction in the patient for several reasons. First of all, if the disorder was familial amyloid polyneuropathy the patient and his family should have been made aware of that fact. They may wish to avail themselves of genetic counseling. Secondly, if this was a form of AL amyloid a more extensive search for a myeloma should have been undertaken, certainly including a bone marrow examination and a radiologic bone survey or a bone scan. In addition, the distinction of AL from AF amyloidosis has potential therapeutic implications. There has been some success in treating patients with AL amyloidosis and patients with other neuropathies related to plasma-cell dyscrasias with plasma exchange[35] and with antineoplastic agents.[29,36]

To this end a biopsy of some tissue affected by amyloidosis should have been performed. I assume that the diagnostic procedure in this case was a sural-nerve biopsy or a muscle biopsy, or both. Although nerve was the only tissue definitely involved in this patient, biopsy of other tissues, including muscle, abdominal fat pad, rectum, gingiva, and skin, is often also diagnostic. In cases of amyloid polyneuropathy a muscle biopsy is the most sensitive technique. The tissue obtained can be subjected to a series of chemical tests aimed at determining the type of the amyloid involved. The procedure recommended by Cohen and Skinner,[32] at the Boston University School of Medicine, is a potassium permanganate test. Potassium permanganate modifies the molecular conformation of secondary AA amyloid so that it no longer stains with Congo red. This test therefore allows distinction between secondary (AA) amyloid and the other forms. If the amyloid is resistant to potassium permanganate (i.e., still stains with Congo red) one should perform immunohistochemical staining with specific antiserum to prealbumin, which will identify the AF form of amyloid. If the specimen is resistant to potassium permanganate and fails to stain with anti-AF antibody then the amyloid must be of the AL type. It is now possible to skip the potassium permanganate test since antibodies have become available against A kappa, A lambda, AA, and prealbumin. Therefore, the precise nature of the amyloid can be determined by using immunohistochemical techniques on biopsy material. If a large enough sample of tissue is available (usually autopsy material is required) a definitive diagnosis of the amyloid type can be made by fibril isolation from unfixed tissue followed by sequence analysis. An evaluation of this type has been carried out by Dalak as and Cunningham,[37] at the National Institutes Health, in characterizing the amyloid in 15 patients with so-called sporadic amyloid polyneuropath meaning a form not obviously familial or related to plasma-cell dyscrasia. The case under discussion may be an example of sporadic amyloid polyneuropathy. In 11 of these 15 cases the amyloid proved to be AL lambda, in 1 it was AL kappa, and in the 3 remaining cases it was prealbumin (i.e., AF). In other words, 80 per cent of the patients were found to have AL amyloid and 20 per cent were found to have familial amyloid. The assumption, of course, is that in those AF cases either the family history was not complete, as in this case, or the disease was the result of a mutation. Therefore, on the basis of those findings it is statistically more likely that this patient had AL amyloidosis than AF amyloidosis. However, this is only guesswork, and only immunohistochemical analysis of biopsy material can resolve this issue definitively.

My final diagnosis is amyloid polyneuropathy, either the AL type (80 per cent probability) or the AF Type 1 (20 per cent probability).

Dr. Hedley-Whyte: Dr. Shahani investigated this man's peripheral nerves electrophysiologically.

Dr. Bhagwan T. Shahani: The electrophysiologic investigations consisted of motor and sensory-nerve conduction studies, study of late responses, and special studies of the function of unmyelinated nerve fibers of small diameter. The nerve conduction studies were performed in the right tibial, left peroneal, and left ulnar nerves. There was slight slowing, with the maximum motor-nerve conduction velocities being 32, 38, and 47 m per second, respectively. There was considerable reduction in the amplitude of compound muscle-action potentials, produced by stimulating distal parts of these nerves, although their duration was within normal limits. We were unable to record sensory-nerve action potentials from median, radial, and sural nerves, suggesting that this neuropathy had affected large sensory-nerve fibers, at least in the distal segments.

The needle electromyographic examination showed evidence of spontaneous brief potentials. There were fibrillations and positive sharp waves in the medial gastroen-emius and the tibialis anterior muscles as well as in the distal intrinsic hand muscles. The proximal muscles, such as the deltoid in the arm and the vastus lateralis in the leg, did not show evidence of active denervation. The minimal latencies of F responses, recorded from the flexor hallucis brevis (FHB), gastroenemius soleus (GS), and exten-sor digitorum brevis, had prolonged latencies (65 to 77 msec in FHB and 34 to 39 msec in GS). Finally, we studied sympathetic skin responses (SSR), which were absent in the hands and feet, suggesting substantial involvement of unmyclinated nerve fibers of small diameter. In summary, the electrophysiologic studies suggest a generalized senso-rimotor peripheral neuropathy with involvement of nerve fibers of small diameter.

DR. HEDLEY-WHYTE: Dr. Adams, you followed this patient. Will you comment on your impression?

DR. RAYMOND D. ADAMS: We were impressed by how much more the pain, tempera-ture, and autonomic function were affected than the motor function. That finding was strongly in favor of amyloid polyneuropathy.

I would take issue with Dr. Samuels on one point. We have seen small-fiber pain–temperature loss in the arms and head, a pseudosyringomyelic syndrome, in adults with Tangier disease. I have seen three cases of that disorder, but I have not observed such diffuse involvement of the feet and legs as well as the arms and trunk in that disease.

DR. HEDLEY-WHYTE: Dr. Pineda, will you give the medical students' diagnosis in this case?

DR. ALLAN E. PINEDA: The medical students' diagnosis was amyloid polyneu-ropathy of either the primary or the familial type. They were unable to be more specific.

CLINICAL DIAGNOSIS

Amyloid polyneuropathy.

DR. MARTIN A. SAMUELS' DIAGNOSIS

Amyloid polyneuropathy, either AL type or AF Type I.

PATHOLOGICAL DISCUSSION

DR. HEDLEY-WHYTE: The diagnostic procedure was a sural-nerve biopsy. Examination of the 1-μm–thick epon sections of the specimen revealed a severe neuropathy, with marked loss of myelinated fibers, endoneurial fibrosis, and clumping of Schwann cells (Fig. 1). The teased-nerve preparations disclosed wallerian degeneration of occasional fibers (Fig. 2). In the paraffin sections of the nerve occasional clumps of amorphous material stained with Congo red (Fig. 3) and exhibited the apple-green color charac-teristic of amyloid viewed under polarized light (Fig. 4). For the most part the amyloid

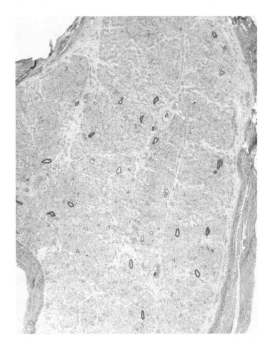

FIG 1 One-μm–Thick Epon Section. Revealing Severe Loss of Myelinated Fibers (Toluidine Blue Stain, ×200).

was not found in blood-vessel walls. Electron-microscopical examination showed that the amyloid consisted of masses of finely fibrillar material 8 to 10 nm in diameter (Fig. 5). Electron-microscopical study also revealed severe loss of unmyelinated fibers as well as myelinated fibers.

Dr. Samuels referred to the possibility of characterizing the amyloid immunohistochemically. Sections were sent to Dr. Marinos C. Dalakas for this purpose, but unfortunately no amyloid was present in these sections.

Coimbra and Andrade[38,39] have pointed out that the extent of destruction of the nerve in amyloid neuropathy is out of proportion to the amount of visible amyloid. The mechanism appears to be axonal degeneration rather than segmental demyelination. Vascular amyloidosis may also occur, with focal infarction, as described by Asbury and Johnson.[40] Thomas and King[41] reported four cases of amyloid neuropathy—three sporadic and

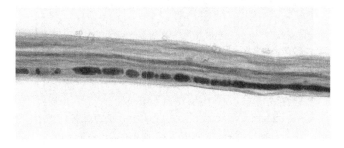

FIG 2 Teased-Fiber Preparation. Revealing Degenerating Myelin Ovoids along a Single Intemode.

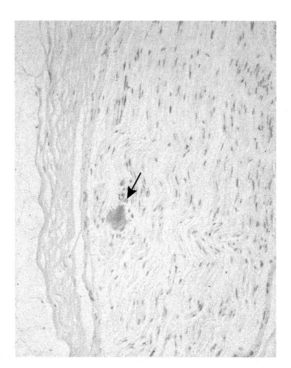

FIG 3 Longitudinal Section of the Nerve, Revealing a Patch of Amorphous Material (Arrow) within the Endoneurium (×125).

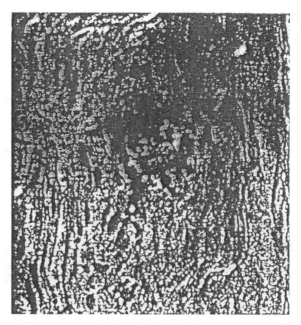

FIG 4 Amorphous Material Seen in Figure 3 Viewed with Polarized Light. Showing the Characteristic Appearance of Amyloid (·500)

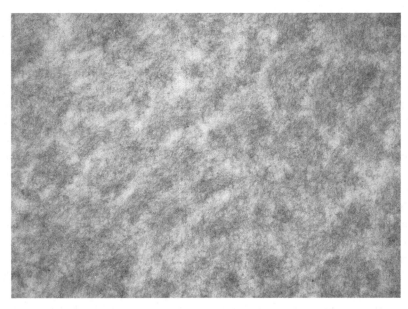

FIG 5 Electron Micrograph Showing the Characteristic Amyloid Fibrils (×37,500).

one familial—and noticed that the density of unmyelinated axons was grossly reduced. In their series the amyloid fibrils were 7 nm in diameter and were usually found in the endoneurium, often associated with capillaries. Dyck and Lambert[42] reported dissociated sensation in association with amyloidosis and described three persons in two kinships with dominantly inherited amyloidosis. In biopsy specimens unmyelinated fibers were almost absent, a finding that correlated with the loss of C-fiber potentials. Coimbra and Andrade[38,39] examined five sural-nerve biopsy specimens and found loss of unmyelinated as well as myelinated fibers. Amyloid can affect the peripheral nervous system by extrancural compression (for example, by deposition in ligaments, giving rise to the carpal-tunnel syndrome),[43] by accumulation in endoncurial vessels, or by extravascular endoneurial deposition, as seen in the patient under discussion. The various types of amyloid can be differentiated in tissue immunohistochemically, as described by Feurle et al.[44]; they found albumin related to AF amyloid in two familial cases of amyloidosis and immunoglobulin light-chain amyloid in one sporadic case.

The residual myelinated fibers are represented by black rings. The perineurium and epineurium are normal.

Adjacent to the thickly myelinated fiber are two thinly myelinated fibers.

In summary, this patient had amyloidosis of the peripheral nerves. Dr. Brown, do you have any followup findings?

DR. ROBERT H. BROWN: Additional clinical studies in this case have included x-ray examination of the bone and a bone scan, which showed no evidence of multiple myeloma or plasmacytoma. Examination of a muscle-biopsy specimen demonstrated weak reactivity with thioflavine T. suggesting intramuscular amyloid. No reaction was seen with antibodies to human light-chain immunoglobulins. The patient's serum has been analyzed by Dr. Maria J.M. Saraiva in the laboratory of Dr. DeWitt Goodman at the

College of Physicians and Surgeons, Columbia University. Dr. Saraiva has extensively investigated amyloid proteins from several Portuguese kindreds with systemic amyloidosis and amyloid polyneuropathy. As first reported by Costa et al.,[45] she has demonstrated that the amyloid protein in these families is prealbumin or transthyretin (TTR), in which she has identified a single amino acid substitution of methionine for valine in position 30.[46] The normal and mutant TTR genes apparently behave as codominant alleles; the mutant TTR is deposited as amyloid in tissues such as peripheral nerves. Dr. Saraiva[47] can now screen for this abnormality in serum, using immunoblotting after partial purification of TTR. With this technique she has demonstrated in preliminary investigations that the TTR protein in the patient under discussion is abnormal in a pattern suggestive of a single amino acid substitution. Thus, it appears likely that this patient, who is of Italian descent, has a disorder related to hereditary Portuguese amyloidosis. Studies are now in progress to determine whether other, asymptomatic members of the family carry this gene and to identify the specific amino acid substitutions in this family's transthyretin.

DR. ADAMS: It has been observed that ischemic disorders in nerves can damage the small fibers, and I wonder if this type of polyneuropathy has an ischemic element.

DR. HEDLEY-WHYTE: In some cases of amyloid polyneuropathy in which the amyloid has been present in the blood-vessel walls, infarcts have been found within the nerve. In this case amyloid was not seen within vessel walls.

DR. SAMUELS: The striking feature in this biopsy specimen is the relative paucity of amyloid in the presence of considerable axonal damage. For this reason it is difficult for me to accept a purely mechanical theory of nerve compression. Engel's idea that the amyloid itself is not responsible for the nerve damage but that it is some co-produced "assassinating" molecule is appealing when one views biopsy findings of this type.

DR. HEDLEY-WHYTE: The initial frozen sections in this case failed to reveal any amyloid. It happened to be present in the pieces that we used for epon embedding, and it was present when the biopsy specimen was processed further through paraffin.

DR. SAMUELS: Dr. Dalakas told me that he has been most successful in seeking amyloid with a muscle biopsy. That fact has made him believe even more strongly that it is not the mass of amyloid that causes the trouble, since the amyloid is nearly always in the muscle, but there is never clinical evidence of a myopathy in these cases.

ANATOMICAL DIAGNOSIS

Amyloid polyneuropathy.

ADDENDUM

DR. ADAMS: The patient is no longer able to work. His neuropathy has worsened slightly, mainly in the sensory sphere. His renal function remains good.

DR. HEDLEY-WHYTE: A subsequent muscle biopsy revealed severe denervation atrophy but no amyloid when examined with Congo-red staining.

REFERENCES

1. von Rokitansky K. Handbuch der pathologischen Anatomic. Vienna: Draumuller and Seidel, 1842.

2. Virchow R. Die Cellularpathologic in ihrer Begründung suf physiologische und pathologische Gewebelehre. Berlin: Hirschwaid. 1858.

3. Wilks S. Cases of lardaceous disease and some allied affections, with remarks. Guys Hosp Rep (Series 3) 1856: 2:103–32.

4. Adams W. Mollities ossium. Trans Pathol Soc Lond 1872: 23:186–8.

5. Koenigstein H. Über Amyloidose der Haut. Arch Dermatol Syphilol 1925: 148:330–83.

6. de Andrade C. A peculiar form of peripheral neuropathy: familial atypical generalized amyloidosis with special involvement of the peripheral nerves. Brain 1952; 75:408–27.

7. Shaumberg HH, Spencer PS. Human tosic neuropathy due to industrial agents. In: Dyck PJ, Thomas PK. Lambert EH. eds. Peripheral neuropathy. 2nd ed. Vol. 2. Philadelphia: WB Saunders. 1984:2115–32.

8. Glenner GG. Amyloid deposits and amyloidosis: the β-fibrilloses. N Engi J Med 1980: 302:1283–92. 1333–43.

9. Cohen AS, Rubinow A. Amyloid neuropathy. In: Dyck PJ, Thomas PK, Lambert EH. eds. Peripheral neuropathy. 2nd ed. Vol. 2. Philadelphia: WB Saunders. 1984:1866–98.

10. Kyle RA, Greipp PR. Amyloidosis (AL): clinical and laboratory features in 229 cases. Mayo Clin Proc 1983: 58:665–83.

11. Morcle RC, Wisniewski HM, Lossinsky AS. Pathogenesis of ocuritic and amyloid plaques in scrapie—ultrastructural study of early changes in the cortical neuropil. In: Samuel D, Algeri S, Gershon S, Grimm VE, Toffano G. eds. Aging of the brain. New York: Raven Press. 1983:61–79.

12. Glenner GG. Alzheimer's disease: the commoness form of amyloidosis. Arch Pathol Lab Med 1983; 107:281–2.

13. Dalakas MC, Papadopoulos NM. Paraproteins in the spinal fluid of patients, with paraproteinemic polyneuropathies. Ann Neurol 1984; 15:590–3.

14. Hansotia P, Gani K, Friedenberg W. Cerebrospinal fluid monoclonal gammopathy in multiple myeloma and Waldenström's macroglöbulinemia. Neurology (NY) 1983: 33:1411–15.

15. Weiss AH, Smith E, Chrissoff N, Kochiva S. Cerebrospinal fluid paraproteins in multiple myeloma. J Lab Clin Med 1965: 66:280–93.

16. Clarke E. Cranial and intracranial myelomas. Brain 1954; 77:61–81.

17. French JD. Plasmacytoma of the hypothalamus: clinical-pathological report of a case. J Neuropathol Exp Neurol 1947; 6:265–70.

18. Moosy J, Wilson CB. Solitary intracranial plasmacytoma. Arch Neurol 1967: 16:212–16.

19. Siager UT, Taylor WF, Opfell RW, Myers A. Leptomeningeal myeloma. Arch Pathol Lab Med 1979; 103:680–2.

20. Kelly JJ Jr, Kyle RA, O'Brien PC, Dyck PJ. The natural history of peripheral neuropathy in primary systemic amyloidosis. Ann Neurol 1979; 6:1–7.

21. Latov N, Godfrey M, Thomas Y, et al. Neuropathy and anti-myclin-associated glycoprotein IgM M proteins: T cell regulation of M protein secretion in vitro. Ann Neurol 1985; 18:182–8.

22. Kelly JJ Jr, Kyle RA, Miles JM, Dyck PJ. Osteosclerotic myeloma and peripheral neuropathy. Neurology (NY) 1983: 33:202–10.

23. Kelly JJ Jr, Kyle RA, Miles JM, O'Brien PC, Dyck PJ. The spectrum of peripheral neuropathy in myeloma. Neurology (NY) 1981; 31:24–31.

24. Takatsu M, Hays AP, Latov N, et al. Immunofluorescence study of patients with neuropathy and IgM M proteins. Ann Neurol 1985; 18:173–81.

25. Nobile-Orazio E, McIntosh C, Latov N. Anti-MAG antibody and antibody compleaes: detection by radioimmunoassay. Neurology (NY) 1985; 35:988–92.

26. Freddo L, Ariga T, Saito M, Macala LC, Yu RK, Latov N. The neuropathy of plasma cell dyscrasia: binding of IgM M-proteins to peripheral nerve-glycolipids. Neurology (NY) 1985: 35:1420–4.

27. Freddo L, Hays AP, Sherman WH, Lasov N. Asonal neuropathy in a patient: with IgM M-protein reactive with nerve endoncurium. Neurology (NY) 1985; 35:1321–5.

28. Hafier DA, Johnson D, Kelly JJ, Panitch II, Kyle R, Weiner HL. Monoclonal gasnenopathy and neuropathy: myclin-associated glyeoprotein reactivity and clinical characteristics. Neurology (NY) 1986: 36:75–8.

29. Trotter JL, Engel WK, Ignaczak FT. Amyloidosis with plasma cell dyserasia: an overlooked cause of adult onset sensorimotoe neuropathy. Arch Neurol 1977; 34:209–14.

30. Colantuoni V, Romano V, Bensi C. et al Cloning and sequencing of a full length cDNA coding for human retunol-binding protein Nucleic Acids Res 1983: 11:7769–76.

31. Lima AB, Martins da Silva A. Clinical evaluation of late onset cases in Type I (Andrade) amyloid neuropathy. In: Glenner GG, ed. Amyloid and amyloidosis. Amsterdam: Eacerpea Medica. 1980:99–105.

32. Cohen AS, Skinner M. The diagnosis of amyloidosis. In: Cohen AS, ed. Laboratory diagnostic procedures in the rheumatic diseases. 3rd ed. Orlando. Fla.: Grune & Stration. 1985:377–99.

33. Libbey CA, Rubinow A, Shirahams T, Deal C, Cohen AS. Familial amyloid polyneuropathy: demonstration of prealbumin in a kinship of German/English ancestry with onsel in the seventh decade. Am J Med 1984; 76:18–24.

34. Lessell S, Wolf PA, Benson MD, Cohen AS. Scalloped pupils in familial amyloidosis. N Engl J Med 1975: 293:914–15.

35. Sherman WH, Olarte MR, McKieman G, Sweeney K, Latov N, Hays AP. Plasma exchange treatment of peripheral neuropathy associated with plasma cell dyscrasia. J Neurol Neurosurg Psychiatry 1984: 47:813–19.

36. Dalakas MC, Flaum MA, Rick M, Engel WK, Grainick HR. Treatment of polyneuropathy in Waldenström's macroglobulinemia: role of paraproteinemia and immunologic studies. Neurology (NY) 1983; 33:1406–10.

37. Dalakas MC, Cunningham GG. Characterisation of amyloid deposits in biopsies of 15 patients with "sporadic" (nonfamilial or plasma cell dyscratic) amyloid polyneuropathy. Acta Neuropathol (Berlin) 1986: 69:66–72.

38. Coimbra A, Andrade C. Familial amyloid polyneuropathy: an electron microscope study of the peripheral nerve in five cases. I. Interstitial changes. Brain 1971; 94:199–206.

39. Idem. Familial amyloid polyneuropathy, an electron microscopic study of peripheral nerve in five cases II. Nerve fibre changes. Brain 197–12.

40. Arbury AK, Johnson PC. Pathology of peripheral nerve. Philadelphia: Saunders. 1978.

41. Thomas PK, King RHM. Peripheral nerve changes in amyloid neuropa. Brain 1974; 97:395–406.

42. Dyck PI, Lambert EH. Dissociated sensation in amyloidosis: compaction potential, quantitative histologic and teased-fiber, and microscopic studies of sural nerve biopsies. Arch Neurol 1969; 507.

43. Bastian PO. Amyloidosis and the carpal tunnel syndrome. Am J Clin Neurol 1974; 61:711–17.

44. Feurle GE, Linke RP, Kuhn E, Wagnet A. Clinical value of immune chemistry with AF-antibody in the diagnosis of familial amyloid neuropathy. J Neurol 1984: 231:237–43.
45. Costa PP, Figuera AS, Bravo FR. Amyloid fibril protein related to albumin in familial amyloidotic polyneuropathy. Proc Natl Acad Sci US 1978: 75:4499–503.
46. Saraiva MJM, Birken S, Costa PP, Goodman DS. Amyloid fibril protein in familial amyloidotic polyneuropathy. Portuguese type: definition of molecular abnormality in transthyretin (prealbumin). J Clin Invest 74:104–19.
47. Saraiva MJM, Costa PP, Goodman DS. Biochemical marker in familial amyloidotic polyneuropathy. Portuguese type: family studies of transthyretin (prealbumin)-methionine-30 variant. J Clin Invest 1985:76:2171–7.

Perspectives and Updates

This is a case in which it is obvious that the diagnosis is amyloid polyneuropathy, but the details of the type of amyloid prove to be the key question. The amyloid story in neurological disease has become an extremely complex and contentious one. A great deal of evidence correlates the accumulation of amyloid β protein with Alzheimer disease and with amyloid angiopathy, though the ultimate cause-and-effect relationship remains elusive.

This case revolves around the cause of a late-onset symmetrical pseudosyringomyelic neuropathy with some autonomic features in a patient of Italian ancestry whose family history of neurological disease was equivocal. It was quite clear that he did not have secondary (AA) amyloid and it was also very unlikely that he had (AL) amyloid. At the time of the case discussion in 1986, I was unaware of any familial amyloid polyneuropathy families of Italian origin. The vast majority of the families were of Portuguese descent, though some of Japanese, Swedish, German and English descent had been discovered by the time of the case discussion. After my discussion, it was mentioned by Dr. Robert H. Brown that serum from the patient had been sent to the laboratories of Drs. Maria J. M. Saraiva and DeWitt Goodman, who had preliminarily identified an abnormal transthyretin (prealbumin) that had a single amino acid substitution of methionine for valine at position 30—a finding identical to that in several Portuguese families they had studied. This suggested that this patient did in fact have familial amyloid polyneuropathy type I (the Andrade type).

Since that time, transthyretin (prealbumin) gene analyses have been performed on an array of European patients with suspected familial amyloid polyneuropathy, including a three-generation Italian family that demonstrated genetic anticipation. In that family, the mutation was in the transthyretin gene in exon 2, position 47, causing a substitution of glycine for glutamate.

As of now over 70 transthyretin gene point mutations are known, each producing its own characteristic though probably not pathognmonic clinical features. This case is another beautiful example of how a careful clinical analysis can lead to a focused genetic evaluation, which can help to prognosticate, to provide valuable information for family members at risk, and to inform decisions around family planning.

At present the precise mechanism whereby amyloid damages nerves remains obscure. Physical damage alone and/or ischemia caused by amyloid infiltration of nerves can sometimes be seen; but more often than not, the amount of amyoid and the degree of ischemia is far less than would explain the severe neuropathy. In a sense, the amyloid story in brain and nerve is similar. There is a clear correlation with the disease but a lack of a cause-and-effect relationship between the amyloid and the illness[1,2,3].

Martin A. Samuels

REFERENCES

1. Pelo E, Da Prato L, Castelli G, Gori F, Pizzi A, Rorricelli F, Marconi G. Familial amyloid polyneuropathy with genetic anticipation. Amyloid 2002; 9: 35–41.
2. Reilly MM, Adams D, Booth DR, Davis MB, Said G, Laubriat-Bianchin M, Pepys MB, Thomas PK, Harding AE. Transthyretin gene analysis in European patients with suspected familial amyloid polyneuropathy. Brain 1995; 118: 849–56.
3. Saraiva, MJM, Costa PP, Goodman DS. Biochemical marker in familial amyloidotic polyneuropathy, Portuguese type. J Clin Invest 1985; 76: 2171–7.

A 26-Year-Old Woman with Dilated Cardiomyopathy and a Stroke

PHEOCHROMOCYTOMA
CPC 15-1988

PRESENTATION OF CASE

A 26-year-old woman was admitted to the hospital because of a question of dilated cardiomyopathy and a stroke.

She was well until six days earlier, when she went out with friends. On the following morning the patient experienced a severe headache and nausea and remained home during the next two days. A friend noticed that she felt "warm." Three days before admission the patient was found lying on her bathroom floor, confused. It was observed that food and drink brought by her friends two days earlier were untouched. Ambulance personnel found a faint pulse at a rate of 150 but could not register a blood pressure. The patient appeared mildly cyanotic, warm, and dry. The pupils were dilated, with a sluggish response to light; she complained only of abdominal pain. An electrocardiographic monitor showed sinus tachycardia. Nearly 2 liters of fluids were administered by vein, and the blood pressure rose to 80 mm Hg systolic. She was taken to another hospital, where another liter of fluid was infused by vein.

On examination the temperature was 38.3°C, the pulse was 130, and the respirations were 18. The blood pressure was 85/60 mm Hg. The patient was minimally cooperative. Ecchymoses were noted over the lower extremities, and there were hematomas at both knees and the left hip. The pupils were 4 mm, equal, and reactive; the optic fundi were normal. The neck was supple. Bilateral basilar crackles were heard. The heart was normal except for sinus tachycardia. The abdomen was relaxed, with markedly diminished bowel sounds; mild, diffuse tenderness was elicited and was more marked on the right side; the liver and spleen were not felt. There was trace peripheral edema bilaterally, without cyanosis or clubbing. Pelvic examination disclosed slight fullness in the right adnexal region, with a mucoid discharge; no tenderness was detected on movement of the cervix. Rectal examination was negative, and a stool specimen gave a + test for occult blood. On neurologic examination the patient was alert and oriented except that she was six months behind as to the date. The cranial nerves were normal except for questionable reduction in rightward gaze. Motor function and pain sensation were intact. There was bilateral dysmetria in the upper extremities. The tendon reflexes were + + and equal, and the plantar responses were flexor.

A specimen of blood drawn during the ambulance ride showed that the hematocrit was 53 percent and the hemoglobin 19 g per 100 ml; the white-cell count was 26,000, with 70 percent neutrophils, 13 percent band forms, 10 percent lymphocytes, and 7 percent monocytes. The glucose was 101 mg per 100 ml (5.61 mmol per liter). The sodium was 147 mmol, the potassium 5.0 mmol, the chloride 111 mmol, and the carbon dioxide 27 mmol per liter. On arrival in the Emergency Ward, after the administration of 2 liters of fluid by vein, the hematocrit was 42 percent, and the white-cell count 22,000. The urea nitrogen was 56 mg per 100 ml (20 mmol per liter), the creatinine 1.9 mg per 100 ml (170 μmol per liter), and the glucose. 117 mg per 100 ml (6.49 mmol per liter). The prothrombin time and partial thromboplastin time were normal, and a test for fibrin-split products was negative. The amylase was 54 U, and the lipase 44 U per liter. Three hours after arrival in the Emergency Ward the urine had a specific gravity of 1.025 and gave positive tests for glucose and ketones; the sediment contained 15 red cells and rare hyaline casts per high-power field. The urea nitrogen was 47 mg per 100 ml (17 mmol per liter), the creatinine 1.7 mg per 100 ml (150 μmol per liter), the calcium 8.2 mg per 100 ml (2.1 mmol per liter), the bilirubin 0.7 mg per 100 ml (10 μmol per liter), the uric acid 11.5 mg per 100 ml (6.84 mmol per liter), the cholesterol 180 mg per 100 ml (47 mmol per liter), the triglyceride 174 mg, and the protein 5.2 g (the albumin 2.8 g and the globulin 2.4 g) per 100 ml. The serum aspartate aminotransferase (SGOT) was 608 U, the lactic dehydrogenase (LDH) 4521 U, and the creatine kinase (CK) 17,348 U per liter. Screening tests on specimens of blood and urine for drugs of abuse were reported to be negative. An electrocardiogram disclosed sinus tachycardia, with nonspecific ST-segment and T-wave abnormalities. X-ray films of the chest, abdomen, ribs, and left hip showed no abnormality. A computed tomographic (CT) scan of the brain (Fig. 1), performed without the administration of contrast material, revealed bilateral cerebellar infarcts, with sparing of some of the right side and of the vermis, as well as left occipital and left posteroparietal infarcts. A lumbar puncture yielded cerebrospinal fluid that contained 17 red cells and no white cells in the fourth tube; the glucose was 96 mg per 100 ml (5.3 mmol per liter), and the protein 57 mg per 100 ml. Nasogastric aspiration yielded bile-stained fluid that gave a negative test for occult blood.

Additional fluids were administered by vein, and increasing dyspnea developed; another x-ray film of the chest showed pulmonary edema. Dopamine and dobutamine were infused, and a Swan-Ganz catheter was inserted; the right atrial pressure was 9 mm Hg, the right ventricular pressure 35/12 mm Hg, the pulmonary arterial pressure 32/20 mm Hg, and the pulmonary-capillary wedge pressure 20 mm Hg; the cardiac output was 3 liters per minute. Determination of oxygen saturations gave no evidence of intracardiac shunting. An echocardiographic study was reported to show enlargement of all four cardiac chambers; minimal mitral regurgitation was seen; the cardiac apex contracted well, but the remaining ventricular areas appeared hypokinetic; the left

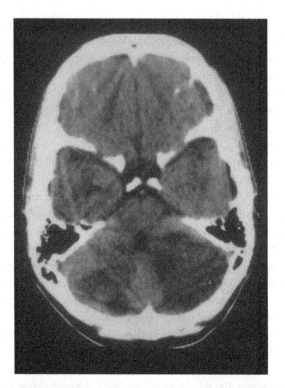

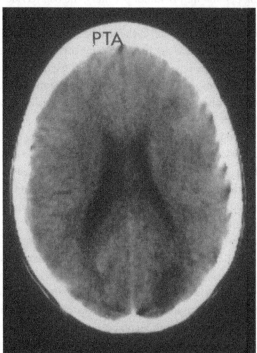

FIG 1 Computed Tomographic Scan Obtained Three Days before Referral to This Hospital, Showing Bilateral Cerebellar (Top) and Parieto-occipital (Bottom) Infarcts.

ventricular ejection fraction was estimated to be 33 percent. Furosemide was administered by vein, with improvement. Repeated electrocardiograms revealed no evidence of
myocardial ischemia or infarction. A serologic test for syphilis and a test for antinuclear
antibodies were negative. Cultures of blood, urine, and cerebrospinal fluid were negative.
The CK fell to 5253 U per liter, and tests for CK-MB were negative. The LDH decreased
to 3850 U, and tests for LDH isoenzymes showed an elevated fraction 2 in excess of fraction 1. On the third hospital day the patient was transferred to this hospital.

The patient was single. She had a history of multiple gynecologic problems of
uncertain nature and was reported to have had parotitis three years before entry. Her
alcohol intake was believed to be small, and she smoked one pack of cigarettes daily.
She used marijuana and cocaine occasionally but denied taking either during the week
before admission. She used a birth-control piil. There was a history of excessive sweating since puberty. There was no past history of hypertension or other cardiovascular or
neurologic problems. She denied intravenous drug abuse, arthralgia, myalgia, hemorrhagic diathesis, paroxysmal symptoms, recent travel, or contact with pets. There was
a history of hypertension in her mother and of nephrolithiasis in her father, but there
was no family history of thyroid, parathyroid, or adrenal disease.

The temperature was 36.7°C, the pulse was 120, and the respirations were 25. The
blood pressure was 100/70 mm Hg.

On examination the patient was an alert, confused, anxious woman who appeared
tired. No ecchymoses, hematomas, or signs of sepsis were seen, and no lymphadenopathy was palpated. The neck was supple; the jugular venous pressure was normal, and
the carotid pulses were ++ bilaterally, without bruits; the thyroid gland was not felt.
The lungs were clear. The heart was normal; no murmur, S4, S3, or pericardial friction
rub was heard. The breasts were normal. Abdominal examination was negative; bowel
sounds were present, and no organs or masses were palpated. There was no peripheral
edema, clubbing, or cyanosis, and no Homans sign was found; the peripheral pulses
were full. Rectal examination was negative except that a stool specimen gave a + test for
occult blood. On neurologic examination the patient was alert and responsive but confused and disoriented as to time and place. Her speech was slightly slurred. Difficulty
in right-left discrimination was noted throughout the examination. The cranial nerves
were normal except that the patient perceived light but could not count fingers or
name objects. Motor function appeared intact except for questionable right pronator
drift. Sensation was preserved except that all modalities felt "different" in the left upper
extremity, and position sense in the toes was poor. Bilateral dysmetria was observed
on the finger-to-nose test. The tendon reflexes were hypoactive throughout, and the
plantar responses were flexor.

The hematocrit was 34.8 percent; the white-cell count was 10,800, with 68 percent
neutrophils, 27 percent lymphocytes, and 5 percent monocytes. The prothrombin time
was 10 seconds, with a control of 10.9 seconds; the partial thromboplastin time was
33.6 seconds. The urea nitrogen was 11 mg per 100 ml (3.9 mmol per liter), the glucose
95 mg per 100 ml (5.3 mmol per liter), the conjugated bilirubin 0.4 mg per 100 ml
(7 μmol per liter), the total bilirubin 0.8 mg per 100 ml (10 μmol per liter), the calcium
8.3 mg per 100 ml (2.1 mmol per liter), the phosphorus 3.3 mg per 100 ml (1.1 mmol

per liter), and the protein 5.5 g (the albumin 2.8 g and the globulin 2.7 g) per 100 ml. The sodium was 140 mmol, the potassium 3.5 mmol, the magnesium 1.9 mmol, the chloride 104 mmol, and the carbon dioxide 25 mmol per liter. The SGOT was 71 U, the LDH 430 U, the CK 358 U, the 5' nucleotidase 4 U, and the amylase 220 U per liter (normal, 53 to 123). The LDH isoenzymes showed an elevation in fraction 2 greater than in fraction 1, and the CK isoenzymes revealed less than 1 percent-MB band. The chorionic gonadotropin was less than 5 mIU per milliliter. The thyroxine was 6.0 μg per 100 ml (77 nmol per liter), and the free thyroxine index 1.9; the triiodothyronine resin uptake was 32 percent, and the thyroid-stimulating hormone 4.3 μU per millili-ter. An electrocardiogram showed a normal rhythm at a rate of 97, with delayed R-wave progression in Leads V_1 and V_2 and nonspecific ST-segment and T-wave abnormalities. An x-ray film of the chest, performed with portable technique, revealed that the lungs were clear except for streaky densities in the retrocardiac area; the heart and medi-astinum appeared normal; a pulmonary-artery line terminated in the right interlobar artery. A cranial CT scan, performed without the administration of contrast material, disclosed large areas of attenuation within the left cerebellar hemisphere, left occipi-tal lobe, and posterior left parietal lobe; a questionable area of low attenuation was also noted within the right cerebellar hemisphere; the fourth ventricle was small and appeared partially compressed; the remaining ventricles were enlarged; no evidence of intracranial hemorrhage was seen; the visible portions of the orbits and paranasal sinuses appeared normal. The total hemolytic complement (CH50) was 104 U per milliliter; the C3 was 117 mg, and the C4 26 mg per 100 ml. A neurologic consultant noted that the patient denied visual problems, although she had difficulty in directing her eyes to the side requested and experienced or reported distorted visual images. The pupils were 5 mm and were equal and reactive. Upward gaze was intact; there was difficulty in sustaining leftward gaze; no definite nystagmus was seen. The face was symmetric; speech was slightly slurred. On the finger-to-nose test she was ataxic, more so on the right side. There was slight weakness of the right grip, with pronation of the right arm. The tendon reflexes were + and equal, and the plantar responses were flexor. Urgent cardiac catheterization showed that the right atrial mean pressure was 3 mm Hg, the right ventricular pressure 30/3 mm Hg, the pulmonary arterial pressure 30/10 mm Hg, and the pulmonary-capillary wedge pressure 11 mm Hg; the cardiac output was 4.6 liters per minute. Multiple biopsy specimens were obtained from the right ventricular endomyocardium. A portable echocardiogram showed no valvular abnormality; the left ventricle was markedly hypokinetic at the base and midventricu-lar level, and function at the apex was hyperkinetic; the overall left ventricular size was at the upper limit of normal; no intraventricular thrombus was seen.

An indwelling catheter was inserted into the bladder, methylprednisolone was administered by vein, and dobutamine was continued by intravenous drip. On the sec-ond hospital day the patient's condition was more stable. The blood pressure ranged from 100/65 to 105/70 mm Hg. The temperature was normal and remained so. On examination the patient was alert and oriented. A right homonymous hemianopia was observed. Lateral gaze was full, although it was still difficult to elicit leftward gaze; upward gaze was limited. The right grip remained slightly weak. Position sense was impaired in the right first toe. The hematocrit was 38.6 percent, the white-cell count 16,000, and the platelet count 180,000. The urea nitrogen was 15 mg per 100 ml. (5.4 mmol per liter), and the glucose 120 mg per 100 ml (6.7 mmol per liter). The SGOT was 53 U, the LDH 412 U, the CK 207 U, and the amylase 179 U per liter. LDH isoenzymes again disclosed an elevation in fraction 2 greater than in fraction 1; CK isoenzymes showed less than 1 percent MB band. Another electrocardiogram revealed a normal rhythm at a rate of 95 and was unchanged. A repeated x-ray film of the chest showed no change. A gated blood-pool study, performed after the intravenous injection of ^{99m}Tc, showed that the right atrium and right ventricle appeared normal in size and contraction; hypokinesis of the upper septal and proximal anterolateral walls of the left ventricle and akinesis of the proximal posterolateral wall were demonstrated; mild dilatation of the left ventricle was observed; the ejection fraction was calculated to be within 40 and 44 percent. The patient was weaned from dobutamine, and the pulmonary-artery line was removed.

On the third hospital day the blood pressure ranged between 100/70 and 120/85 mm Hg, and the pulse varied from 84 to 120. Examination of the heart remained negative. A right homonymous hemianopia persisted; extraocular movements were full, without nystagmus. Joint position sense was intact at the right first toe, but several errors were noted at the left first toe. The abdomen was slightly tender in both lower quadrants. The urea nitrogen was 19 mg per 100 ml (6.8 mmol per liter), and the glucose 93 mg per 100 ml (5.2 mmol per liter). The LDH was 334 U, and the CK 94 U per liter. Another electrocardiogram demonstrated sinus tachycardia at a rate of 105, with improvement in the nonspecific ST-segment and T-wave abnormalities. Another x-ray film of the chest again disclosed subsegmental atelectasis at the base of the left lung; the remaining lung fields and cardiomediastinal silhouette appeared normal. Ranitidine was begun.

On the following day the patient's condition was improved. She still experienced difficulty with leftward gaze, and a right homonymous hemianopia was again observed. The heart and lungs were normal; very mild tenderness was present in both lower abdominal quadrants. The blood pressure and pulse were normal and remained so thereafter. The hematocrit was 37.3 percent, and the white-cell count 13,900. Another electrocardiogram revealed a normal rhythm at a rate of 80, without important change. A repeated cranial CT scan, performed without the intravenous administration of contrast material, again showed left occipital and bilateral cerebellar infarcts, all of which appeared unchanged; the lateral ventricles appeared smaller; there was no evidence of intracranial hemorrhage.

On the fifth hospital day the patient's condition was further improved; she was able to wash and feed herself in a clumsy fashion and to walk to the bathroom with a stationary walker. Minimal ataxia persisted on the finger-to-nose test; there was still difficulty in sustaining leftward gaze, with a right homonymous hemianopia. Stool specimens continued to give + tests for occult blood. The urea nitrogen was 15 mg per 100 ml (5.4 mmol per liter), and the glucose 94 mg per 100 ml (5.2 mmol per liter). Microscopical examination of the biopsy specimens from the right ventricular endomyocardium (Fig. 2 to 4) showed multifocal myocyte necrosis; scattered myocytes were hypereosinophilic, with focal disruption of their sarcolemmal membranes, and

Table 1. Analysis of 24-Hour Urine Specimens.

Collection	Volume	Vanilmandelic Acid	Meta-nephrine	En-nephrine	Norepinephrine	Creatinine
	ml	*mg*	*mg*	*µg*	*µg*	*mg/kg of body wt*
No. 1	1850	10.7	4.1	18	120	907
No. 2	2450	14.2		16	98	1176
No. 3	3750	12.4				
No. 4	4920	17.8				

had blue-staining cytoplasm on modified Mallory trichrome staining. Direct immunofluorescence showed scattered myocytes with positive staining for IgG, IgA, and C3. Indirect immunofluorescence was negative. Congo-red-stained sections showed no evidence of amyloid. No myocyte hypertrophy or interstitial inflammation was seen. The changes were considered diagnostic of multifocal myocyte necrosis; no evidence of myocarditis was observed. The dose of methylprednisolone was gradually tapered. On the seventh hospital day the patient was depressed, although her ability to walk was progressively improved. Examination showed no change except that the abdomen was no longer tender. A right homonymous hemianopia persisted, and she still had difficulty in directing her gaze to the left or sustaining it there. The hematocrit was 37.9 percent, the white-cell count 19,700, and the erythrocyte sedimentation rate 35 mm per hour. The amylase was 198 U, and the CK 77 U per liter. A [1+1]In antimyosin antibody scan showed diffuse uptake of tracer material in the cardiac region, particularly on the anterior projection; the left anterior oblique view demonstrated more intense focal uptake at the cardiac apex; the SPECT (single-photon emission computed tomographic) images revealed intense uptake at the cardiac apex and diffuse uptake in the remaining portions of the left ventricle.

On the eighth hospital day a neuro-ophthalmologic consultant found a right inferior homonymous quadrantanopia, consistent with a left parieto-occipital lesion. The optic fundi appeared normal; no evidence of emboli was seen. The hematocrit was 39.5 percent; the white-cell count was 17,800, with 75 percent neutrophils. The amylase was 195 U, and the lipase 43 U per liter. An ultrasonographic examination of the abdomen disclosed that the pancreas was not enlarged; a solid mass, 6 by 6.5 cm, was seen in the right adrenal gland; mixed echotextures that ranged from high to low density were present within the mass. The results of additional laboratory studies were received (Table 1).

A diagnostic procedure was performed.

DIFFERENTIAL DIAGNOSIS

DR. MARTIN A. SAMUELS[*]: In summary, this young woman who allegedly was previously in good health was found at home confused and dehydrated. Her only medical

---

[*] Chief. Neurology Service, Brockton-West Roxbury Veterans Administration Medical Center: associate professor of neurology. Harvard Medical School. Currently Chair, Department of Neurology, Brigham and Women's Hospital.

history was that of a long problem of profuse sweating, the use of an oral contraceptive, and occasional nasal use of cocaine. She was severely volume-depleted and
was taken to a hospital, where she was found to have had a posterior-fossa stroke and
to have pulmonary edema. An echocardiographic study showed a dilated cardiomyopathy. Over several days her hemodynamic status improved, although it was easily
demonstrable even late in the course that she had both acute and chronic cardiac damage. An endomyocardial biopsy showed multifocal myocyte necrosis, and an abdominal ultrasound examination revealed a large adrenal mass.

This is an exceptional clinicopathological conference. As the discusser I not only
know the diagnosis but also know the patient as well. I was the attending neurologist
on the consultation service when she was in the hospital and had the opportunity to
participate in the decision-making process regarding the management of her care on
a firsthand basis. When it was decided that the issues surrounding this patient's course
were important enough to warrant presentation at a clinicopathological conference a
problem arose. If all the information were given to the prospective discusser the final
diagnosis would have been so obvious that any consideration of the alternatives that
faced the treating physicians would have been inconceivable. However, if the crucial
diagnostic test, the abdominal ultrasound study, were excluded from the case record
the unsuspecting discusser would have found it virtually impossible to reach the correct diagnosis. This case was simply not an ideal one for presentation as a diagnostic
exercise. Nonetheless, the problems raised were of such great general interest that it
seemed appropriate to use the case in this unusual way. Therefore, I shall discuss the
case in the order and manner in which we considered the problems in reality.

I have organized the discussion into a series of questions that were addressed by the
attending physicians during the patient's course in the hospital. This story represents
a dramatic success. The patient is not only alive but also is doing well and cured of the
underlying disease. I am grateful to the attending physicians who allowed me to see
this patient and to discuss the case today on their behalf.

The first question that we faced concerned the nature of the neurologic event. Was
it hypertensive encephalopathy, ischemic encephalopathy, or a stroke? The unequivocal answer to this question is that this patient had a stroke. I shall discuss the details of
that stroke later. She complained of headache and was said by a friend to feel "warm,"
an observation that could have indicated that sweating was observed. This observation
could be construed to describe a paroxysm of hypertension due to a catecholamine
"storm." Indeed, such an event may have occurred, but the patient's neurologic state
on admission was not due to either hypertensive encephalopathy or hypoxic ischemic encephalopathy. Hypertensive encephalopathy nearly always occurs in the context
of malignant hypertension—that is, almost always with papilledema, left ventricular
hypertrophy, and proteinuria. This patient had none of those findings. It is probably
true that hypertensive encephalopathy is caused by a failure of cerebral-vessel auto-
regulation in the very high blood-pressure ranges and thus could occur with a single
paroxysm of hypertension outside the general context of chronic hypertension or the
syndrome of malignant hypertension. However, if such an event had occurred in this
patient and was severe enough to produce this degree of neurologic deficit and the

CT-scan findings described, papilledema certainly should have developed within 12 or at least 24 hours of the onset of the difficulty. The papilledema would have been visible for many days thereafter. The fundi were observed several times during the patient's course, and papilledema was not seen at any time. Of greater importance, the pathologic changes of hypertensive encephalopathy consist of widespread small areas of ischemic injury, not an area of infarction localized to the distribution of a single vessel. If one postulates a paroxysm of hypertension followed by prolonged hypotension due to either dehydration or a systemic exhaustion of catecholamines after the "storm," one is faced with a similar problem. Systemic hypotension produces either a widespread cerebral syndrome with microscopic lesions in characteristic regions (e.g., the deep layers of the cerebral cortex, the basal ganglia, the cerebellar Purkinje cells, and the hippocampus) or with larger lesions in the cerebral border zones. In the absence of a fixed stenosis of cerebral vessels, which is unlikely to be present in a 26-year-old woman, one would not expect a localized infarct in the distribution of a single vessel or in a single border zone. The answer to the first question is thus unequivocally a stroke — in other words, a sudden or rapid event in a known vascular territory due to some sort of cerebrovascular disease.

The second question arises naturally from the first. What was the distribution of the stroke? On clinical grounds the deficit was in the cerebellum, more on the left side, and in the parieto-occipital cortex, also more on the left side. The prolonged period of unconsciousness followed by confusion and inattention probably reflected a disorder of the rostral reticular formation. All these structures are in the distribution of the top of the basilar artery. An alternative hypothesis would be that the stroke was in the posterior border zone and due to hypotension. However, the absence of a lesion in the anterior border zone is against this concept. Not all aspects of the top-of-the-basilar syndrome were present. For example, there was no disorder of convergence (neither weakness nor spasm of convergence was ever seen) or difficulty with vertical gaze. The pupils initially were dilated and poorly reactive but thereafter were noted to be normal. All these features, missing in this patient, are usually seen when the top-of-the-basilar syndrome includes prolonged occlusion of the precommunicating segment of the posterior cerebral artery, also known as the basilar communicating or mesencephalic artery, from which the paramedian arteries usually arise. The recovery from coma and the absence of persistent abnormality of the pupils and eye movements inform us that the process primarily affected the post-communicating segment of the posterior cerebral artery, more on the left side than on the right side. The existence of several of the elements of Balint's syndrome (simultanagnosia, "psychic paralysis of gaze," and abnormalities in visually directed reaching) made it very likely, however, that the lesion in the parieto-occipital region was bilateral, although clearly larger on the left side. In addition, I can state from my examination of the patient that she had alexia without agraphia, a syndrome due to a lesion in the left occipital cortex that extends into the splenium of the corpus callosum.

At this point we should review the neuroradiologic studies.

DR. KENNETH R. DAVIS: The plain CT scan obtained three days before admission to this hospital (Fig. 1) shows bilateral cerebellar low-absorptive abnormalities with a mass effect compressing the fourth ventricle from each side. Bilateral parieto-occipital low-absorptive abnormalities are also evident. The CT scan obtained on the first hospital day shows lower absorptive cerebellar abnormalities and an increase in the mass effect and ventricular size. On the CT scan performed on the fourth hospital day edema from the infarcts is evident. The hydrocephalus had decreased slightly. No extension of the infarction into the thalamus or posterior limb of the internal capsule is seen.

DR. SAMUELS: The third question concerns the nature of the cerebrovascular disease that caused this stroke. A stroke in a young woman always poses a perplexing problem for the neurologist. The precise cause is seldom established. The possibilities include emboli from a cardiac source, thrombosis in situ, and unusual cerebrovascular diseases such as fibromuscular hyperplasia and complex migraine. Furthermore, there is epidemiologic evidence that such events are more frequent in persons who use oral contraceptive agents, particularly those with a history of migraine.[1] Since a cerebral angiographic study was not performed in this case we cannot say that every stone had been turned, but even with an angiographic examination the precise vascular cause of such a stroke can seldom be determined with certainty. Furthermore, the risk of an angiographic study in this patient was probably higher than average because the stroke involved the basilar territory, requiring a more dangerous angiographic study, and may have been due to abnormal vascular reactivity, a process that can be worsened by the infusion of contrast material.

In this patient the most likely possibilities include a cardiac source, top-of-the-basilar embolism, and so-called complex migraine with thrombosis in situ at the top of the basilar artery. Thrombosis in situ at the top of the basilar artery is improbable in view of the involvement of the superior cerebellar artery and the distal posterior cerebellar artery combined with relative sparing of the interposed precommunicating segment of the posterior cerebral artery. The absence of a prior history of migraine and the severity of the cerebellar infarction make the diagnosis of complex migraine very unlikely. I cannot choose among these three major possibilities with the available data. The occurrence of headache and nausea at the onset is consistent with any posterior-fossa stroke or with migraine. On the basis of the ultimate hypothesis of catecholamine toxicity all three of these major vascular disorders—embolism of cardiac origin, thrombosis in situ, and migraine—are possibly exacerbated by excessively high circulating catecholamine levels.

A fourth question confronted the treating physicians. What was the nature of the cardiopulmonary disease? This patient was given a volume of fluids to treat her dehydration and hypotension and rapidly went into congestive heart failure. Hemodynamic data from a Swan-Ganz catheter were obtained before the administration of diuretic therapy; the rightsided pressures were elevated and the pulmonary-capillary wedge pressure was 20 mm Hg, clearly elevated but not high enough to explain the pulmonary edema. There was, therefore, a combination of cardiogenic and noncardiogenic pulmonary edema. An echocardiographic study demonstrated evidence of a dilated cardiomyopathy. The marked elevation of the enzyme levels (CK of 17,348 U, SGOT of 608 U, and LDH of 4521 U per liter) was not of cardiac origin and almost certainly reflected muscle necrosis secondary to the prolonged period of immobility at home before admission. A right ventricular endomyocardial biopsy performed later showed multifocal myocyte necrosis. At this point it would be worthwhile to have the pathologist show us the results of this biopsy.

Dr. James F. Southern: Marked vacuolization of some of the myocardial cells was evident, and some of the nuclei were enlarged and contained nucleoli (Fig. 2). Many of the myocytes were smudgy and degenerated. There was no interstitial inflammation. A modified trichrome stain showed that many of the myocytes, particularly those in a perivascular distribution, had a muddy, purple appearance (Fig. 3). These degenerated myocytes were present around vessels and just under the endocardium. Examination of tissue embedded into plastic showed marked degeneration of myocytes with considerable lipid accumulation, prominent dark-staining mitochondria containing increased iron and calcium, and loss of the contractile mechanism (Fig. 4). No contraction bands were present either within the necrotic cells or as normal artifacts within the viable-appearing myocytes. Such artifacts are seen in most normal myocardial-biopsy specimens.

Dr. Samuels: This type of cardiopulmonary problem is important in both the theory and the practice of neurocardiology. The effects of the nervous system on the "lower" organs have been known for a long time and are encompassed in the general field of psychosomatic or psychophysiologic medicine. The relation between the nervous system and the heart has been particularly thoroughly studied, probably because of the availability of the electrocardiogram as a noninvasive tool for the recognition of cardiac abnormalities seen in the context of neurologic illness. To summarize a large literature briefly, electrocardiographic abnormalities, largely in the form of repolarization changes, are seen in patients with a wide array of neurologic catastrophes.[2] Approximately a quarter of patients with neurologically induced electrocardiographic

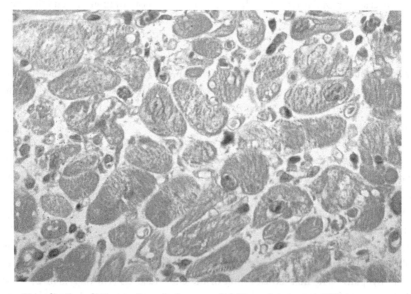

FIG 2 Vacuolization of Myocytes in an Endomyocardial-Biopsy Specimen (×300).

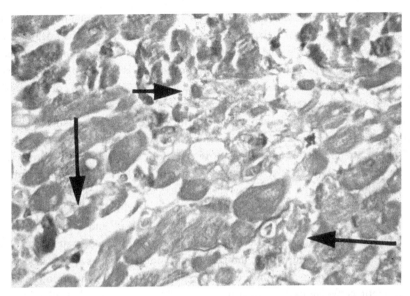

FIG 3 SMUDGY, GRAY–BLUE NECROTIC MYOCYTES (ARROWS) (MASSON'S TRICHROME STAIN, ×220).

changes also have elevation of myocardial enzymes in the peripheral blood, indicating that cardiac damage may occur in this circumstance.[3] In patients who die in this state a characteristic cardiac lesion can be found, known variously as contraction-band necrosis, coagulative myocytolysis, or myofibrillar degeneration. This lesion, which cannot be diagnosed on an endomyocardial biopsy since the procedure itself produces contraction bands as an artifact, is found in four broad categories of circumstances—catecholamine infusion, stress, nervous-system stimulation, and reperfusion.[4]

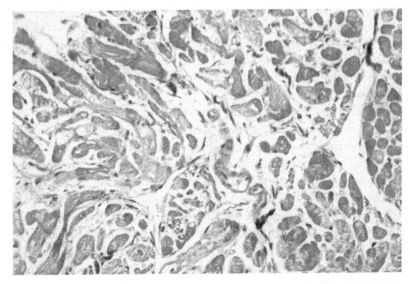

FIG 4 Large Lipid Droplets and Mitochondrial Iron and Calcium Aggregates (Small Granules) (Plastic-Embedded 1-μm Section, ×450).

It has been known at least since 1907 that elevation of catecholamine levels can cause a cardiomyopathy.[5] It has now been established that this disorder can be either a hypertrophic or a dilated cardiomyopathy, probably depending on whether there is chronic hypertension, and that this condition is at least partially reversible.[6] An identical cardiac lesion can be produced by various forms of stress, the effect of which is exacerbated by the concomitant use of certain steroids, but the lesion can also occur spontaneously in extremely stressful circumstances without the administration of steroids.[7,8] This lesion is very arrhythmogenic and may contribute to a tendency for sudden death in stressful circumstances.[9] Examples are death after a vicious attack,[10] death during panic attacks,[11] death during natural catastrophes such as the 1981 Athens earthquake,[12,13] death among racehorses[14] and other domestic[15] and wild animals,[16] death during delirium tremens, the sudden unexpected nocturnal death syndrome, death from asthma,[17] and "voodoo" death.[18] An identical lesion can be produced by stimulation of the nervous system along the outflow tract of the sympathetic limb of the autonomic nervous system anywhere from the amygdala down to the stellate ganglion.[19,20] Autostimulation in the form of epileptic convulsions probably can produce this lesion, possibly explaining the cardiac arrhythmias seen in some patients with complex partial seizures[21] and the increased risk of sudden death in epileptic patients.[22,23] The same lesion is seen in hearts reperfused after periods of ischemia,[24] such as in the areas around myocardial infarction after angioplasty, or after periods on the cardiopulmonary-bypass pump.[25]

A unifying hypothesis can be constructed (Fig. 5) arguing that the final common pathway for all these circumstances involves calcium entry into the cardiac cell, an event that can be mediated by catecholamine action on a receptor-operated calcium channel.[17] Calcium entry may in its own right be toxic to the cell causing the myocyte necrosis,[26] or there may be damage by oxygen free radicals caused by ischemia and reperfusion or by the effects of the metabolism of excessive amounts of catecholamines through toxic intermediates such as adrenochrome.[27,28] Whatever the precise mechanism, it is clear that the nervous system through its innervation of the heart can produce a cardiac lesion that is consistent with the lesion found on the endomyocardial biopsy in this patient.

Furthermore, it is known that the sympathetic nervous system innervates the pulmonary vasculature in a way analogous to its innervation of the heart. Stimulation of the sympathetic limb of the autonomic nervous system probably results in opening of the tight junctions in pulmonary capillaries, leading to the transudation of a high-protein pulmonary-edema fluid. This occurrence results in the production of an exudative alveolar pulmonary edema that is due not to cardiac failure but rather to a direct effect on the pulmonary vasculature by the sympathetic nerves. This effect is probably mediated by the release of neurotransmitters in the catecholamine class, which act to increase the pore size in the pulmonary capillaries and probably also to increase pulmonary-capillary hydrostatic pressure by mediating venoconstriction. This mechanism probably accounts for the so-called neurogenic pulmonary edema that occurs in the context of many neurologic catastrophes.[29]

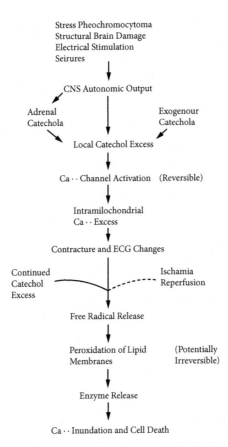

FIG 5 Pathogenetic Scheme for the Development of Neurogenic Cardiac Damage (Reprinted with Permission).[17]

Thus, it is probable that this patient had an at least partially reversible catecholamine cardiomyopathy on which was superimposed an acute event, possibly due to hemorrhage into the catecholamine-producing tumor. This acute event caused a catecholamine "storm," which led to a mixture of cardiac and noncardiac pulmonary edema and was associated in some way with the top-of-the-basilar-artery syndrome, because an embolus arose from the dilated myopathic heart, because the excessive catecholamines resulted in platelet aggregation and thrombosis in situ at the top of the basilar artery, because elevated catecholamine levels resulted in a vasospastic response at the top of the basilar artery loosely known as migraine, or because there was a period of hypotension after the hemorrhage into the tumor that resulted in a border-zone stroke in the terminal arterial territories of the basilar artery.

Could the stroke itself have resulted in the production of enough catecholamines to explain the urinary catecholamine data in this case? It is known that stroke can cause elevated catecholamine levels for several days.[30] However, this patient's vanilmandelic acid (VMA) level rose after admission, with the highest level recorded on the last collection (Table 1). This occurrence would be highly atypical for the pattern of elevation of catecholamines seen after a stroke, in which the levels fall rapidly from the time of admission to normal ranges within a few days. Furthermore, the dilated cardiomyopathy presumably took some time to develop and thus could not have been due exclusively to catecholamine elevation related to the stroke alone. In other words, it may be true that some of the elevation in the catecholamine values noted in this patient was due to the stress of the stroke itself, but the entire syndrome cannot be explained on this basis alone.

What was the relation of the patient's use of cocaine to the development of this problem? Since cocaine is a catecholamine re-uptake inhibitor similar in this respect to the tricyclic antidepressant drugs, it theoretically could have exacerbated the effects of catecholamines[31,32] and as such could have made an otherwise asymptomatic pheochromocytoma become evident. There is, of course, no direct way of proving this hypothesis, but it is likely that the use of cocaine exacerbated the effect of what otherwise might have been a relatively silent tumor.

The last major question that we faced in the care of this patient concerned the nature of the large adrenal mass. Obviously, given the clinical context, everyone agreed that the mass must be removed on the assumption that it was a pheochromocytoma. Any preoperative speculation about the nature of the tumor was therefore only academic. There was, however, some disagreement as to the nature of this tumor. Many observers thought that the slightly elevated urinary catecholamine levels were not characteristic of a pheochromocytoma and that the tumor would be found to be an incidental adenoma or lipoma. Dr. Godine and Dr. Lewis Landsberg, however, believed that the tumor would prove to be a pheochromocytoma, arguing that the relatively slight elevation of the catecholamine levels reflected either internal metabolism of most of the catecholamines by the tumor or partial destruction of the tumor by hemorrhage, the event that presumably caused the catecholamine "storm" that led to the acute cardiopulmonary disorder and indirectly the neurologic ictus. Certainly, an underlying pheochromocytoma, perhaps unmasked by the use of cocaine, could have produced this patient's cardiopulmonary picture on the basis of catecholamine toxicity[33-35] and thus was believed to be the most parsimonious explanation. Under Dr. Godine's careful supervision the patient was treated preoperatively with alpha- and beta-receptor blockers and underwent a successful removal of the adrenal mass.

My final diagnoses are a top-of-the-basilar-artery embolus of cardiac origin, catecholamine cardiomyopathy, and adrenal pheochromocytoma.

CLINICAL DIAGNOSES

Embolic stroke, of cardiac origin.
Catecholamine cardiomyopathy.
Pheochromocytoma of adrenal gland.

DR. MARTIN A. SAMUELS' DIAGNOSES

Top-of-the-basilar-artery embolus of cardiac origin.
Catecholamine cardiomyopathy. Pheochromocytoma of adrenal gland.

PATHOLOGICAL DISCUSSION

DR. SOUTHERN: The surgeons explored the patient using a right posterior transpleural approach. They found an adrenal mass, 8 by 6 by 6 cm, the surface of which appeared to be covered by normal adrenal cortex. The patient's blood pressure rose substantially while the medial aspect of the tumor was being manipulated, and the intravenous administration of nitroprusside was used for blood-pressure control. The mass was removed with little difficulty.

Sectioning of the specimen showed a rim of adrenal cortex, subcortical fibrous tissue, and a large, granular, irregular central mass with areas of hemorrhage and yellow discoloration (Fig. 6). Microscopical examination revealed nests of large polygonal cells with granular, amphophilic cytoplasm that contained occasional eosinophilic globules and open, uniform nuclei, without mitotic activity (Fig. 7). There were extensive areas of fibrosis. Focal old hemorrhage and recent hemorrhage with organization were also observed. The diagnosis is a pheochromocytoma that had undergone extensive hemorrhagic infarction.

A number of pheochromocytomas have presented clinically with hypotension or even sudden death, especially in children.[36–42] This type of presentation may occur after only relatively minor abdominal trauma.[38,43] A similar event appears to have occurred in this case — that is, hemorrhage into a pheochromocytoma, an ensuing adrenal medullary "storm," and widespread myocardial necrosis due to an excess of

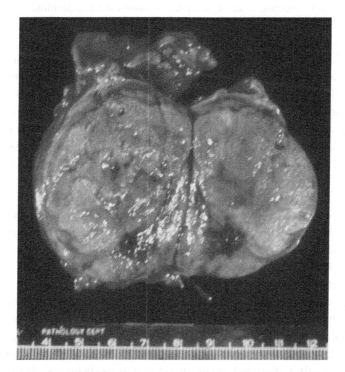

FIG 6 Sectioned Surfaces of the Pheochromocytoma, with Necrosis and Hemorrhage.
A rim of normal adrenal cortex can be seen above the tumor

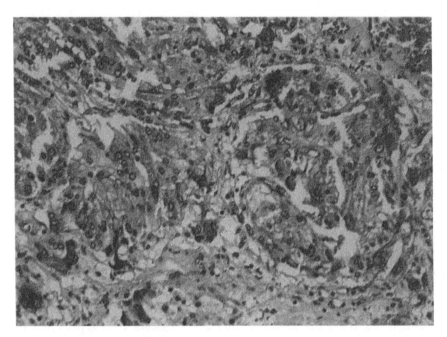

FIG 7   Nests of Tumor Cells, Some of Which Contain Hyaline Droplets (×90).

catecholamines, resulting in acute heart failure with cardiac dilatation. The episode of hyperamylasemia also may have been due to the action of catecholamines released from the adrenal tumor on the pancreatic vascular bed.[44]

The effects of both endogenous and exogenous catecholamines on the myocardium have been reviewed extensively.[45,46] The designation "toxic myocarditis" has been used in many references on the subject.[6,45,46] Similarly, a diagnosis of myositis has been made on examination of catechol-induced ischemic changes in skeletal muscle.[47] However, since the inflammation seen is in response to the myocyte necrosis[48] those designations should be avoided. Many reports of pheochromocytoma-induced cardiomyopathy note that the physiologic effects are reversible after removal of the tumor.[6,37,49–52]

Contraction-band necrosis is commonly accepted as the characteristic histologic feature of catechol toxicity.[4,45,46] Contraction bands may be seen in the acute period after myocardial infarction, during severe stress reactions, and after the administration of catecholamines or sympathomimetic agents, including cocaine,[46,53] but the contraction bands disappear progressively thereafter. The endomyocardial biopsy in this patient was performed between five and seven days after her crisis, and no contraction bands were present in the necrotic cells. Of interest was the absence of contraction bands in the viable myocytes as well, since contraction bands are a normal biopsy artifact.[54] The absence of contraction bands in both the viable and the necrotic myocytes may have been due to the chronic effects of catecholamines, decreasing the density and down-regulating the sensitivity of adrenergic receptors in tissues.[55–57] These effects may also have been responsible for the patient's premorbid normotensive state.[50] The presence of myocyte necrosis in the myocardium immediately under the endocardium seen in this case is not found in lesions caused by cardiac arrest on an ischemic basis. The only other situation in which I have seen this distribution of necrosis is in biopsy specimens obtained within several days after cardiac transplantation, during which both total cessation of flow in intracardiac vessels and absence of diffusion of oxygen from intraluminal blood occur. For that reason we concluded that the subendocardial necrosis could not be explained on the basis of simple cardiac arrest. We interpreted the histologic changes in the biopsy specimen as due to catecholamine excess, with the differential diagnosis including pheochromocytoma, the administration of sympatho-mimetic agents, and thyrotoxicosis.

I wonder if the brain lesions might have been due to cerebral-artery spasm, since vascular spasm in peripheral, coronary, and cerebral arteries has been induced with sympathomimetic agents, either intentionally as in the treatment of epistaxis or as an unintended complication of use of these agents.[53] Spasm could have caused either transient impairment of circulation[58] or infarcts. Also, shock may have had an effect on the watershed regions of the cerebral circulation, especially if catechol-induced vaso-spasm was present concurrently. This controversy must remain moot, since no histo-logic or radiologic evidence favoring any of these mechanisms is available.

Dr. Mandel E. Cohen: I have a question about death as a result of panic or anxiety attacks. We have studied several hundred patients with anxiety or panic attacks with-out any deaths. Also, in a 20-year followup study, done with Dr. Edwin O. Wheeler and others at this hospital in 1950, deaths in patients with these attacks were less than the expected number in various control groups.[59] On the basis of our data I tell my patients that anxiety-panic states will not kill them, will not give them heart trouble, and will not lead to the so-called psychosomatic diseases.

Dr. Samuels: A couple of studies have suggested an excessive mortality rate from cardiovascular causes among patients with anxiety disorders.[11] It is true that the num-ber of patients is small, and I consider the association between panic attacks and sud-den death only tentative.

Dr. Godine, do you wish to comment?

Dr. John E. Godine: There was a difference of opinion about the nature of the adre-nal mass but uniform agreement that the patient should be prepared for operation with recognition of the possibility that the tumor would prove to be a pheochromo-cytoma. She was treated with phenoxybenzamine and subsequently, because of tachy-cardia, with propranolol.

This patient had no history of paroxysmal symptoms and no documented hyperten-sion either before admission or while in the hospital awaiting the operation. She did report excessive sweating with minor provocation over at least 10 years. When Dr. Ashby C. Moncure manipulated the medial side of the tumor in the operating room, the patient became acutely hypertensive despite the blockade with alpha- and beta-receptors.

Dr. Scully: Dr. Palacios, do you have any comments?

Dr. Igor F. Palacios: This patient presented us with an interesting differential diagnosis of a dilated cardiomyopathy. Although the endomyocardial biopsy demon-strated areas of myocyte necrosis, the diagnosis of acute myocarditis was ruled out by the absence of a cellular infiltrate surrounding the necrotic myocytes. The areas of myocyte necrosis were compatible with a disease that could result in high levels of circulating catecholamines, such as a pheochromocytoma. A more difficult question to answer is whether the dilated cardiomyopathy was of recent onset or was chronic. I believe that it was acute in view of the absence in the specimen of chronic changes such as interstitial fibrosis and myocyte hypertrophy. Furthermore, the ventricular dysfunction was only transient. A repeated echocardiographic study performed before the operation demonstrated normal size and function of both ventricles and no evidence of cardiac hypertrophy. She recently underwent a gated blood-pool scan, which showed normal motion of the left ventricular wall and normal right and left ventricular function.

ANATOMICAL DIAGNOSES

Pheochromocytoma of left adrenal gland, with hemorrhagic infarction.
  Catecholamine-induced dilated cardiomyopathy.

ADDENDUM

DR. GODINE: When seen four months after the operation the patient still had a right homonymous field defect but had noticed gradual improvement in some aspects of cognitive function — e.g., mathematical ability. She reported a reduction in her long-standing sweating. The results of repeated assays of urine for catecholamines have been normal.

REFERENCES

1. Collaborative Group for the Study of Stroke in Young Women. Oral contraceptives and stroke in young women: associated risk factors. JAMA 1975; 231:718–22.
2. Samuels MA. Electrocardiographic manifestations of neurologic disease. Semin Neurol 1984; 4:91–9.
3. Dimant J, Grob D. Electrocardiographic changes and myocardial damage in patients with acute cerebrovascular accidents. Stroke 1977; 8:448–55.
4. Karch SB, Billingham ME. Myocardial contraction bands revisited. Hum Pathol 1986; 17:9–13.
5. Josué O. Hypertrophic cardiaque causée par l'adrénaline et la toxine typhique. C R Soc Biol (Paris) 1907; 63:285–6.
6. Imperato-McGinkey J, Gautier T, Ehlers K, Zallo MA, Goldstein DS, Vaughan ED Jr. Reversibility of catecholamine-induced dilated cardiomyopathy in a child with a pheochromocytoma. N Eagl J Med 1987; 316:793–7.
7. Selye H. The chemical prevention of cardiac necroses. New York: Ronald Press, 1958.
8. Meerson FZ. Pathogenesis and prophylaxis of cardiac lesions in stress. Adv Myocardiol 1983; 4:3–21.
9. DeSilva RA. Central nervous system risk factors for sudden cardiac death. Ann NY Acad Sci 1982; 382:143–61.

10. Cebelin MS, Hirach CS. Human stress cardiomyopathy. Hum Pathol 1980; 11:123–32.

11. Coryell W, Noyes R Jr, House JD. Mortality among outpatients with anxiety disorders. Am J Psychiatry 1986; 143:508–10.

12. Trichopoulos D, Katsouyanni K, Zavitsanos X, Tzonou A, Dalla-Vorgia P. Psychological stress and fatal heart attack: the Athens (1981) earthquake natural experiment. Lancet 1983; 1:441–3.

13. Voridis EM, Mallios KD, Papantonis TM. Hober monitoring during 1981 Athens earthquakes. Lancet 1983; 1:1281–2.

14. Gelberg HB, Zachary JF, Everia JI, Jensen RC, Smetzer DL. Sudden death in training and racing thoroughbred horses. J Am Vet Med Assoc 1985; 187:1354–6.

15. King JM, Roth L, Haschek WM. Myocardial necrosis secondary to neural lesions in domestic animals. J Am Vet Med Assoc 1982; 180:144–8.

16. Richter CP. On the phenomenon of sudden death in animals and man. Psychosom Med 1957; 19:191–8.

17. Drislane FW, Samuels MA, Kozakewich H, Schoen FJ, Strunk RC. Myocardial contraction band lesions in patients with fatal asthma: possible neurocardiologic mechanisms. Am Rev Respir Dis 1987; 135:498–501.

18. Cannon WB. "Voodoo" death. Psychosom Med 1957; 19:182–90.

19. Porter RW, Kamikawa K, Greenhoot JH. Persistent electrocardiographic abnormalities experimentally induced by stimulation of the brain. Am Heart J 1962; 64:815–9.

20. Klouda MA, Brynjolfsson G. Cardiotoxic effects of electrical stimulation of the stellate ganglia. Ann NY Acad Sci 1969; 156:271–80.

21. Blumhardt LD, Smith PEM, Owen L. Electrocardiographic accompaniments of temporal lobe epileptic seizures. Lancet 1986; 1:1051–5.

22. Jay GW, Leestma JE. Sudden death in epilepsy: a comprehensive review of the literature and proposed mechanisms. Acta Neurol Scand [Suppl] 1981; 82:1–66.

23. Leestma JE, Kalelkar MB, Teas SS, Jsy GW, Hughes JR. Sudden unexpected death associated with seizures: analysis of 66 cases. Epilepsia 1984; 25:84–8.

24. Braunwald E, Kloner RA. Myocardial reperfusion: A double-edged sword? J Clin Invest 1985; 76:1713–9.

25. Schoen FJ, Bernhard WF, Khuri SF, Koster JK Jr, Van Devanter SJ, Weintraub RM. Pathologic findings in postcardiotomy patients managed with a temporary left ventricular assist pump. Am J Surg 1982; 143:508–14.

26. Dhalla NS, Pierce GN, Panagia V, Singal PK, Beamish RE. Calcium movements in relation to heart function. Basic Res Cardiol 1982; 77:117–39.

27. Singal PK, Kapur N, Dhillon KS, Beamish RE, Dhalla NS. Role of free radicals in catecholamine-induced cardiomyopathy. Can J Physiol Pharmacol 1982; 60:1390–7.

28. Rona G. Catecholamine cardiotoxicity. J Mol Cell Cardiol 1985; 17:291–306.

29. Malik AB. Mechanisms of neurogenic pulmonary edema. Circ Res 1985; 57:1–18.

30. Myers MG, Norris JW, Hachinski VC, Sole MJ. Plasma sorepinephrine in stroke. Stroke 1981; 12:200–4.

31. Masuda Y, Matsuda Y, Levy MN. The effects of cocaine and metanephrine on the cardiac responses to norepinephrine infusions. J Pharmacol Exp Ther 1980; 215:20–7.

32. Matsuda Y, Masuda Y, Levy MN. The effects of cocaine and metanephrine on the cardiac responses to sympathetic nerve stimulation in dogs. Circ Res 1979; 45:180–7.

33. Kline IK. Myocardial alterations associated with pheochromocytomas. Am J Pathol 1961; 38:539–51.

34. Van Vliet PD, Burchell HB, Titus JL. Focal myocarditis associated with pheochromocytoma. N Engl J Med 1966; 274:1102–8.

35. Reichenbach DD, Benditt EP. Catecholamines and cardiomyopathy: the pathogenesis and potential importance of myobbrillar degeneration. Hum Pathol 1970; 1:125–50.

36. Stenström G, Waldenström J. Positive correlation between urinary excretion of catecholamine metabolites and tumour mass in pheochromocytoma: results in patients with sustained and paroxysmal hypertension and multiple endocrine neoplasia. Acta Med Scand 1985; 217:73–7.

37. Shaw TR, Rafferty P, Tait GW. Transient shock and myocardial impairment caused by phaeochromocytoma crisis. Br Heart J 1987; 57:194–8.

38. Andersen PT, Basdsgaard SE, Larsen BP. Repetitive bleeding from a pheochromocytoma presenting as an abdominal emergency: case report. Acta Chir Scand 1986; 152:69–70.

39. Buist RJ. Phaeochromocytoma presenting as an acute abdomen. Br Med J 1985; 291:1724–5.

40. Friedman E, Mandel M, Kattnelson D, Sack J. Pheochromocytoms and hydralazine-induced myocardial ischaemia in a 14-year-old boy. Eur J Pediatr 1986; 145:318–20.

41. Ciobotaru M, Eisenman A, Veisler A, Freud M. Pheochromocytoma of the organ of Zuckerkandl presenting as shock. 1st J Med Sci 1985; 21:517–9.

42. Lamberts SWJ, Bruining HA, Alexiev T, van Essen LH, DeGreef WJ, Oosterom R. "Hypotension" as a presenting symptom in fatal and near-fatal pure adrenaline-secreting phaeochromocytomas. Neth J Med 1984; 27:385–8.

43. Primhak RA, Spicer RD, Variend S. Sudden death after minor abdominal trauma: an unusual presentation of phaeochromocytoma. Br Med J 1986; 292:95–6.

44. Yamanishi J, Nishikawa M, Obomori Y, Furuta Y, Pukuzaki H. Phaeochromocytoma with transient hyperamylasaemia during hypertensive crisis. Br Med J 1985; 291:1171.

45. McAllister HA Jr. Endocrine diseases and the cardiovascular system. In: Silver MD, ed. Cardiovascular pathology. New York: Churchill Livingstone, 1983:1035–57.

46. Fenoglio JJ Jr. The effects of drugs on the cardiovascular system. In: Silver MD, ed. Cardiovascular pathology. New York: Churchill Livingstone. 1983:1085–107.

47. Bhatnagar D, Carey P, Pollard A. Focal myositis and elevated creatine kinase levels in a patient with phacochromocytoma. Postgrad Med J 1986; 62:197–8.

48. Bloom S. Catecholamine cardiomyopathy. N Engl J Med 1987; 317:900.

49. Cho T, Tanimura A, Saito Y. Catecholamine-induced cardiopathy accompanied with pheochromocytoma. Acta Pathol Jpn 1987; 37:123–32.

50. Kanemoto N. Imaoka C. Hiramatzu K. Goto Y. A case of normotensive pheochromocytoma masquerading as a dilated cardiomyopathy. Jpn Circ J 1986; 50:1128–32.

51. Stenström G, Holmberg S. Cardiomyopathy in phaeochromocytoma: report of a case with a 16-year follow-up after surgery and review of the literature. Eur Heart J 1985; 6:539–44.

52. Lam JB, Shub C, Sheps SG. Reversible dilatation of hypertrophied left ventricle in pheochromocytoma: serial two-dimensional echocardiographic observations. Am Heart J 1985; 109:613–5.

53. Isner JM, Estes NAM III, Thompson PD, et al. Acute cardiac events temporally related to cocaine abuse. N Engl J Med 1986; 315:1438–43.

54. Fenoglio JJ Jr, ed. Endomyocardial biopsy: techniques and applications. Boca Raton, Fla.: CRC Press. 1982:33–44.

55. Tsujimoto G, Hashimoto K, Hoffman BB. Effects of pheochromocytoma on cardiovascular alpha adrenergic receptor system. Heart Vessels 1985; 1:152–7.

56. Jones CR, Hamilton CA, Whyte KF, Elliott HL, Reid JL. Acute and chronic regulation of alpha 2-adrenoceptor number and function in man. Clin Sci 1985; 68:Suppl 10:129S–132S.

57. Tsujimoto G, Honda K, Hoffman BB, Hashimoto K. Desensitization of postjunctional alpha 1- and alpha 2-adrenergic receptor-mediated vasopressor responses in rat harboring pheochromocytoma. Circ Res 1987; 61:86–98.

58. White PD, Lishman WA, Wyke MA. Phaeochromocytoma as a cause of reversible dementia. J Neurol Neurosurg Psychistry 1986; 49:1449–51.

59. Wheeler EO, White PD, Reed EW, Cohen ME. Neurocirculatory asthenia (anxiety neurosis, effort syndrome, neurasthenia): a twenty year follow-up study of one hundred and seventy-three patients. JAMA 1950; 142:878–89.

Massachusetts General Hospital wishes to acknowledge the generous support of the following sponsors in making possible the continued preparation of the Case Records:

E. R. Squibb & Sons, U.S., and the Squibb Science and Technology Group
The Upjohn Company

Perspectives and Updates

This is one of the most unusual of all of the Cabot Cases, as I was both one of the treating physicians and the discusser. It had been traditional in the Cabot Case series for the patient's problem to be a mystery for the guest discusser. However, the problems raised in this patient's illness (issues in neurocardiology) were in my own field of expertise, and it was decided by the CPC team (Robert Scully, the editor, Eugene Mark and William F. McNeely, associate editors, and Betty U. McNeely, the assistant editor) that an exception would be made. Of course when I was helping to care for the patient I did not know the ultimate diagnosis, but by the time of my CPC discussion, I knew the results of all of the investigations and the patient's clinical state. This model was later expanded in the *New England Journal of Medicine* in a series of clinical decision-making exercises, which remain quite popular in the current iteration of the journal.

Over the 23 years since my discussion of this case, I have remained very interested in neurovisceral disease and would now make slightly different observations about this patient's condition, though the main lessons remain the same. The two major issues to be reconsidered in light of new information are the etiology of the cerebral ischemic event in the distribution of the posterior circulation of the brain and the nature and cause of the dilated cardiomyopathy.

In the CPC discussion I say unequivocally that the event was a stroke and postulate a cardiac source embolism to the top of the basilar artery. In retrospect I wonder how I could have been so certain. That sort of hubris has been softened considerably with the passing of time; perhaps one of the few advantages of aging. A stroke caused by an embolism arising in the dilated left ventricle remains a possibility, but two other considerations would now be entertained. One is the possibility of a reversible cerebral vasoconstriction syndrome (RCVS), the Call-Fleming syndrome. It is now recognized that RCVS is associated with exposure to stimulants (cocaine and catecholamines from a pheochromocytoma are two such possibilities). RCVS is a spectrum from a probably asymptomatic vasospastic state, through a severe and sudden "thunderclap" headache, to cerebral infarction and cerebral and subarachnoid hemorrhage. Patients are usually treated with calcium channel blockers and many do well, but certainly cerebral infarction and subarachnoid hemorrhages can be the outcome in severe cases.

A second possibility would be cerebral autoregulatory dysfunction, often noted clinically and by imaging techniques to be predominantly in the white matter of the posterior portions of the brain, hence the popular term "reversible posterior leukoencephalopthy" (RPLE). As the syndrome has expanded, it has become clear that it may not be restricted to the posterior circulation, may involve both white and gray matter, and may not be reversible. A newer term, "posterior reversible encephalopathy syndrome" (PRES), attempts to address some of these concerns. Posterior predominance is not required; however, it is the most common pattern. Though the finding can sometimes be appreciated by CT scanning, MRI is much more sensitive, accounting for increased recognition of the syndrome in many clinical contexts since the MRI era began.

The underlying pathogenesis probably involves dysfunction of the endothelial cells that constitute the blood-brain barrier. The endothelial damage can be barotrauma, toxic or immune-mediated. The posterior predominance may simply reflect the fact that the anterior circulation has a backup vascular regulatory system (the sympathetic nervous system) whereas the posterior circulation does not, leaving it more vulnerable to the syndrome. Many formerly separate syndromes are probably explained by this mechanism, including hypertensive encephalopathy, toxemia of pregnancy, and related disorders such as hemolysis with elevated liver function tests and low platelets (HELLP), thrombotic thrombocytopenic purpura (TTP), hemolytic uremic syndrome (HUS), and calcineurin (e.g., cyclosporine, tacrolimus) toxicity. The syndrome of post–carotid endarterectomy hemisphere swelling may be a unilateral form of an identical pathogenesis whereby barotraumas caused by the restitution of normal blood flow to a chronically low-pressure circulation can force water through the endothelial tight junctions (the blood-brain barrier). Though this condition is potentially reversible, there is no doubt that some patients suffer permanent ischemic strokes and/or hemorrhages, usually in the posterior portions of the brain, including the cerebellum. Complications of brain swelling may also occur. In retrospect, this patient could have suffered from severe PRES caused by the catecholamine storm of a pheochromocytoma combined with cocaine exposure.

With regard to the cardiac disease, in retrospect this patient may well have had the takotsubo-type cardiomyopathy, so named in 1990 by Sato and colleagues in Japan because of the appearance of the heart by echocardiography and/or ventriculography, which simulates the shape of the Japanese octopus-trapping pot, the *takotsubo*. This group of disorders (also known as left ventricular apical ballooning, cardiac stunning, and broken heart syndrome) has been increasingly recognized because of the widespread use of echocardiography. Three major theories of its pathogenesis have vied for prominence: coronary vasospasm, myocarditis, and direct catecholamine cardiotoxicity. Data from many sources strongly favor catecholamine toxicity as the inciting factor, which may secondarily cause neurogenic inflammation (myocarditis) and coronary vasospasm. The characteristic takotsubo shape is caused by the distribution of β1 and 2 receptors in the heart. When the predominant catecholamine is norepinephrine (as would occur when psychological stress or a central nervous system lesion has led to the release of norepinephrine by sympathetic nerve terminals into the heart), the left ventricular apex dilates, and the base contracts, producing the characteristic shape. However, when the dominant catechoamine is epinephrine (as would occur with cocaine use or pheochromocytoma), the reverse may occur, producing the so-called inverted takotsubo. Combinations of the two mechanisms—as would have occurred in this case (cocaine, pheochromocytoma, and stroke)—can produce various shapes of the left ventricle, including regional wall motion abnormalities and global hypokinesis. The vast majority of patients with takotsubo-type cardiomyopathy are women; they generally recover completely, as did this patient. Most spontaneous cases occur in much older women, but the pheochromocytoma combined with cocaine use produces the perfect storm for this type of cardiac process to develop. The fact that this process completely disappeared on follow-up echocardiography after the pheochromocytoma was removed supports the hypothesis that it was, in fact, the mechanism of the dilated cardiomyopathy in this patient. Though most patients with takotsubo-type cardiomyopathy recover completely, some suffer complications, which include embolism from the transiently dysfunctional left ventricle, left ventricular free wall rupture, and potentially lethal cardiac arrhythmias because of affection of the cardiac conducting system by this predominantly subendocardial catecholamine-mediated process. The catecholamines probably act on a receptor-operated calcium channel, which in turn produces profound changes in the electrocardiogram (i.e., cerebral T waves). Calcium-activated oxygen free radical damage may then ensue, resulting in cardiac necrosis marked by cardiac enzyme release.

Thus, with the view through the retrospectoscope, I would now say that this patient, because of a pheochromocytoma and the use of cocaine, developed a catecholamine-induced dilated cardiomyopathy, which may indeed have generated an embolism to the top of the basilar artery. However, it is also possible that the brain disease was an independent effect of the catecholamine toxicity, either via the mechanism of cerebrovascular spasm or by producing an endothelial disorder of cerebral vessels (i.e., PRES), with a consequent stroke. This case was a landmark one in that it foreshadowed three new syndromes: takotsubo-type cardiomyopathy, posterior reversible encephalopathy syndrome, and reversible cerebral vasoconstriction syndrome. It also served an important pedagogical function by using the CPC format in a new way by working through the case in the order in which the clinicians actually did their work, rather than facing it as an unknown.

In any case, all's well that ends well. The pheochromocytoma was successfully removed and the patient improved.[1,2,3,4]

Martin A. Samuels

REFERENCES

1. Samuels MA. The brain-heart connection. Circulation 2007; 116:77–84.
2. Sato H., Tateishi H, Uchida T. Takotsubo-type left ventricular dysfunction due to mulitivessel coronary spasm. In: Kodama K, Haze K, Hori M, eds. Clinical aspects of myocardial injury: from ischemia to heart failure. Tokyo, Japan: Kagakuhyoronsha Publishing; 1990:56–64.
3. Call GK, Fleming MC, Sealfon S, Levine H, Kistler JP, Fisher CM. Reversible cerebral segmental vasoconstriction. Stroke 1988; 19:1159–70.
4. Singhal AB, Hajj-Ali RA, Topcuoglu MA, Fok J, Bena J, Yang D, Calabrese LH. Reversible cerebral vasoconstriction syndromes: analysis of 139 cases. Arch. Neurol 2011; 68:1005–12.

A 35-Year-Old Man with Changed Mental Status and Multiple Intracerebral Lesions

NEUROSYPHILIS

CPC 32-1991

PRESENTATION OF CASE

A 35-year-old man was admitted to the hospital because of the gradual onset of a change in mental status and left-sided neurologic abnormalities.

The patient was well until four or five months earlier, when he began to experience difficulty in finding his way while driving his car over familiar routes. During ensuing months he had increasing problems in carrying out activities that were dependent on previously acquired information and also experienced difficulty in organizing new memories. Two or three weeks before admission he began to have episodes of lightheadedness and became aware of unsteadiness of gait, with inversion of the left foot while walking and a tendency to fall to the left side. Examination by a neurologist showed focal left-sided abnormalities, and a cranial magnetic resonance imaging (MRI) scan was reported to be abnormal. The patient was referred to this hospital.

The patient was right-handed and sold automotive supplies. Several weeks before admission he had experienced an exacerbation of chronic low-back pain, as well as pain in the left shoulder and chest wall that was ascribed by a physician to a "muscle strain." He recalled having mild headaches in recent weeks. He had traveled to Florida on several occasions in the preceding two years and to Spain, Guyana, Venezuela, and the Caribbean area one year before entry: during his trips he was careful to avoid taking local food or water and had little contact with natives. He had gained approximately 9 kg in weight during the two months preceding entry and ascribed the gain to a decrease in physical activity. He had used alcohol and marijuana in past years. His wife, children, and parents were in good health. There was no history of fever, chills, sweats, cough, disease of the ears or paranasal sinuses, recent dental procedures, exposure to tuberculosis, previous skin lesions, ingestion of raw meat, intravenous drug abuse, homosexual activity, sexual promiscuity, or transfusion of blood products. There was no family history of neurologic disease.

The temperature was 37.0°C, the pulse was 76, and the respirations were 18. The blood pressure was 120/70 mm Hg.

On examination the patient appeared well but slightly overweight. No rash or lymphadenopathy was found. The head was normal, with good dentition. The neck was supple: the carotid pulses were full and equal, and no bruits were heard. The lungs, heart, abdomen, extremities, and genitalia were normal.

On neurologic examination the patient was abulic but alert and fully oriented: his speech was fluent, without dysarthria or paraphasic errors: he calculated well, spelled "world" backward, and named two of three common objects after three minutes. Cranial-nerve functions were intact. Motor power was graded 5/5 throughout. Sensation was normal in response to pinprick. Coordination was normal except for inversion of the left foot and impairment of rapid alternating movements of the left hand and foot. The tendon reflexes were + + and equal except that the ankle jerks were +; bilateral Babinski signs were present.

The urine was normal. The hematocrit was 39.9 percent; the white-cell count was 5500, with 53 percent neutrophils, 38 percent lymphocytes, 6 percent monocytes, 2 percent eosinophils, and 1 percent basophils. The mean corpuscular volume (MCV) was 89 μm^3 per cell, the mean corpuscular hemoglobin (MCH) 31.9 pg per red cell, and the mean corpuscular hemoglobin concentration (MCHC) 35.5 percent. The platelet count was 197,000. and the erythrocyte sedimentation rate 15 mm per hour. The prothrombin time was 10.5 seconds, with a control of 10.9 seconds: the partial thromboplastin time was 30.4 seconds. The urea nitrogen was 5.4 mmol per liter (15 mg per 100 ml). The sodium was 143 mmol, the potassium 3.8 mmol, the chloride 106 mmol, and the carbon dioxide 29.7 mmol per liter. An electrocardiogram and an x-ray film of the chest were normal. A cranial MRI scan (Fig. 1) revealed extensive edema of the white matter in the right frontal lobe and in the right-sided deep white-matter tracts, extending into the right temporal lobe, midbrain, and pons: after the intravenous administration of gadolinium there were multiple foci of enhancement adjacent to the basal cisterns, at the stem of the right sylvian fissure, at the posterior margin of the right gyrus rectus, in the inferior right putamen, at the anterior portion of the right cingulate gyrus, at the lateral margin of the right pontomesencephalic junction, and in the left uncus.

Carbamazepine was begun, with intermittent doses of acetaminophen. The patient remained afebrile. On the second hospital day physical examination showed a tendency to topple to the right on Romberg's test. On the following day the patient's condition was unchanged. The glucose was 5.83 mmol per liter (105 mg per 100 ml). A test for antibodies to cytomegalovirus (CMV) was positive: a test for antibodies to human immunodeficiency virus (HIV) was negative. A lumbar puncture yielded clear, colorless cerebrospinal fluid that contained 6 red cells and 72 white cells per cubic millimeter of which 3 percent were neutrophils, 92 percent lymphocytes, and 5 percent large cells with dark-blue cytoplasm and folded nuclei; the glucose was 2.0 mmol per liter (36 mg per 100 ml), and the protein 2.76 g per liter (276 mg per 100 ml): the chloride was 118 mmol per liter; microscopical examination of stained specimens of the fluid showed no acid-fast bacilli or other microorganisms; a test for cryptococcal antigen was negative; cytologic

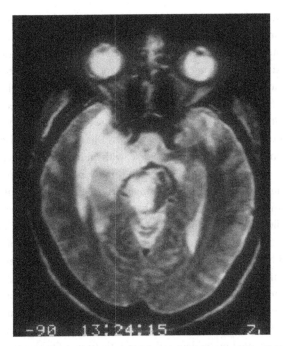

FIG 1 T_2-Weighted MRI Scan through the Basal Cisterns. Revealing Extensive T_2 Bright-Signal Abnormality in the Right Medial Temporal Lobe and Midbrain.

examination disclosed many lymphocytes and rare monocytoid cells, consistent with a reactive process; no evidence of malignant-tumor cells was found; tests for lymphocyte surface markers showed a predominance of T-cell markers, with occasional cells positive for kappa light chain and a few cells with questionable staining for lambda: a culture yielded no microorganisms: the concentration of IgG in the cerebrospinal fluid was 81 mg (normal. 0 to 8.6), and the albumin 161 mg per 100 ml (normal. 11 to 48): four or five monoclonal bands were seen in a specimen of the cerebrospinal fluid that was concentrated less than 31-fold; the director of the Immunology Laboratory raised the question of contamination by serum. A neuro-ophthalmologic consultant found no abnormality except for a tendency to substitute saccades for pursuit and inability to suppress the vestibulo-ocular reflex with visual fixation.

On the fourth hospital day a tuberculin skin test (PPD. 5 TU) was negative, and a skin test with candida antigen was positive at 48 hours. Tests for toxoplasma antibodies, heterophil agglutinins, and antinuclear antibodies were negative. Serum immuno-electrophoresis showed normal IgG. IgA. and IgM precipitin arcs: agarose-gel electrophoresis was normal. The concentration of IgM was 276 mg per 100 ml. A computed tomographic CT scan of the thorax, performed without the intravenous administration of contrast material, showed clear lungs and no enlargement of mediastinal lymph nodes. A CT scan of the abdomen, performed after the oral administration of contrast material, revealed that the liver, spleen, pancreas, and kidneys appeared grossly normal: no evidence of lymphadenopathy was detected. An ultrasonographic examination of the testes disclosed areas of decreased echogenicity throughout the left testis, with a possible left hydrocele: the right testis appeared normal. An ultrasonographic examination of the abdomen showed that the spleen was enlarged, with equivocal nonhomogeneity in its echotexture: both kidneys, the liver, and the gallbladder appeared normal, as did the head and body of the pancreas: the pancreatic tail was not well seen. On the sixth hospital day x-ray films of the lumbar spine revealed a Schmorl's nodule in the inferior end plate of the first lumbar vertebra: no other abnormality was detected.

On the seventh hospital day the patient had nausea and a mild headache. On physical examination he was less alert; slight weakness was noted in the distal parts of the left upper extremity: his gait appeared worse, with an increased tendency to fall now to the right side on walking. Another CT scan (Fig. 2), performed before and after the intravenous administration of contrast material, again revealed multiple contrast-enhancing lesions: edema of the white matter and a mass effect were evident, and there was a mild right-to-left midline shift. The carcinoembryonic antigen (CEA) was less than 0.5 ng per milliliter. Another lumbar puncture was contemplated but was postponed because of the cerebral edema and midline shift. Later in the day the patient was confused, and his speech was noticed to be dysarthric. A urologic consultant found no abnormality. Dexamethasone was begun after a consultation with the Infectious Disease Unit. On the following day the patient was improved subjectively and objectively: he still showed a tendency to fall to the right side. A radionuclide bone scan revealed no evidence of metastatic tumor. On the ninth hospital day

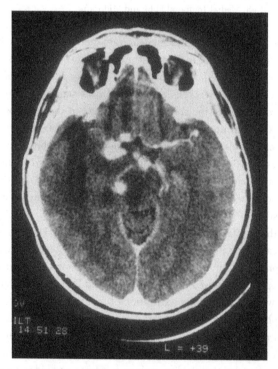

FIG 2 Contrast-Enhanced CT Scan Obtained on the Seventh Hospital Day. Demonstrating Multiple Basal-Meningeal Enhancing Lesions as Well as Persistent Right Hemispheric and Midbrain Edema.

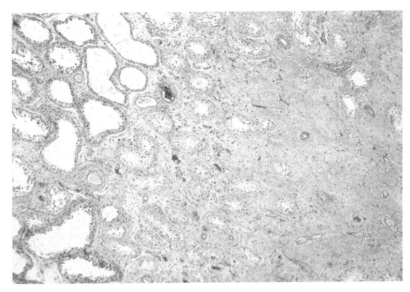

FIG 3 Orchidectomy Specimen (×320).

Seminiferous tubules are separated by interstitial fibrous tissue on the left side. Broad areas of fibrosis obscure the normal testicular architecture on the right side.

the patient was again alert and oriented, with an improved gait. A test for human chorionic gonadotropin was negative. A left radical orchidectomy was performed. Microscopical examination of the excised specimen (Fig. 3 and 4 revealed zonal fibrosis that involved the seminiferous tubules and interstitium and perivascular infiltrates of mononuclear cells; no evidence of a malignant tumor, vasculitis, or vascular occlusion was observed.

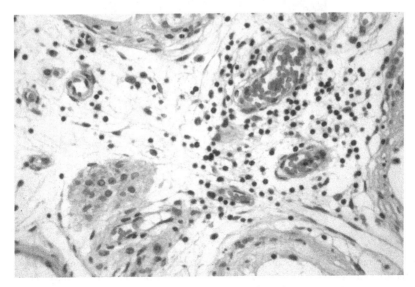

FIG 4 Perivascular Mononuclear-Cell Infiltrate in the Testis (×800).

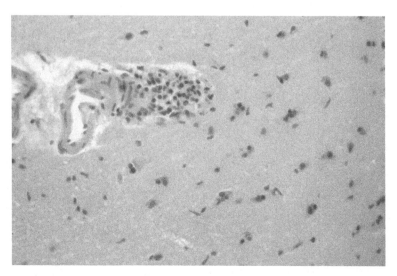

FIG 5 Eccentric Paravascular Cluster of Mononuclear Cells in the Corpus Striatum (×800).

On the 11th hospital day a telephone call to the Centers for Disease Control revealed that tests on the blood and cerebrospinal fluid for cysticercosis were negative. A right frontal stereotactic biopsy of the corpus striatum was performed. Microscopical examination of the specimen (Fig. 5) showed mild gliosis and focal paravascular chronic inflammation that was believed to be consistent with, but not diagnostic of, granulomatous inflammation: no granulomas or necrosis was seen: clusters of histiocytes,

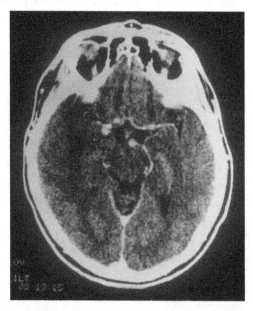

FIG 6 Contrast-Enhanced CT Scan. Obtained after Steroid Therapy, Showing Diminished Size of the Basal-Cistern Enhancing Lesions as Well as Almost Complete Resolution of the Right Hemispheric and Midbrain Edema.

and lymphocytes were located eccentrically around arteries microscopical examination of stained specimens revealed no acid-fast bacilli or other microorganisms: no evidence of atypia or a malignant tumor was detected.

Rod-shaped nuclei (arrowheads), characteristic of microglia, are scattered in the parenchyma.

On the 14th hospital day the patient had no symptoms, and physical examination revealed no change in the neurologic findings. The hematocrit was 37.9 percent, the white-cell count 9800, and the platelet count 220,000. The prothrombin time was 8.7 seconds, with a control of 11.0 seconds; the partial thromboplastin time was 24.2 seconds. The urea nitrogen was 5.4 mmol per liter (15 mg per 100 ml), and the glucose 5.9 mmol per liter (106 mg per 100 ml). The alpha-feto-protein was less than 10 IU per milliliter. A lumbar puncture again yielded clear, colorless cerebrospinal fluid that contained 17 red cells and 10 white cells per cubic millimeter, of which 2 percent were neutrophils and 98 percent lymphocytes; the glucose was 3.5 mmol per liter (63 mg per 100 ml), and the protein 0.76 g per liter (76 mg per 100 ml); microscopical examination of a stained specimen of the fluid showed no microorganisms; cytologic examination revealed small lymphocytes and rare monocytoid cells; the findings were believed to be consistent with a reactive process. On the 16th hospital day a repeated contrast-enhanced cranial CT scan (Fig. 6) disclosed a marked decrease in the enhancing abnormalities to approximately a third of their previous size; the white-matter edema and the midline shift had resolved.

A diagnostic report was received.

DIFFERENTIAL DIAGNOSIS

DR. MARTIN A. SAMUELS[*]: This straightforward case becomes a difficult problem when a circa 1530 disease is subjected to circa 1990 technology. The clinicopathological conference (CPC) has two sides. Its major focus, of course, is to demonstrate the clinical method and to create a venue in which the student can learn the art of diagnostics through the example of experienced clinicians. The other side is the art and science of discovering the diagnosis with the use of methods unavailable to the treating physicians.

I have discussed five previous cases at these exercises. In preparing this case I reviewed my own CPC experience, with the following diagnoses: meningioma of the foramen magnum; Paget's disease with extramedullary hematopoiesis compressing the spinal cord: porphyria; amyloid neuropathy; and pheochromocytoma; those are some of the most classic disorders in the history of medicine. I was missing only one. The ultimate irony is that my personal experience with the disease that I think this patient had is far less than my experience with discussing CPCs at the Massachusetts General Hospital. Despite this irony I used the experience that I have had.

The case of a 35-year-old man with an apparent chronic granulomatous meningitis and periarteritis is presented. Every imaginable test, even including a brain

* Chief of neurology. Brigham and Women's Hospital; associate professor of neurology. Harvard Medical School. Currently Chair, Department of Neurology, Brigham and Women's Hospital.

biopsy and an orchidectomy, is listed except one—the serologic test for syphilis. My CPC experience told me that this was indeed a critical clue. It is. I am sure, a case of neurosyphilis.

It is ironic how difficult it has become to think of neurosyphilis in an immunocompetent person in 1990. Arguably the most important disease in the history of humankind, unequivocal descriptions of it appear in the medical literature from the time of the return of Columbus from the New World. Some observers have held that the disease had a New World origin, citing evidence of syphilitic lesions found in skeletal remains in pre-Columbian American Indians, whereas others have argued that the illness was brought to the New World by the European explorers, pointing out that many outbreaks of what was called leprosy before the voyage of Columbus were thought to be highly contagious, sexually-transmitted diseases, probably in fact representing syphilis. In 1530 Dr. Philippus Aureolus Theophrastus Bombastus von Hohenheim, who called himself Paracelsus, a name he gave himself to reflect his view that he was even greater than Celsus, the renowned first-century Roman physician, wrote a detailed description of syphilis and argued that it could be treated with mercury, a remarkable and accurate observation made almost 400 years before the discovery of Salvarsan. In 1909 Dr. Paul Ehrlich, allegedly on his 606th attempt, discovered the arsenical treatment arsphenamine. The "magic bullet," as Ehrlich called it, seemed to be effective against a whole range of illnesses, including syphilis. This discovery probably marks one of the first collaborations between a pharmaceutical firm (Hoechst) and a medical scientist aimed at developing a specific disease cure. Under the trade name Salvarsan, meaning "preserving health," the pharmaceutical firm released 65,000 doses free to physicians around the world, an amazing philanthropic gesture that unfortunately has not proved to be a popular precedent. After the discovery by Dr. J.F. Mahoney in 1943 that the responsible organism. *Treponema pallidum*, was exquisitely sensitive to penicillin the prevalence of the disease plummeted, only to return recently in immunocompromised persons usually ill with human immunodeficiency virus (HIV) infection. When I was a medical student, from 1967 through 1971. I was told by my teachers that syphilis, the great masquerader, the disease that taught more doctors medicine, had filled more journal pages, and had made more professors than all other diseases combined, had vanished forever from the earth. Now nearly all experienced physicians can recognize the disease in patients with the acquired immunodeficiency syndrome (AIDS), with its characteristic foreshortened stages and more malignant course. Classic syphilis in an immunocompetent host remains a relatively uncommon illness, although its prevalence may be rising in recent years. No wonder the physicians caring for this patient had such a difficult time.

Now I shall turn to the details of this man's presentation and test results. He presented with a few months' history of a nonspecific encephalopathy and some vague signs pointing to trouble in the right hemisphere. An MRI scan was performed. Dr. Carbonneau, will you show the findings?

DR. ROBERT CARBONNEAU: The MRI scan of the brain (Fig. 1), performed on the day of admission, shows a low T_1, high T_2 signal abnormality involving the right basal ganglia, anterior cingulum, gyrus rectus, pontomesencephalic junction, and left uncus.

There is prominent deep white-matter edema in the right frontal and temporal lobes extending into the midbrain and pons. A gadolinium-enhanced image demonstrates multiple enhancing lesions predominantly located at the meningocortical junction adjacent to the basal cisterns.

DR. SAMUELS: After this study treatment with carbamazepine was begun, presumably to prevent seizures, and the patient was given acetaminophen, presumably for headache, although nothing is specifically stated about either of these problems in the case record.

Next a lumbar puncture was performed and showed a pleocytosis (72 white cells per cubic millimeter, most of which were lymphocytes and reactive cells) and a very high protein level (276 mg per 100 ml, with 59 percent albumin and 29 percent IgG). The spinal fluid protein level is usually less than 45 mg per 100 ml in adults, with 45 percent albumin and 10 percent IgG. Furthermore, four to five monoclonal bands were seen in the spinal fluid. It is not specifically stated that these bands were not seen in the serum, but I shall assume that they were so-called oligoclonal bands, a finding that implies that there is production of IgG within the central nervous system. Only reactive cells were noted on cytologic examination of the spinal fluid, and tests for lymphocyte surface markers did not suggest a malignant clone responsible for the lymphocytes found in the cerebrospinal fluid. The cerebrospinal fluid findings may be summarized as showing inflammation with breakdown of the blood–brain barrier and local production of IgG, with no evidence of a malignant tumor. A neuro-ophthalmologist detected only saccadic pursuit, a nonspecific finding most consistent with an encephalopathic state, and presumably did not find an Argyll Robertson pupil, a finding usually seen in parenchymatous neurosyphilis. When present in its classic form as a small, irregular pupil with light-near dissociation it is virtually pathognomonic of parenchymatous neurosyphilis, usually the tabetic form.

On the fourth hospital day the physicians embarked on an extensive search for an underlying malignant tumor and found only decreased echogenicity in the left testis. Dr. Carbonneau, will you show us the testicular ultrasound study?

DR. CARBONNEAU: The ultrasound images show diffuse patchy hypoechogenicity of the left testis, without evidence of testicular enlargement. The right testis is normal.

DR. SAMUELS: The spleen appeared slightly enlarged on the ultrasound study but not on the CT scan, and the lumbar-spine film showed only a Schmorl's nodule in the first lumbar vertebra. I reviewed those studies earlier with Dr. Carbonneau but did not think that they were critical in making the diagnosis, and there is no need for us to see them now.

Between the fifth and seventh hospital days the patient's condition deteriorated, and two CT scans were performed. Dr. Carbonneau, will you demonstrate the findings?

DR. CARBONNEAU: The contrast-enhanced CT scan obtained on the seventh hospital day (Fig. 2) shows no change in the multiple enhancing lesions. The low attenuation in the deep white-matter structures is slightly more extensive than the corresponding T_2 bright signal that was seen on the earlier MRI scan. The contrast-enhanced CT scan, performed two days later, displays further progression of white-matter low attenuation, with extension into the subcortical white matter of the right frontal and temporal lobes. There is new low attenuation in the right thalamus, with a suggestion of slight compression and displacement of the third ventricle from right to left. At the level of the basal cisterns the enhancing lesions appear more prominent. The suprasellar and perimesencephalic cisterns are partially effaced, indicating impending brain-stem compression at the level of the tentorial incisura.

In summary, these two CT scans show a pattern of disease progression manifested by slight enlargement of the enhancing lesions, increasing white-matter edema and mass effect, shrinkage of the basal cisterns, and impending brain-stem compression at the level of the tentorial incisura.

DR. SAMUELS: After that latest study treatment with dexamethasone was begun, and there apparently was a dramatic improvement, supporting the hypothesis that the patient had primarily vasogenic cerebral edema. This type of edema responds best to steroids.

Next a radical orchidectomy was performed, followed shortly thereafter by a stereotactic brain biopsy. Dr. Sobel, will you review the pathological findings in these two specimens.[1]

DR. RAYMOND A. SOBEL: The first specimen was the left testis with 6 cm of spermatic cord. The testis was of normal size. Sectioning revealed poorly defined, firm, yellow-white areas interspersed with unremarkable testicular tissue. Examination of frozen and permanent sections revealed areas of fibrosis, with effacement of the normal architecture and atrophic tubules. Scattered mononuclear-cell infiltrates were present within and near the borders of the fibrotic areas (Fig. 3 and 4). No granulocytes and only small numbers of plasma cells were present. Vasculitis, giant cells, and areas of necrosis were absent, and there was no evidence of a neoplasm. Examination of seminiferous tubules away from the abnormal areas showed normal spermatogenesis.

A stereotactic biopsy of enhancing lesions in the corpus striatum was performed by Dr. Brooke Swearingen. Two cores of brain tissue, 0.1 cm in diameter, were received for frozen and permanent sections. The architecture of the corpus striatum was intact, and there were scattered perivascular lymphocytes and monocytes. Only rare plasma cells and granulocytes were seen. The vessel walls were intact; giant cells and necrosis were absent. There were prominent reactive astrocytes, and increased numbers of rod cells or reactive microglia were found in the parenchyma (Fig. 5). Stains for gram-positive and gram-negative organisms, acid-fast bacteria, and fungi were negative. These mild abnormalities are nonspecific but are consistent with the presence of an inflammatory process in the adjacent basilar leptomeninges.

DR. SAMUELS: On the 14th hospital day a repeated lumbar puncture showed improvement in the leak in the blood–brain barrier, as expected on the basis of the clinical and CT findings. The protein level was only 76 mg per 100 ml, but there was still evidence of inflammation, with 10 white cells per cubic millimeter, again mostly lymphocytes. Cytologic examination again revealed only reactive cells, without evidence of a malignant tumor. Gamma globulin and albumin levels were not measured in this second cerebrospinal fluid specimen. On the 16th hospital day another CT scan was performed. Dr. Carbonneau, will you show us the last in the series of imaging studies?

DR. CARBONNEAU: The final contrast-enhanced CT scan after steroid therapy shows marked resolution in the previously described abnormalities (Fig. 6). The right-frontal-lobe and the right-temporal-lobe white matter was normal. The low-attenuation changes in the right lenticular nucleus, right thalamus, midbrain, and pons had resolved. The enhancing lesion at the border of the right putamen and external capsule is still evident, but the right-cingulate-gyrus lesion is no longer visible. The basal enhancing meningeal lesions are markedly decreased in size. The basal cisterns are well delineated, indicating a decrease in the overall edema and mass effect in the interval. Hence, after the steroid therapy there had been marked resolution of the brain edema and a slight decrease in the size of the enhancing basal meningeal lesions.

Dr. Samuels: There were several pertinent negative evaluations in this case. There was no evidence of a malignant tumor despite an extensive search. The negative x-ray studies and CT scan of the chest and the absence of lymphadenopathy make the diagnosis of sarcoidosis very unlikely. Cultures of the blood and spinal fluid were negative. There was no serologic evidence of HIV infection, cryptococcosis, toxoplasmosis, systemic lupus erythematosus, or cysticereosis. The negative tuberculin skin test with a concomitant positive candida skin test and a normal x-ray film of the chest makes tuberculosis of the nervous system very unlikely.

In summary, we are faced with the clinical, CT, MRI, spinal fluid, and brain-biopsy findings of chronic granulomatous meningitis and periarteritis. In addition, examination of the testis showed evidence of a burned-out orchitis. Fungal or tuberculous meningitis could produce a similar picture, but it is usually more acute or subacute, with evidence of systemic disease. In the rare case of cryptococcal or tuberculous meningitis without evidence of systemic disease there is either a positive cryptococcal serologic test or a positive tuberculin skin test or more cells and a lower glucose level are found in the cerebrospinal fluid. Furthermore, systemic steroid therapy probably would have made both of these conditions worse, whereas dexamethasone made this patient dramatically better. Sarcoidosis can produce a granulomatous meningitis, usually at the base of the brain and in particular around the infundibulum. This patient's unexplained weight gain could have been due to involvement of the satiety-control centers in the hypothalamus, but that abnormality is not specific for sarcoidosis and could occur with any basilar process involving the hypothalamus or infundibulum, or both. Nearly all patients with central nervous system sarcoidosis have bilateral hilar lymphadenopathy, a finding that was absent in this case. Even in the rare case of pure nervous system sarcoidosis, so much local production of IgG within the central nervous system would not be expected. The diagnosis of brucellosis is probably the closest fit to this man's problem other than syphilis. It can produce an encephalopathy with considerable edema and granulomatous inflammation, orchitis, and even lowback pain due to brucella osteomyelitis, which can appear radiologically identical to a Schmorl's nodule, a finding in this case. However, brucellosis is a disease that is seen virtually exclusively in inhabitants of the Middle East, mostly of Kuwait and Saudi Arabia, or in veterinarians or food processors elsewhere in the world. On epidemiologic grounds it is very unlikely that this patient had brucellosis.

The diagnosis simply must be neurosyphilis of the meningeal, gummatous type.

The natural history of syphilitic infection in an otherwise normal host is well known. Ten days to 10 weeks after an initial exposure to the organism a chancre appears, and the organism can be seen with use of dark-field microscopical examination. With or without treatment the chancre heals without a trace in less than a month. About half the persons infected enter the secondary stage of spirochetemia, characterized by a rash involving the palms and soles, joint symptoms, and often meningismus. Sometimes a striking meningitis occurs referred to as "acute symptomatic syphilitic meningitis," with hundreds of cells in the spinal fluid, an elevated spinal fluid protein level, and hypoglycorrhachia. In most patients with syphilitic meningitis, which occurs in about 25 percent of all infected persons, however, the meningeal involvement is asymptomatic and recognizable only by lumbar puncture. If the organism invades the central nervous system, it usually does so within 3 to 18 months of inoculation. In many persons the meningitis subsides without treatment, whereas in others it persists and may result in the various syndromes of tertiary neurosyphilis. The precise syndrome that develops is presumably related to the chronicity of the infection. The earliest forms of tertiary neurosyphilis are meningeal and meningovascular; the later forms, paretic and tabetic, are due to eventual infiltration of the organisms from the Virchow–Robin spaces into the surrounding brain. A gumma—a syphilitic granuloma—can occur at any stage of the disease, but the location of the gumma in the brain again reflects the chronicity of the infection. Gummatous meningitis occurs in the early phases of tertiary syphilis, whereas parenchymatous gummas are seen later. In his classic book *Pathology for Students and Practitioners* Kaufmann[1] wrote, "The lesion produced by cerebral syphilis is a basal, gummatous meningitis. This is composed of circumscribed solitary or multiple inflammatory foci, or of a more diffuse specific tissue reaction in the meninges." Our 1990 imaging studies seem a perfect match for Kaufmann's description, with inflammatory nodules following the courses of arteries. This man apparently had gummatous meningitis and periarteritis, which places his initial infection about 8 to 12 years before admission.

The serologic tests for syphilis fall into two categories. One consists of the nontreponemal tests, which are based on detecting in the patient's serum or cerebrospinal fluid so-called reagin antibodies (IgM or IgG) directed against a cardiolipin–lecithin antigen produced by the interaction of the treponeme with the host tissues. These tests include the Venereal Disease Research Laboratory (VDRL), Hinton, Kolmer, and Kahn tests. The second category of tests consists of the so-called treponemal tests, which are based on detection of the presence of antibodies directed specifically against treponemal antigens. They include *T. pallidum* immobilization (TPI) and fluorescent treponemal-antibody absorption (FTA-ABS) tests.

The nontreponemal tests are inexpensive and readily available but are less sensitive than the treponemal tests. The nontreponemal tests are the last to turn positive after the onset of infection and the first to turn negative after treatment, making them useful as a measure of successful treatment, although the degree of spinal fluid cellularity remains the most reliable method of gauging the success of treatment. In late neurosyphilis the serum nontreponemal tests are negative in as many as a third of the cases. The cerebrospinal fluid nontreponemal tests may be positive despite a negative serum nontreponemal test, but even a negative cerebrospinal fluid nontreponemal antibody test does not exclude neurosyphilis. Biologically false positive nontreponemal antibody tests are common with aging, various rheumatic diseases, and endocarditis.

The most widely available treponemal test is the FTA-ABS test. It is the most sensitive—that is, it is the first to become positive and the last to become negative. It may remain positive despite adequate therapy even for the rest of the patient's life, making it useless as a measure of successful treatment. A positive FTA-ABS test with a titer of more than 1:2 rules out a biologically false positive nontreponemal antibody test. As many as 10 percent of patients with late neurosyphilis have a negative FTA-ABS test. There is virtually no use for a cerebrospinal fluid FTA-ABS test. Of the treponemal tests, the "gold standard" is the TPI test, against which all other tests are compared, but it is difficult to perform and available in only a few laboratories. Newer tests are based on the detection of a 19S IgM antibody directed against *T. pallidum* and provide evidence of active disease in the serum or cerebrospinal fluid.

Treponemal tests may be positive in patients with diseases caused by organisms that are members of other species in the genus treponema—namely, yaws, pinta, and bejel. Yaws is caused by *T. pertenue* and is common in the Caribbean. Latin America, Central Africa, and the Far East. It is usually associated with a very obvious skin eruption (the mother yaw), and late disease is typically benign, without any of the neurologic effects seen in syphilis. Pinta is caused by *T. carateum* and is limited to the skin and would not be a consideration in this case. Bejel is caused by a variant of *T. pallidum* and often presents with an oral lesion or, in its secondary stage, with a generalized rash. Late disease resembles benign syphilis. Although this man was known to have traveled through some of the areas where these diseases are endemic, the malignant neurologic course was inconsistent with the other known treponemal diseases.

Other spirochetes (that is, members of the family Spirochaetaceae) known to cause human neurologic disease are members of the genuses leptospira and borrelia. Leptospirosis may produce an aseptic meningitis, but not with the degree of granuloma formation and edema noted in this case. Furthermore, most patients with leptospirosis have some abnormality of liver or kidney function, or both, neither of which was evident in the case under discussion. *Borrelia burgdorferi* is known to cause the tick-borne Lyme disease. It may be associated with an aseptic meningitis but usually after the recognition of the characteristic skin lesion, erythema chronicum migrans, and never with the degree of granuloma formation and edema observed in this case.

In summary, I believe that this patient had tertiary gummatous meningeal syphilis. I think that the laboratory test was a VDRL slide test followed by a specific treponemal antibody test, probably the FTA-ABS, after which he was treated with penicillin.

Dr. Edward P. Richardson, Jr.: Are there any comments or questions?

Dr. Mandel E. Cohen: I have seen a couple of hundred cases of central nervous system syphilis, and in the days when we did routine blood tests for syphilis we did not miss the diagnosis of paresis or other types of central nervous system syphilis in Boston. I wonder whether we should resume routine blood tests to aid in the diagnosis of the rare case.

CLINICAL DIAGNOSES

? Granulomatous process in basilar meninges.

? Tumor metastatic to brain.

? Primary central nervous system lymphoma.

DR. MARTIN A. SAMUELS' DIAGNOSIS

Neurosyphilis, meningeal gummatous type.

PATHOLOGICAL DISCUSSION

DR. RICHARDSON: Dr. Gruber, will you tell us about your observations of this patient?

DR. MICHAEL L. GRUBER: We considered infectious granulomatous diseases such as toxoplasmosis, cryptococcosis, tuberculosis, and cysticercosis, as well as sarcoidosis, metastatic tumor, principally malignant melanoma and testicular, renal, and lung cancer, and primary central nervous system lymphoma.

It was decided to proceed with a stereotactic brain biopsy. A pre-biopsy CT scan with contrast enhancement demonstrated marked diminution of the size of the brain masses. This change has been described in other patients with meningovascular syphilis. A double dose of contrast material was required to enable the neurosurgeon to visualize the lesion and obtain a biopsy specimen.

On repeated spinal fluid examination the VDRL and the FTA-ABS tests were strongly positive. The patient was provided with 24 million units of penicillin per day, given by vein over a period of two weeks, followed by penicillin G benzathine (Bicillin) on a weekly basis for a total of four doses. An MRI scan performed two months after completion of the antibiotic treatment revealed no residual disease. When last seen he was well, had resumed work, and appeared to have no neurologic deficits.

This case underscores the need to consider neurosyphilis in the differential diagnosis of disappearing lesions of the central nervous system. Despite the marked decline in the frequency of neurosyphilis over the past three decades in this country, new cases continue to appear, both sporadically and as a complication of AIDS. Since neurosyphilis is a treatable condition, it is important not only to consider the diagnosis but also to reinstitute the routine use of VDRL serologic testing and spinal fluid examination when clinically indicated.

DR. SOBEL: After learning the serologic findings we reevaluated the surgical specimens for possible clues to the correct diagnosis. In the testis the lesion was largely inactive, but the small number of inflammatory cells, particularly plasma cells, might have suggested a previous infection rather than a traumatic lesion or infarct. In old syphilitic lesions in the testis and other organs, intimal thickening in small arteries may indicate that obliterative arteritis had been present previously, but such features were not found in this case. The testicular lesion is best interpreted as the diffuse fibrotic form of testicular syphilis rather than as a gumma.[2,3]

Perivascular inflammation, conspicuous rod cells or microglia, and reactive astrocytosis are characteristic of parenchymal neurosyphilis.[4,5] There is considerable current interest in the immunologic functions of microglia,[6] and the long-recognized prominence of these cells in neurosyphilis may indicate an important immunopathologic role in this disease. Examination of the brain-biopsy specimen disclosed no classic endarteritis obliterans, plasma cells, or necrosis, so that even in retrospect the findings are appropriately considered nonspecific. We cannot comment about basilar meningeal involvement because leptomeninges were not present in the biopsy sample.

Warthin–Starry stains for treponema were subsequently performed on both the orchidectomy and the brain-biopsy specimens. Because the disease was largely inactive, no organisms were demonstrated in the testis. In the brain the interpretation of this stain was complicated by staining of normal neural structures, and we were unable to demonstrate organisms unambiguously with that technique.

We rarely encounter neurosyphilis in surgical neuropathological material, particularly in needle-biopsy specimens of the brain. Recent literature suggests that there has been a resurgence of the diverse manifestations of neurosyphilis,[7,8] and that concurrent HIV infection may alter the pathobiology of the disease.[9,10] The latter suggestion is exemplified particularly in a case of the rare so-called quaternary form of neurosyphilis in a patient with AIDS reported by Morgello and Laufer.[11]

Various manifestations of syphilis have been discussed at these exercises,[12] but orchidectomy and brain biopsy were not the usual diagnostic procedures for the diagnosis of neurosyphilis. For all of us the less-than-optimal sequence of events leading to the correct diagnosis in this case was a humbling experience. The case certainly emphasizes that as clinicians, radiologists, and pathologists we must still consider syphilis in the differential diagnosis when confronted with a diagnostically challenging case.

ANATOMICAL DIAGNOSIS

Tertiary syphilis, with parenchymatous neurosyphilis and fibrosis of left testis.

REFERENCES

1. Kaufmann E. Pathology for students and practitioners. Reimann S. trans Philadelphia: P. Blakiston's, 1929.
2. Morgan AD. Inflammation and infestation of the testis and paratesticular structures. In: Pugh RCB, ed. Pathology of the testis. Oxford, England: Blackwell Scientific, 1976:98–101.
3. Persaud V, Rao A. Gumma of testis. Br J Urol 1977: 49:142.
4. Merritt HH, Adams RD, Solomon HC. Neurosyphilis. New York: Oxford University Press, 1946:180–93.
5. Harriman DGF. Bacterial infections of the central nervous system. In: Blackwood W. Corselfis JAN, eds. Greenfield's neuropathology. 3rd ed. London: Edward Arnold. 1976:238–68.

6. Streit WJ, Graeber MB, Kreutzberg G. Functional plasticity of microglia, a review. GLIA 1988: 1:301–7.

7. Simon RP, Neurosyphilis. Arch Neurol 1985: 42:606–13.

8. Burke JM, Schaberg DR. Neurosyphilis in the antibiotic era. Neurology 1985: 35:1368–71.

9. Johns DR, Tierney M, Felsenstein D. Alteration in the natural history of neurosyphilis by concurrent infection with the human immunodeficiency virus. N Engl J Med 1987: 316:1569–72.

10. Richards BW, Hessburg TJ, Nussbaum JN. Recurrent syphilitic uveitis N Engl J Med 1989: 320:62.

11. Morgello S, Laufer H. Quaternary neurosyphilis in a Harrian man with human immuno-deficiency virus infection. Hum Pathol 1989: 20:808–11.

12. Case Records of the Massachusetts General Hospital Case 15–1984, N Engl J Med 1984: 310:972–81.

The Massachusetts General Hospital wishes to acknowledge the generous support of the following sponsors in making possible the continued preparation of the Case Records:

E. R. Squibb & Sons, U.S., and the Squibb Science and Technology Group
The Upjohn Company

Perspectives and Updates

Over the course of my 12 Cabot Cases, I have had the opportunity to analyze some of the most infamous and influential human diseases, but it can be convincingly argued that this one leads the pack. As I noted in the CPC discussion, syphilis has been known for centuries and was clearly described as long ago as the 16th century. Some of the most important breakthroughs in therapeutics occurred around this disease, including the use of mercury, arsenic, and penicillin. The arsenical compound arsphenamine was probably the first example of a designer drug, scientifically developed by a physician (Paul Ehrlich) and a pharmaceutical company (Hoechst). Using the trade name Salvarsan, Hoechst released 65,000 doses free to physicians around the world. This is especially ironic in light of our current era of intense distrust, bordering on phobia, when it comes to collaborating with the pharmaceutical industry to develop new drugs.

With 20 years of perspective; two interlocking issues arise in thinking about this case: the new face of syphilis in the HIV era and the difficulty in diagnosing an entity, no matter how typical, when it appears out of the expected context.

Since the beginning of the penicillin era, syphilis had been on the decline over the entire globe. Then, in the 1990s, its incidence began to rise again, largely but not entirely related to the epidemic of HIV infection. Because HIV and syphilis have common risk factors and perhaps because each facilitates infection by the other, the incidence of syphilis in all of its forms has increased. However, many younger physicians have seen syphilis only in HIV-infected people. Much of the data are equivocal, but it is probably true that HIV infection increases the virulence of the infection with syphilis and may accelerate the transition time from one stage to another. A new, more aggressive necrotizing stage of syphilis (quaternary syphilis) has become extant. There is little doubt that treatment of syphilis is more difficult in HIV-infected patients (as measured by the time that it takes to achieve a 50 percent reduction in spinal fluid pleocytosis and serological test intensity), and there are clearly more penicillin-resistant cases of syphilis than in the pre-HIV era. Neurosyphilis in the early phases of the infection may or may not be more common, but it is unequivocally more difficult to recognize clinically because of its phenomenological similarity to HIV encephalitis and other infections seen in compromised hosts. One of the more interesting aspects of this problem is that the incidence of syphilis, including neurosyphilis, in non-HIV-infected people is also on the rise. The highest risk group comprises men who have sex with men. The net effect is that the clinician must have a high index of suspicion for neurosyphilis, particularly in those infected with HIV but in others as well. In 1991, when I discussed this case, I said that I had had more experience discussing Cabot Cases for the *New England Journal of Medicine* (five at that time) than I had with neurosyphilis. My teachers would not have said the same, and sadly I can no longer say it either. The great masquerader has returned with a vengeance.

We like to believe that diagnostic skills are scientific, in which we follow algorithms, all drawn from carefully obtained evidence using randomized controlled trials. In truth, we make diagnoses in a manner similar to other cognitive processes. We make an estimate based on the case's initial features and then gradually hone that impression by using collateral data from the history, exam, and laboratory. These processes are not sequential but parallel. The great clinician has the experience to recognize a large number of patterns and also the flexibility to alter the initial impression when faced with conflicting data. The art is to know when to adhere to the initial impression when a piece of additional data is conflicting (a false positive) and when to change course when the new piece of information is sufficiently compelling and reliable to make the original hypothesis indefensible. One of the most challenging situations arises when one sees a pattern out of context. For me and the generation behind me, syphilis is a disease of those who are HIV-infected or perhaps men who have sex with men. This was the pitfall into which the treating doctors fell in this case. Yet the clinical picture strongly suggested neurosyphilis. It is truly ironic that testicular and brain biopsies were required to make a diagnosis that Charcot would have made in the blink of an eye.

Martin A. Samuels

REFERENCES

1. Marra CM. Update on neurosyphilis; Curr Infect Dis Rep 1999; 11: 127–34.
2. Marra CM. Normalization of CSF abnormalities after neurosyphilis therapy: does HIV status matter? Clin Infect Dis 2004; 38:1001–6.
3. Kent ME, Romanelli F. Re-examining syphilis: an update on epidemiology, clinical manifestations and management. Ann Pharmacother 2008; 42:226–36.

A 71-Year-Old Man with A Rash and Severe Sensorimotor Neuropathy

PARAPROTEINEMIC NEUROPATHY

Allan H. Ropper and Ann C. Mckee

CPC 21-1993

ARTICLE

A 71-year-old man was admitted to the hospital because of a rash, diffuse muscle weakness, and respiratory failure.

There was a long history of insulin-dependent diabetes mellitus and alcoholism. The patient had been in stable health until two or three months before entry, when a diffuse maculopapular erythematous rash developed. It improved with prednisone therapy but flared when the dose was tapered, with the onset of difficulty in walking and arising from a chair. Twenty-six days before admission he experienced sudden right flank pain and was admitted to another hospital.

On physical examination a diffuse erythematous scaling rash was present; no costovertebral-angle tenderness was found. The urine was normal. The laboratory values during this admission and the later admission are presented in Table 1, Table 2, Table 3, and Table 4. Radiographs of the chest and abdomen were normal. An ultrasonographic examination of the abdomen and kidneys and an intravenous pyelographic examination were negative.

Benzodiazepine, ranitidine, and methylprednisolone (125 mg every eight hours) were administered, with disappearance of the flank pain, followed by the onset of "stinging" pains that "shot down the legs." The patient subsequently became unable to move his extremities, sit up, or draw a deep breath. On the sixth hospital day the rash and weakness were improved, and prednisone (20 mg twice daily) was substituted for methylprednisolone. On the next day the patient experienced diffuse myalgia and arthralgia and was unable to stand because of weakness of the legs; methylprednisolone was promptly resumed. On the ninth hospital day dyspnea developed and was associated with leukocytosis. Hypoxemia developed, and pulmonary infiltrates were demonstrated on radiologic examination on the 12th hospital day. Ceftriaxone was administered. Microscopical examination of a biopsy specimen of the skin showed findings consistent with pyoderma gangrenosum, and examination of a biopsy specimen of bone marrow

N Engl J Med 1993; 328:1550-1558 | May 27, 1993

Table 1 Hematologic Values

Variable	26 Days before Admission	14 Days before Admission	12 Days before Admission	At Admission
Hematocrit (%)	30.8			31.6
White-cell count (per mm³)	14,900	24,200		11,800
Differential count (%)				
Neutrophils				94
Lymphocytes				1
Monocytes				4
Metamyelocytes				1
Platelet count (per mm³)				130,000
Erythrocyte sedimentation rate (mm/hr)	70		123	40
Mean corpuscular volume (μm³/cell)	98			94
Ferritin	Elevated			
Prothrombin time				Normal
Partial-thromboplastin time				Normal
Iron	Normal			
Iron-binding capacity	Reduced			
Vitamin B$_{12}$	Normal			
Folic acid	Normal			

revealed 15 percent plasma cells, a finding consistent with multiple myeloma. On the 26th hospital day the patient was transferred to this hospital, receiving methylprednisolone (20 mg by vein every eight hours), ranitidine, allopurinol, furosemide, antibiotics, and pancuronium bromide and morphine sulfate as required.

The temperature was 36.4 °C, the pulse 64, and the blood pressure 205/105 mm Hg; the patient was undergoing mechanical ventilation at a rate of 12 breaths per minute.

On physical examination the patient was sedated but arousable, with occasional spontaneous movements. On neurologic examination he blinked his eyelids on verbal command; he moved his eyes fully and furrowed his brow bilaterally. The right pupil was eccentric, 2 mm in diameter, and reactive to light; the left pupil was 1.5 mm and minimally reactive. Diffuse tremulous movements of the jaw were noted. The extremities were flaccid and areflexic, with no response to noxious stimuli.

The urine gave a ++++ result for glucose and negative results for protein and ketones; the specific gravity was 1.015; the sediment contained 2 white cells and 15 red cells per high-power field. A specimen of arterial blood, drawn while the patient

Table 2 Serum Laboratory Values*

Variable	26 Days before Admission	12 Days before Admission	At Admission
Urea nitrogen (mg/dl)	28	105	128
Creatinine (mg/dl)	2.1	2.3	1.2
Glucose (mg/dl)			184
Protein (g/dl)			4.5
Albumin			1.6
Globulin			2.9
Calcium			Normal
Phosphorus			Normal
Bilirubin			Normal
IgA (mg/dl)		1135	819
IgG			Normal
Sodium (mmol/liter)			152
Potassium (mmol/liter)			4.3
Chloride (mmol/liter)			111
Carbon dioxide (mmol/liter)			30
Alanine aminotransferase (U/liter)			83
Aspartate aminotransferase (U/liter)			68
Lactate dehydrogenase (U/liter)†			438
Alkaline phosphatase (U/liter)			175
Creatine kinase			Normal
Amylase	Normal		Normal
Lipase	Normal		

*To convert values for urea nitrogen to millimoles per liter, multiply by 0.357; to convert values for creatinine to micromoles per liter, multiply by 88.4; to convert values for glucose to millimoles per liter, multiply by 0.05551.
†Measured in a hemolyzed specimen.

was undergoing mechanical ventilation with 60 percent oxygen, showed that the partial pressure of oxygen was 99 mm Hg, the partial pressure of carbon dioxide 36 mm Hg, and the pH 7.55. An electrocardiogram disclosed sinus bradycardia at a rate of 59, with nonspecific ST-segment and T-wave abnormalities. Radiographs of the chest showed a right pleural effusion. A computed tomographic (CT) cranial scan revealed severe central and peripheral cerebral atrophy. A skeletal survey and an ultrasonographic examination of the kidneys were negative. A CT scan of the abdomen and pelvis (Figure 1) showed thickening of the rectal wall and perirectal soft tissues and poor renal opacification; edema and stranding of the subcutaneous tissues, retroperitoneum, and presacral space, small bilateral pleural effusions, and a small amount of ascitic fluid were observed.

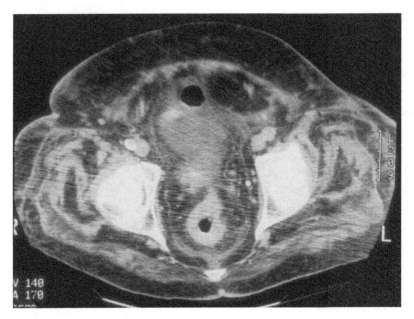

FIG 1 CT Scan of the Lower Pelvis, Demonstrating a Small Amount of Ascites.

Conduction studies of five motor nerves revealed compound motor-action potentials of very low amplitude, normal distal latencies, and a slight reduction in maximal motor-conduction velocities. Sensory-nerve action potentials were unobtainable in either sural nerve or in the left median and ulnar nerves. Blink-reflex latencies

Table 3 Cerebrospinal Fluid Findings on Admission

Variable	Finding
Initial pressure	185 mm
Appearance of fluid	Clear, slightly xanthochromic
Cell count (per high-power field)	
Red cells	2
White cells	3
White-cell differential count (%)	
Lymphocytes	40
Mononuclear cells	60
Glucose (mg/dl)*	171
Protein (mg/dl)	288
Albumin	190
IgG	48.3
Cytologic examination	No malignant-tumor cells
Cryptococcal antigen	Negative
Cultures (bacterial, microbacterial, fungal, viral)	Negative

*To convert value to millimoles per liter, multiply by 0.05551.

Table 4 Miscellaneous Laboratory Variables with Negative Findings during Admission

Thyroid-stimulating hormone	Antinuclear antibodies
Plasma cortisol	Rheumatoid factor
Haptoglobin	Antineutrophilic cytoplasmic antibodies
Urobilinogen	Cryoprotein
Porphobilinogen	Bence Jones protein
CH_{50}	Hepatitis-B surface antigen and antibody
C3	Antibodies to Jo-1
C4	Antineuronal nuclear antibodies
Carcinoembryonic antigen	Antibodies to myelin-associated glycoprotein
Serum viscosity	Antibodies to GM_1 ganglioside
Angiotensin-converting enzyme	Heavy metals in 24-hour urine specimen
Prostate-specific antigen	Cytologic examination of bronchial washings, urine, and sputum
Aldolase	

were normal. Electromyographic examination of multiple proximal and distal muscles showed abundant fibrillations and positive sharp waves; no voluntary activity was elicited from most limb muscles.

Microscopical examination of a biopsy specimen of bone marrow showed scattered plasma cells, with rare cytologic atypia and benign-appearing lymphoid aggregates but no evidence of plasma-cell myeloma. Immunofluorescence studies revealed no evidence of a clonal B-cell population. Microscopical examination of a quadriceps-muscle-biopsy specimen showed myonecrosis, denervation, and regeneration, without evidence of vasculitis or active myositis. Examination of a sural-nerve-biopsy specimen disclosed marked depletion of myelinated nerve fibers, a moderate reduction in axons, and myelin ovoids, indicative of acute axonopathy. A test for viral hepatitis C antibodies was positive; the β_2-macroglobulin was 6.9 U (normal, 0.7 to 3.4). Serum immunoelectrophoresis showed a normal IgG precipitin arc, an abnormal IgA arc, and no visible IgM arc. Agarose-gel electrophoresis revealed several bands in the gamma globulin zone; one of the bands appeared to be an IgA lambda M component, and another was an IgG kappa M component in low concentration.

No Bence Jones protein was detected in a 50-fold concentrated urine specimen.

Early in the hospital course the patient had marked autonomic instability, with a heart rate that ranged between 30 and 90 beats per minute; intermittent hypotension was managed with intravenous infusions of norepinephrine, which were followed by bouts of hypertension. Plasmapheresis was performed on five occasions, followed by questionable transitory recovery of slight movement about the shoulder girdles and elbows. Melphalan and an adreno corticosteroid medication were administered, without a decrease of the IgA level to normal. During the final week of life Staphylococcus aureus sepsis, paralytic ileus, and perforation of the urinary bladder occurred.

On the 50th hospital day the patient was alert and responded appropriately to single commands. Partial bilateral ptosis, slight limitation of upward gaze, and mild weakness of the orbicularis oculi muscles were present; the pupils were normal. The intrinsic hand and distal forearm muscles were wasted. There was 2/5 power in the deltoid and biceps muscles and in the intrinsic muscles of the left hand; no movement was detected in the other upper-extremity muscles or in the legs; the patient was areflexic. Loss of sensory responses to all stimuli extended to the levels of the mid-forearm and upper thighs.

On the 54th hospital day the patient died.

Dr. Allan H. Ropper[*]: This elderly man's basic problems were an unusual paraproteinemia and weakness due to a generalized neuropathy.

His health was stable until a maculopapular rash developed and prednisone was prescribed. Soon after the dose was tapered the first neurologic symptom, proximal weakness, occurred. On admission to another hospital for flank pain the patient reported stinging pain that shot down his legs, probably signifying a disturbance of sensory roots or ganglia. The weakness was steroid-responsive. Generalized weakness is often not evident or is disregarded in the presence of other medical diseases. When finally recognized, proximal weakness, in particular, is frequently attributed to the general debility caused by an underlying disease or to a myopathy, although neuropathies are a far more common cause of proximal weakness. Also, the patient had autonomic instability, with variations in the heart rate and blood pressure early in the illness. The triad of generalized weakness, sensory symptoms, and dysautonomia suggests a polyneuropathy rather than a myopathy, a myelopathy, or brain disease. The tempo of the progression and the subsequent electrophysiologic features will be useful in the differential diagnosis.

The flaccid, areflexic, complete limb paralysis observed on neurologic examination confirmed the clinical impression of a peripheral neuropathy. He had "no response to noxious stimuli," presumably because of paralysis but also because of severe sensory loss since he was awake and voluntarily able to blink and move his eyes. Although no measurements were made, his continued respiratory failure in the absence of parenchymal lung disease was probably also neuromuscular and related to the generalized paralysis. There are three signposts of the tempo of the neuropathy. His initial proximal weakness occurred at least one month before he entered the first hospital. Soon thereafter he was too weak to sit up or move his extremities. When he entered this hospital two months after the first weakness he was quadriplegic. This rate of progression indicated subacute generalized sensorimotor neuropathy with a more acute deterioration over a period of one or two weeks.

The electrophysiologic tests showed a severe axonal polyneuropathy (low-amplitude muscle potentials and abundant fibrillation potentials) without demyelination, since there were normal distal latencies, only minimally reduced conduction velocities, and normal blink reflexes. Several days before his death the presence of muscle wasting in the hands and forearms corroborated the axonal nature of the polyneuropathy. The

Chief of Neurology, St. Elizabeth's Hospital, Boston; professor of neurology, Tufts University School of Medicine. Currently Vice Chair of Neurology, Brigham and Women's Hospital.

best evidence for a demyelinating neuropathy was the inability to contract voluntarily some muscles that could be stimulated electrically, perhaps suggesting proximal conduction block. The inability to elicit sensory-action potentials in any nerve tested signified a sensory neuropathy distal to the dorsal-root ganglia, although not necessarily sparing the sensory roots. There were no inexcitable motor nerves. A sural-nerve biopsy showed severe large-fiber loss, which was apparently primarily axonal.

Except for the inflammatory demyelinating neuropathies, such as the Guillain-Barre syndrome, most polyneuropathies are related to medical diseases, with different causes of axonal and demyelinating forms. There are numerous causes of subacute axonal neuropathy (Table 5). The common metabolic causes of neuropathies due, for example, to diabetes or alcoholism, as well as countless other causes are not associated with this severe and relatively rapid paralysis and respiratory failure. Acute toxic neuropathy, such as that due to heavy metals, would be unlikely to progress so much under observation and was excluded by laboratory testing. Renal-failure neuropathy, which can be surprisingly rapid but infrequently so severe, occurs with renal failure more profound than occurred in this case.

Table 5 Analysis of a Motor-Sensory Polyneuropathy

Acute Disease (Days to Weeks)	
Demyelinating	*Axonal*
Guillain-Barré syndrome	Toxin-induced neuropathy
Arsenical polyneuropathy	Porphyria
	Critical-illness polyneuropathy
	Axonal Guillain-Barré syndrome
Subacute Disease (Weeks to Two Months)	
Guillain-Barré syndrome or chronic inflammatory demyelinating polyneuropathy*	Toxin- or drug-induced neuropathy
	Nutritional polyneuropathy
	Uremic polyneuropathy
	Lyme disease neuropathy
Paraproteinemic polyneuropathy	Paraneoplastic polyneuropathy
	Myeloma neuropathy
	Paraproteinemic polyneuropathy
Chronic Disease	
Chronic inflammatory demyelinating polyneuropathy*	Diabetic polyneuropathy
	Nutritional polyneuropathy
	Uremic polyneuropathy
Paraproteinemic polyneuropathy	Familial neuropathy
	Paraneoplastic polyneuropathy
	Paraproteinemic polyneuropathy

*Includes the symptomatic forms of this disorder, such as those with underlying lymphoma or systemic lupus erythematosus.

Intermittent acute porphyria must be considered, especially in view of the early autonomic instability, but the other cardinal features of porphyria or a preceding history were absent, as was porphobilinogen. Sarcoidosis and autoimmune diseases that may be associated with subacute inflammatory neuropathies were excluded by the absence of consistent laboratory or clinical features. Paracarcinomatous neuropathies are rarely so severe, and there was no evidence of cancer in this patient.

This patient's illness simulated the Guillain-Barre syndrome, the most common form of severe areflexic paralysis with a raised spinal fluid protein level[1-3]. However, that syndrome is an acute, monophasic illness with its progression arbitrarily limited to four weeks, although "chronic Guillain-Barre syndrome," now called "chronic inflammatory demyelinating polyneuropathy," typically advances over a longer period or relapses[4]. The tempo of this patient's illness was more nearly that of the subacute Guillain-Barre syndrome, which develops over four to eight weeks and may be steroid-responsive[5-7]. From a purely syndromic point of view this patient's illness fits into the category of the subacute Guillain-Barre syndrome.

These inflammatory demyelinating polyneuropathies share the features of conduction block, conduction slowing or other electrophysiologic signs of demyelination, and spinal-fluid "albuminocytologic dissociation" (elevated protein content without cells). The axonal features in this case are unusual, although there is an "axonal" Guillain-Barre syndrome, which designates a severe, rapidly progressive polyneuropathy with many electrically inexcitable nerves, few sensory features, and normal or nearly normal spinal fluid protein[8]. In many cases of what appears to be axonal Guillain-Barre syndrome it is initially demyelinating, and an electromyographic study obtained late in the course, as it was in this case, may be misleading. There were no signs of demyelination to support the typical form of the disease, and there were no inexcitable motor nerves, the progression was too slow, the sensory loss was too severe, and the cerebrospinal fluid protein level was too high for the axonal variant[9]. However, the resemblance of the findings in this case to a subacute Guillain-Barre syndrome is pivotal, because many subacute neuropathies, with or without demyelinating features, are associated with underlying systemic diseases. Rapid fluctuations as a result of changes in steroid dose have also been markers for underlying disease on occasion, although idiopathic chronic inflammatory demyelinating polyneuropathy has often responded to steroids as well. In this patient the slow evolution to profound weakness and the clinical changes with steroids compel a search for an underlying disease as the cause of the polyneuropathy.

The second major feature of the illness was an unusual IgA-lambda M component with a concentration of 1135 mg per deciliter. In view of the association of 10 percent of neuropathies with paraproteins[10] (Table 5), this paraprotein may be an important marker for a systemic disease. It had a role in the overall illness, because pyoderma gangrenosum, a nonspecific lesion typically associated with ulcerative colitis, can result from monoclonal or biclonal gammopathies, the majority of which are IgA, as in this patient[11-13].

Paraproteinemia can also be a marker for lymphoma, which in turn is rarely associated with a neuropathy resembling chronic inflammatory demyelinating polyneuropathy, but there was no evidence of lymphoma in this case. Since most

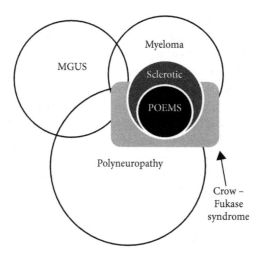

FIG 2 Interrelation between Polyneuropathy and Gammopathies.

paraproteinemias of this small magnitude do not progress to myeloma, another consideration is a polyneuropathy due to a monoclonal gammopathy of undetermined significance (MGUS). Both axonal and demyelinating neuropathies have been described with what used to be called "benign monoclonal gammopathy" (Figure 2). They tend to be chronic, predominantly sensory, distal, and mild, generally unlike the picture in this case[10,14]. Paraproteinemic neuropathies have been divided into IgM and non-IgM (IgA and IgG) categories, because half of IgM neuropathies have a characteristic insidious, predominantly sensory syndrome, with a greatly elevated spinal fluid protein level and a specific antiglycolipid antibody against myelin surface antigen, a myelin-associated glycoprotein. The non-IgM group, however, may be associated with severe weakness, and this patient conceivably had an atypical MGUS-related axonal polyneuropathy. The distinction from other paraproteinemic neuropathies depends on the absence of a biologically more complex disease, such as a plasma-cell dyscrasia.

Polyneuropathies are associated with multiple myeloma in 3 to 5 percent of the patients, although many more patients have electrophysiologic evidence of nerve disease (Figure 2)[15,16]. The most distinctive pattern in myeloma neuropathy is a sensory and autonomic syndrome due to amyloid deposition, which does not apply in this case. The other myeloma neuropathies include a distal axonal polyneuropathy with mild weakness and a sensory polyneuropathy closely resembling the paraneoplastic syndrome of Denny-Brown, both of which can occur with or without amyloid deposition. In occasional cases the disorder simulates the Guillain-Barre syndrome or chronic inflammatory demyelinating polyneuropathy. The axonal polyneuropathy of myeloma tends to affect elderly men, and in some cases it has been predominantly motor and very severe, as in this patient, with the neuropathy obscuring the underlying multiple myeloma[15-17]. The typical myeloma neuropathy is gradually progressive, distally predominant, and mild, sparing cranial nerves. It is associated with only minimal elevation of the cerebrospinal fluid protein level and is seen in cases of florid disease with high levels of paraprotein, usually over 3 g per deciliter. In many ways the axonal syndrome resembling the Guillain-Barre syndrome and the medical context in this patient resemble myeloma neuropathy, but it is difficult to make the diagnosis of multiple myeloma in this case.

Features against the diagnosis of myeloma in this case include the low concentration of paraprotein, the absence of bone pain, lytic bone lesions, hypercalcemia, and Bence Jones light chains, the normal IgG level, and the negative second bone marrow biopsy. The spinal fluid protein level was also considerably higher than is usual for myeloma neuropathies. The renal failure was mostly prerenal, a finding inconsistent with myeloma nephropathy. In favor of myeloma are the diagnosis of myeloma on the first bone marrow examination, the persistent, greatly elevated sedimentation rate, the normocytic anemia, and the unchanged paraprotein levels after treatment with melphalan, prednisone, and plasma exchange. "Smoldering" myeloma[18] requires a paraprotein level above 3 g per deciliter, but the bone lesions, renal failure, and other typical manifestations of myeloma do not develop for months or years.

There is a distinctive neuropathy associated with sclerotic myeloma or plasmacytoma. Few patients with myeloma have osteosclerotic lesions, but over half of those with sclerotic lesions have neuropathy. Furthermore, the paraprotein is usually an IgA or IgG in small concentrations, almost always with a lambda light chain,[19–21] whereas only a third of M proteins from multiple myeloma or MGUS have a lambda light chain. Of all the neuropathies with plasma-cell dyscrasias, the type associated with sclerotic myeloma is most likely to become severe, and the cerebrospinal fluid protein level tends to be very high, often over 200 mg per deciliter. Electrophysiologic studies may show demyelination with some axonal features, but a primarily axonal process with secondary segmental demyelination has been described[22] most often and might result in findings similar to those in this case.

The osteosclerotic myeloma neuropathy tends to be associated with edema and involvement of systemic organs. One particular constellation that has been highlighted consists of polyneuropathy, organomegaly or lymphadenopathy, endocrinopathy, and skin changes, mainly hyperpigmentation but also sclerodermatous thickening or papular angiomas, given the acronym POEMS[21] to signify the polyneuropathy, organomegaly, endocrinopathy, M protein, and skin changes (Figure 2). POEMS, strictly speaking, requires osteosclerotic myeloma and the four other features, but few of the patients have more than two or three of these features and the syndrome or fragments of it may occur without sclerotic myeloma. From my experience with several patients who had IGM-lambda paraproteins and skin changes, but not osteosclerotic myeloma, I cannot agree with recent studies that equate POEMS with osteosclerotic myeloma[23].

The eponym "Crow-Fukase syndrome"[24–26] does not require all the components of POEMS, occurs without sclerotic bone lesions, and includes clinical features of the syndrome beyond POEMS (Figure 2), such as fluctuating azotemia, soft-tissue and limb edema, lymphocytic infiltrates in muscle, steroid responsiveness of the neuropathy, a low serum paraprotein level, and mild bone marrow plasmacytosis,[24–27] all of which were present in this case. The two central features of the Crow-Fukase syndrome are the polyneuropathy and the lambda paraproteinemia.

May we review the radiologic findings?

Dr. Giles W. Boland: The abdominal and pelvic CT scan (Figure 1), obtained with the intravenous administration of contrast material, shows small pleural effusions and a small amount of ascites. Widespread strands of soft-tissue density consistent with edema are most notable in the subcutaneous tissues, the retroperitoneum, the abdominal and pelvic mesentery, and the presacral space. There is rectal-wall thickening, which is also consistent with edema.

Dr. Ropper: In addition to its peculiar distribution, this patient's edema was not due to congestive heart failure, water overload, or renal failure, since the sodium was 152 mmol per liter and the urea nitrogen was 128 mg per deciliter, whereas the creatinine was 1 to 2 mg per deciliter, suggesting dehydration. The small pleural effusions and ascites may have been part of the POEMS edema syndrome[28,29].

The most frequent initial findings in the Crow-Fukase syndrome[25] are related to the polyneuropathy and edema. Nail clubbing and hyperhidrosis are common but were absent in this patient. Glucose intolerance occurs in about a third of the cases. Gynecomastia and impotence, which are present in two thirds of the patients with the Crow-Fukase syndrome, are not mentioned in this case. In 95 percent of cases of the syndrome there is either an IgG or IgA lambda M component, and in about 10 percent it becomes biclonal, as it eventually did in this patient. The other hematologic characteristics of the Crow-Fukase syndrome were also present in this case: no skeletal lesions in a third to half of the cases; a low concentration of paraprotein; and normal concentrations of other immunoglobulin subclasses.

The plasma-cell excess in the Crow-Fukase syndrome varies from a mild monoclonal plasmacytosis to frank myeloma. In Japan, where myeloma is uncommon, half the patients with the Crow-Fukase syndrome have no bone lesions but do have increased numbers of plasma cells in the marrow[24,25]. Most non-Japanese patients, in contrast, have plasma-cell dyscrasias, evenly divided among sclerotic, lytic, and mixed myeloma[25]. The polyneuropathy seems to be tied to the other parts of the syndrome solely by the lambda IgA or IgG paraprotein rather than by the plasma-cell disorder. Furthermore, most patients without bone lesions have also had Castleman's disease of the lymph nodes.

In view of the findings on the first bone marrow biopsy in this case a myeloma or plasma-cell excess is very likely, probably with monoclonal lambda-producing cells. I believe that the axonal polyneuropathy was related to the paraprotein and plasma-cell disorder, and in combination with other clinical features I would link the illness to the Crow-Fukase syndrome. The case may be unique in the extreme axonal nature of the electrophysiologic findings. If this is all correct, then despite the low concentration of paraprotein and the negative second bone marrow examination this man probably had multiple myeloma. Neuropathological examination probably revealed a widespread polyneuropathy with a predominant loss of large fibers, including autonomic fibers, in view of the cardiovascular instability. If inflammation was present, it would establish the illness as a secondary inflammatory polyneuropathy.

Peripheral neuropathy associated with paraproteinemia.

Subacute large-fiber axonal polyneuropathy, with IgA-lambda light-chain myeloma.

Dr. Ann C. McKee: The examination of the specimen from the right sural nerve biopsy specimen revealed marked depletion of myelinated nerve fibers, with a normal appearance of the remaining myelin. Staining with Bodian's silver method demonstrated a marked reduction in the number of axons. Teased-fiber preparations showed no evidence of segmental demyelination. The internodal lengths did not vary, and there was no evidence of well-myelinated internodes alternating with thinly myelinated internodes, as would be expected in segmental demyelination with remyelination. There were numerous clusters of myelin ovoids, providing unequivocal evidence of active axonal degeneration (Figure 3). Evaluation of 1-micrometer epon-embedded sections (Figure 4) confirmed the severe loss of nerve fibers, with abundant connective tissue.

The findings at general autopsy were multiple myeloma with atypical plasma cells in the vertebral bone marrow, a monoclonal production of IgA lambda, and a single microscopic tumor nodule in the vertebral bone marrow.

Microscopical examination of the brain and spinal cord revealed slight lymphocytic infiltration of the leptomeninges of the brain stem and spinal cord but no evidence of a plasma-cell infiltrate or lymphoma. At the midbrain level, mild myelinated nerve-fiber loss and lymphocytic infiltration of the third cranial nerve were seen. Staining with the Bielschowsky silver method showed a reduced number of axons and occasional degenerating axons. At the root exit zone of the vagus nerve we found a small cluster of lymphocytes and severe depletion of myelinated fibers.

Examination of the posterior columns of the cervical and thoracic spinal cord showed gliosis, demyelination, and active wallerian degeneration, most severe in the fasciculus gracilis. Examination of the anterior horn cells at all levels showed pronounced central chromatolysis, with rounding of the cell-body periphery (changes

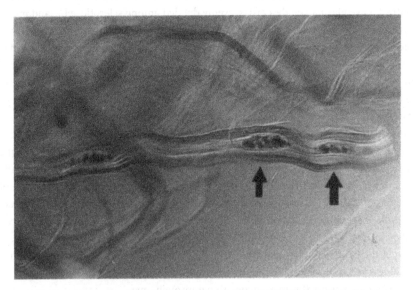

FIG 3 Active Axonal Degeneration Readily Apparent on Teased-Fiber Preparation of the Sural-Nerve-Biopsy Specimen, Showing Numerous Macrophages Containing Axonal and Myelin Debris (Arrows) (×180).

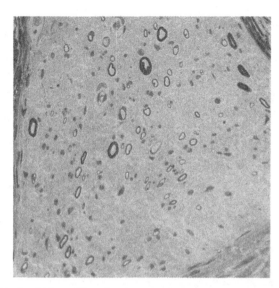

FIG 4 Section of the Sural-Nerve-Biopsy Specimen (1 micrometer, Embedded in Epon), Showing Depletion of Nerve Fibers and Abundant Connective Tissue (×360).

indicating severe axonal injury) and mild wallerian degeneration in the lateral corti-cospinal tracts with astrocytosis and macrophage infiltration. At all levels of the spinal cord there was moderate loss of myelinated nerve fibers and axons from the anterior and posterior roots. The sciatic nerve had extensive nerve-fiber loss, with scattered clusters of lymphocytes and occasional macrophages (Figure 5). The lymphocytic infil-tration was principally endoneurial and perivenular. Immunoperoxidase studies of the

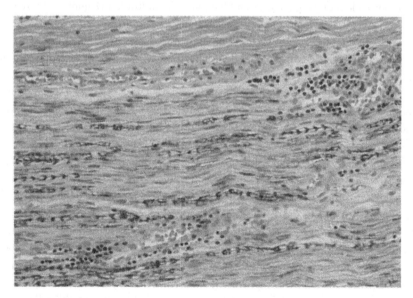

FIG 5 Extensive Perivascular Lymphocytes and Occasional Macrophages in the Endoneurium and Perineurium of the Sciatic Nerve (Luxol Fast Blue-Hematoxylin and Eosin Stain, ×180).

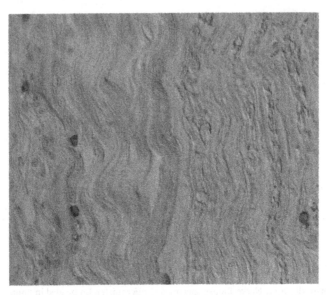

FIG 6 Immunoperoxidase-Stained Section of the Sciatic Nerve, Demonstrating Lymphocytes, Positively Stained for the T-Cell Marker UCHL1, Surrounding a Capillary in the Perineurium and Scattered throughout the Endoneurium (×480).

inflammatory infiltrate disclosed predominant T cells and occasional macrophages (Figure 6). Examination with Bielschowsky's silver stain revealed severe loss of axons, frequent beading of axons, and occasional axonal spheroids and varicosities. In the dorsal-root ganglia there were scattered nodules of Nageotte (indicators of ganglion-cell loss) and focal lymphocytic infiltrates. Examination of the sympathetic ganglia also showed loss of ganglion cells and lymphocytic infiltration (Figure 7). There was severe denervation atrophy of all the skeletal muscles sampled.

These findings indicate an extensive inflammatory polyneuritis, and the absence of pathological evidence of segmental demyelination and the unequivocal presence of active axonal degeneration indicate a primary axonopathy.

The regional pattern of alterations most closely resembles that seen in the Guillain-Barre syndrome. The involvement of the 3rd and 10th cranial nerves, motor and sensory peripheral nerves, and sensory and autonomic ganglia[30–32] as well as the presence of endoneurial and perivascular inflammatory cells, specifically T cells and macrophages, is characteristic of that disorder[32,33]. In this case, however, nerve-fiber degeneration was axonal and not directed at the myelin sheath, unlike the vast majority of cases of the Guillain-Barre syndrome. Although the demyelinating polyneuropathy of the Guillain-Barre syndrome may be accompanied by secondary wallerian degeneration,[34,35] only 11 cases of this syndrome with a primary axonopathy and little or no preceding demyelination have been reported[8,35]. Furthermore, in 9 of those 11 cases the diagnosis of a primary axonopathy was made on the basis of electrophysiologic studies, and electrophysiologic evidence of demyelination disappears in the presence of severe secondary axonal degeneration[38]. Two patients with a diagnosis of the axonal variant of the Guillain-Barre syndrome have had histologic evaluation.

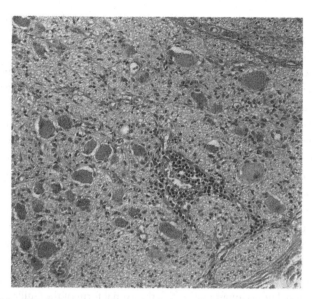

FIG 7 Loss of Ganglion Cells and Lymphocytic Infiltration in a Sympathetic Ganglion (Luxol Fast Blue-Hematoxylin and Eosin Stain, ×180).

Peroneal-nerve biopsies performed on day 30 in one patient disclosed acute axonopathy with little inflammation,[37] and examination at autopsy of another patient 26 days after the onset of symptoms[8] revealed axonal degeneration and occasional regeneration in the vagus nerves and cervical and lumbar nerve roots and axonal degeneration in the superficial peroneal and phrenic nerves; central chromatolytic changes were found in the cervical and sacral anterior horn cells. In contrast to the case under discussion, there was minimal lymphocytic infiltration. If the disorder in this case represents the axonal variant of the Guillain-Barre syndrome, not only is it unusual in its clinical presentation, but it is also the first reported case of an inflammatory polyneuropathy in this syndrome.

The other primary diagnostic consideration is a neuropathy associated with myeloma, in which there is usually segmental demyelination with secondary axonal degeneration[16,17]. In one study,[39] however, sural-nerve biopsies in four of five patients revealed only axonal degeneration. Inflammation is typically absent[16,17] and, when present, is generally minimal, consisting of scattered epineurial lymphocytes,[16,17] abnormal collections of plasma cells,[16,17] or histiocytic granulomas[41]—features absent in the case under discussion. Inflammation and neuronal loss may be found in the dorsal-root ganglia in myeloma-associated neuropathy, but they are usually limited[17]. The typical pathological features of the polyneuropathy associated with osteosclerotic myeloma are also axonal degeneration and segmental demyelination,[19,43] which some investigators believe are secondary to axonal attenuation[45]. Unlike the endoneurial and pericapillary infiltrates in this case, only mild lymphocytic infiltrates largely limited to the epineurium have been described[17,48].

This case, then, has features of both the Guillain-Barre syndrome and the neuropathy associated with myeloma, particularly the osteosclerotic form, but it is not typical of either entity. Although the case is best described as a primary axonal polyneuritis arising in association with IgA lambda myeloma, its precise classification must await future insights.

Axonal polyneuritis associated with IgA lambda multiple myeloma.

Dr. Ropper: The clinical and pathological features of this axonal polyneuritis with myeloma are unusual, if not unique. I concluded that this illness was too aberrant to be the axonal variant of the Guillain-Barre syndrome, because the weakness progressed and fluctuated subacutely over weeks and because the characteristic inexcitable nerves on electrophysiologic testing were absent. Moreover, the idiopathic or postinfectious Guillain-Barre syndrome is a clinical diagnosis, not a pathological diagnosis, and the presence of a major underlying disease that is known to be associated with polyneuropathy stretches the use of the term.

The most interesting finding, the presence of endoneurial lymphocytic infiltrates, indicates that there are several pathologically distinct acute immune polyneuropathies, one of which is the classic Guillain-Barre syndrome. These polyneuropathies are as follows: the most common typical inflammatory perivascular demyelination that has the appearance of an allergic process (classic Guillain-Barre syndrome)[31]; demyelination with minimal or no inflammation[30,32]; the axonal form of the Guillain-Barre syndrome, which is essentially noninflammatory; and as in this case an inflammatory process with active degeneration of axons as shown by myelin ovoids.

Therefore, an important feature, endoneurial inflammation, is shared with the Guillain-Barre syndrome, but it may be best to classify this patient's disease among the paraproteinemic illnesses because of the dissimilarity to any previous clinical or pathological case and the compelling connection between the polyneuropathy and the myeloma. An axonal polyneuropathy is more likely to be associated with myeloma than with the Crow-Fukase syndrome; however, most of the patients in the largest series of cases of the Crow-Fukase syndrome had some inexcitable nerves, particularly in the legs, and a number of the patients were found to have a pure axonal process on nerve biopsy[26]. The pathological findings in this case are atypical for either disease, although in occasional cases of paraproteinemic or paramyelomatous neuropathies there have been inflammatory changes,[18] and they are rarely seen in osteosclerotic myeloma[48]. These crossover cases between paraproteinemic and inflammatory axonal neuropathies are one way to relate the polyneuropathy, lambda paraproteinemia, aberrant myeloma, and systemic features. An immunologic effect of the paraprotein was possibly responsible for the nerve damage.

REFERENCES

1. Guillain G, Barre JA, Strohl A. Sur un syndrome de radiculonevrite avec hyperalbuminose du liquide cephalo-rachidien sans reaction cellulaire: remarques sur les caracteres cliniques et graphiques des reflexes tendineux. Bull Soc Med Hop Paris 1916; 40:1462–70.
2. Ropper AH, Wijdicks EFM, Truax BT. Guillain-Barre syndrome. Philadelphia: F.A. Davis, 1991.
3. Ropper AH. The Guillain-Barre syndrome. N Engl J Med 1992; 326:1130–6.
   Web of Science | Medline

4. Dyck PJ, Arnason B. Chronic inflammatory demyelinating polyradiculoneuropathy. In: Dyck PJ, Thomas PK, Lambert EH, Bunge R, eds. Peripheral neuropathy. 2nd ed. Vol. 2. Philadelphia: W.B. Saunders, 1984:2101–14.

5. Oh SJ. Subacute demyelinating polyneuropathy responding to corticosteroid treatment. Arch Neurol 1978; 35:509–16.
Web of Science | Medline

6. Hughes R, Sanders E, Hall S, Atkinson P, Colchester A, Payan P. Subacute idiopathic demyelinating polyradiculoneuropathy. Arch Neurol 1992; 49:612–16.
Web of Science | Medline

7. Hughes RAC. Guillain-Barre syndrome. London: Springer-Verlag, 1990.

8. Feasby TE, Gilbert JJ, WF Brown WF. An acute axonal form of Guillain-Barre polyneuropathy. Brain 1986; 109:1115–26.
CrossRef | Web of Science | Medline

9. AH Ropper AH. Severe acute Guillain-Barre syndrome. Neurology 1986; 36:429–32.
Web of Science | Medline

10. Kelly JJ, Kyle RA, O'Brien PC, Dyck PJ. Prevalence of monoclonal protein in peripheral neuropathy. Neurology 1981; 31:1480–3.
Web of Science | Medline

11. Powell FC, Schroeter AL, Su WP, Perry HO. Pyoderma gangrenosum and monoclonal gammopathy. Arch Dermatol 1983; 119:468–72.
CrossRef | Web of Science | Medline

12. van der Sluis I. Two cases of pyoderma (ecthyma) gangraenosum associated with the presence of an abnormal serumprotein (β2-A-paraprotein): with a review of the literature. Dermatologica 1966; 132:409–24.
CrossRef | Medline

13. Reboul M-C, Coiffet J, Forestier J-Y, Cambazard F, Coeur P, Colomb D. Pyoderma gangrenosum et gammapathie biclonale d'origine myelomateuse probable. Ann Dermatol Venereol 1981; 108:951–8.
Web of Science | Medline

14. Gosselin S, Kyle RA, Dyck PJ. Neuropathy associated with monoclonal gammopathies of undetermined significance. Ann Neurol 1991; 30:54–61.
CrossRef | Web of Science | Medline

15. Kelly JJ. Polyneuropathies associated with plasma cell dyscrasias. Semin Neurol 1987; 7:30–9.
CrossRef | Web of Science | Medline

16. Kelly JJ, Kyle RA, Miles JM, O'Brien PC, Dyck PJ. The spectrum of peripheral neuropathy in myeloma. Neurology 1981; 31:24–31.
Web of Science | Medline

17. Victor M, Banker BQ, Adams RD. The neuropathy of multiple myeloma. J Neurol Neurosurg Psychiatry 1958; 21:73–88 .
CrossRef | Web of Science | Medline

18. Kyle RA, Greipp PR. Smoldering multiple myeloma. N Engl J Med 1980; 302:1347–9.
Free Full Text | Web of Science | Medline

19. Iwashita H, Ohnishi A, Asada M, Kanazawa Y, Kuroiwa Y. Polyneuropathy, skin hyperpigmentation, edema, and hypertrichosis in localized osteosclerotic myeloma. Neurology 1977; 27:675–81.
Web of Science | Medline

20. Bardwick PA, Zvaifler NJ, Gill GN, Newman D, Greenway GD, Resnick DL. Plasma cell dyscrasia with polyneuropathy, organomegaly, endocrinopathy, M protein, and skin changes: the POEMS syndrome: report on two cases and a review of the literature. Medicine (Baltimore) 1980; 59:311–22.
Web of Science | Medline

21. Kelly JJ, Kyle RA, Miles JM, Dyck PJ. Osteosclerotic myeloma and peripheral neuropathy. Neurology 1983; 33:202–10.
Web of Science | Medline

22. Ohi T, Nukada H, Kyle RA, Dyck PJ. Detection of an axonal abnormality in myeloma neuropathy. Ann Neurol 1983; 14:120, abstract.
Web of Science

23. Miralles GD, O'Fallon JR, Talley NJ. Plasma-cell dyscrasia with polyneuropathy: the spectrum of POEMS syndrome. N Engl J Med 1992; 327:1919–23.
Free Full Text | Web of Science | Medline

24. Takatsuki K, Sanada I. Plasma cell dyscrasia with polyneuropathy and endocrine disorder: clinical and laboratory features of 109 reported cases. Jpn J Clin Oncol 1983; 13:543–55.
Web of Science | Medline

25. Nakanishi T, Sobue I, Toyokura Y. The Crow-Fukase syndrome: a study of 102 cases in Japan. Neurology 1984; 34:712–20.
Web of Science | Medline

26. Crow RS. Peripheral neuritis in myelomatosis. BMJ 1956; 2:802–4.
CrossRef | Web of Science | Medline

27. Trentham DE, Masi AT, Marker HW. Polyneuropathy and anasarca: evidence for a new connective-tissue syndrome and vasculopathic contribution. Ann Intern Med 1976; 84:271–4.
Web of Science | Medline

28. Tanaka O, Oshawa T. The POEMS syndrome: report of three cases with radiographic abnormalities. Radiologe 1984; 24:472–4.
Web of Science | Medline

29. Loeb JM, Hauger PH, Carney JD, Cooper AD. Refractory ascites due to POEMS syndrome. Gastroenterology 1989; 96:247–9.
Web of Science | Medline

30. Haymaker W, Kernohan JW. The Landry-Guillain-Barre syndrome: a clinicopathologic report of fifty fatal cases and a critique of the literature. Medicine (Baltimore) 1949; 28:59–141.
Web of Science | Medline

31. Asbury AK, Arnason BG, Adams RD. The inflammatory lesion in idiopathic polyneuritis: its role in pathogenesis. Medicine (Baltimore) 1969; 48:173–215.
CrossRef | Web of Science | Medline

32. Honavar M, Tharakan JKJ, Hughes RAC, Leibowitz S, Winer JB. A clinicopathological study of the Guillain-Barre syndrome: nine cases and literature review. Brain 1991; 114:1245–69.
CrossRef | Web of Science | Medline

33. Hughes R, Atkinson P, Coates P, Hall S, Leibowitz S. Sural nerve biopsies in Guillain-Barre syndrome: axonal degeneration and macrophage-associated demyelination and absence of cytomegalovirus genome. Muscle Nerve 1992; 15:568–75.
CrossRef | Web of Science | Medline

34. Vallat JM, Hugon J, Tabaraud F, Leboutet MJ, Chazot F, Dumas M. Quatre cas de syndrome de Guillain-Barre avec lesions axonales. Rev Neurol (Paris) 1990; 146:420–4.
Web of Science | Medline

35. van der Meche FGA, Meulstee J, Kleyweg RP. Axonal damage in Guillain-Barre syndrome. Muscle Nerve 1991; 14:997–1002.
CrossRef | Medline

36. Zochodne DW, Feasby TE, Brown WF, Gilbert JJ, Koopman WJ, Hahn AF. lnexcitable motor nerves in Guillain-Barre polyneuropathy. Can J Neurol Sci 1985; 12:205–205, abstract.
Web of Science

37. Feasby TE, Gilbert JJ, Brown WF. Acute "axonal" Guillain-Barre polyneuropathy. Neurology 1987; 37:357.
Web of Science | Medline

38. van der Meche FGA, Oomes PG, Kleyweg RP, Banffler JRJ, Meulstee J. Axonal Guillain-Barre. Neurology 1991; 41:1530–1.
Medline

39. Walsh JC. The neuropathy of multiple myeloma: an electrophysiological and histological study. Arch Neurol 1971; 25:404–14.
Web of Science | Medline

40. Vital C, Vallat JM, Deminiere C, Loubet A, Leboutet MJ. Peripheral nerve damage during multiple myeloma and Waldenstrom's macroglobulinemia: an ultrastructural and immunopathologic study. Cancer 1982; 50:1491–7.
CrossRef | Web of Science | Medline

41. Hesselvik M. Neuropathological studies on myelomatosis. Acta Neurol Scand 1969; 45:95–108.
Web of Science | Medline

42. Mayo CM, Daniels A, Barron KD. Polyneuropathy in the osteosclerotic form of multiple myeloma. Trans Am Neurol Assoc 1968; 93:240–2.
Medline

43. Gherardi R, Baudrimont M, Kujas M. Pathological findings in three non-Japanese patients with the POEMS syndrome. Virchows Arch A Pathol Anat Histopathol 1988; 413:357–65.
CrossRef | Medline

44. Ohnishi A. Geographical patterns of neuropathy: Japan. In: Asbury AK, Gilliatt RW, eds. Peripheral nerve disorders. Vol. 4, Neurology. London: Butterworths, 1984:303–19.

45. Ohi T, Kyle RA, Dyck PJ. Axonal attenuation and secondary segmental demyelination in myeloma neuropathies. Ann Neurol 1985; 17:255–61.
CrossRef | Web of Science | Medline

46. Semble EL, Challa VR, Holt DA, Pisko EJ. Light and electron microscopic findings in POEMS, or Japanese multisystem syndrome. Arthritis Rheum 1986; 29:286–91.
CrossRef | Web of Science | Medline

47. Bergouignan FX, Massonnat R, Vital C. Uncompacted lamellae in three patients with POEMS syndrome. Eur Neurol 1987; 27:173–81.
CrossRef | Web of Science | Medline

48. Morley JB, Schwieger AC. The relation between chronic polyneuropathy and osteosclerotic myeloma. J Neurol Neurosurg Psychiatry 1967; 30:432–42.
CrossRef | Web of Science | Medline

49. Carrier H, Guillaud-Barbaret C, Chazot G, Bady B, Schott B. Les neuropathies des gam-mapathies monoclonales: immunofluorescence et immunomarquage en microscopie electronique d'immunoglobulines a structure amyloide. Acta Neuropathol (Berl) 1978; 44:77–81.
CrossRef | Web of Science | Medline

CITING ARTICLES (1)

1. Cohnen M, Uppenkamp M, Meusers P, Brittinger G. POEMS-Syndrom. *Medizinische Klinik* 1998; 93:11: 678–82.
CrossRef

Perspectives and Updates

I consider this to be another case of a paraproteinemic neuropathy, similar to CPC case 7–2010, which can also be found in this book. At the time of the discussion in 1993, the condition now recognized as POEMS was called Crowe-Fukase syndrome and was difficult to differentiate from the broad category of paraproteinemic neuropathies. For those interested in the "inside baseball" of the CPCs, I now must acknowledge that I negotiated with the neuropathologists to avoid having them call the case one of axonal Guillain-Barré syndrome (GBS). I still believe I was correct, because the diagnosis of GBS would have required neglecting the IgA-lambda monoclonal protein and the overt multiple myeloma with atypical plasma cells in the vertebral bone marrow. Furthermore, the patient had unexplained edema that was similar to the ascites in the better characterized case of POEMS, 7–2010, mentioned above.

Nonetheless a careful reading of the last paragraph of the pathology discussion shows that it tries to strike a compromise between paraproteinemic neuropathy and GBS while acknowledging that the case was not typical of either entity. My addendum at the time of publication of the CPC was a polemic about why this was not GBS.

This is probably a relatively unique case. It is unlike axonal GBS because there are extensive endovascular infiltrates that are more typical of demyelinating GBS. I use the histopathology slides in lectures that I give on the subject of GBS inorder to indicate that an acute postinfectious polyneuropathy can show severe axonal degeneration (Fig. 3) with extensive infiltration of perivascular T lymphocytes and macrophages (Fig. 5). Since that earlier discussion, several articles have been published on the opposite configuration, a pauci-inflammatory GBS that may be demyelinating[1] or axonal.[2]

Allan H. Ropper

REFERENCES

1. Ropper AH, Adelman L. Early Guillain-Barré syndrome without inflammation. Arch Neurol 1992;49:979.
2. Honovar M, Tharakan JK, Hughes RAC, et al. A clinico-pathological study of Guillain-Barré syndrome: nine cases and literature review. Brain 1991;114:1245

A 49-Year-Old Man with an Intracranial Mass

PRIMARY CENTRAL NERVOUS SYSTEM LYMPHOMA

CPC 36-1994

PRESENTATION OF CASE

A 49-year-old man was admitted to the hospital because of the finding of an intracranial mass.

The patient had been well until six months earlier, when impotence developed, with absence of morning erections and diminished libido. He became fatigued and required more sleep, with decreased endurance of physical activity and cold intolerance. Two months before admission he began to experience nocturnal thirst and nocturia. Six weeks before admission he began to have increasing headaches at the vertex and occiput. He noticed that his hearing was diminished, especially on the right side, his gait became more unsteady than usual, and his vision was blurred. During several weeks before admission his thirst became increasingly severe, with polydipsia, polyuria, and anorexia, and he lost 10 kg in weight. Two weeks before admission dysarthria developed.

On the day of admission a cranial magnetic resonance imaging (MRI) examination at another hospital showed a hypothalamic tumor. A computed tomographic (CT) scan of the chest, abdomen, and pelvis was normal. A lumbar puncture yielded clear, acellular cerebrospinal fluid; the protein level was 96 mg per deciliter. The patient was referred to this hospital.

The patient was a mechanic. His wife and child were well. He had had infectious mononucleosis at the age of 18 years, which had persisted for one year. Ten years before admission he sustained frontal head trauma and a brain contusion; he was treated at another hospital during a stay of four months and experienced anosmia and gait instability thereafter. He had a smoking history of 80 pack-years. There was no history of gynecomastia, galactorrhea, mood changes, or risk factors for human immunodeficiency virus (HIV) infection.

The temperature was 37.4°C, the pulse was 88, and the respirations were 18. The blood pressure was 110/70 mm Hg.

On examination the patient appeared fatigued. General physical examination was negative except for slightly small testes and a female escutcheon; no gynecomastia was found.

On neurologic examination the patient was alert and fully oriented, with mild dysarthria. The eyes were normal except for moderate horizontal nystagmus, which was more prominent on gaze to the left. Facial movement and sensation were intact. There was marked sensorineural hearing loss on the right side; hearing was relatively intact on the left side. The remaining cranial-nerve functions were preserved. The gait was wide-based and unsteady; Romberg's test was negative. Muscle tone was normal throughout; motor power was graded 5/5 except that the left hip flexors were graded 4/5. Sensation was normal. Mild dysmetria and an intention tremor were present in the left arm; no dysdiadochokinesis was observed. The heel-to-shin test was performed well bilaterally. The deep tendon reflexes were +++ and equal except that the ankle jerks were ++; the plantar responses were flexor.

The urine had a specific gravity of 1.003 and was otherwise normal. Blood chemical and endocrine chemical findings are presented in Tables 1 and 2, respectively. Routine hematologic values were normal (hematocrit, white-cell count, platelet count, pro-thrombin time, and partial-thromboplastin time); values were also normal for uric acid, bilirubin, albumin, globulin, calcium, phosphorus, glucose, aspartate aminotrans-ferase, lactate dehydrogenase, creatine kinase, and alkaline phosphatase. Serum immu-noelectrophoresis revealed normal precipitin arcs and normal concentrations of IgG, IgA, and IgM. Agarose-gel electrophoresis showed a low-concentration band in the "slow gamma" region near its origin; the band was not identified by immunofixation, probably because of its low concentration. In a random urine specimen the sodium was 26 mmol, the potassium 16.5 mmol, and the chloride 42 mmol per liter; the osmolal-ity was 103 mOsm per kilogram. A cosyntropin (Cortrosyn) stimulation test showed that the fasting cortisol concentration was 1.7 μg per deciliter (50 nmol per liter); at 30 minutes, it was 8.5 μg per deciliter (240 nmol per liter), and at 60 minutes, 9.5 mg per

Table 1 Blood Chemical Findings.

Variable*	Value
Sodium (mmol/liter)	152
Potassium (mmol/liter)	4.5
Chloride (mmol/liter)	113
Carbon dioxide (mmol/liter)	31.1
Osmolality (mOsm/kg)	308
Angiotensin-converting enzyme (U/liter)	72.6 (normal, 10–50)
Urea nitrogen (mg/dl)†	5
Creatinine (mg/dl)†	0.8
Triglyceride (mg/dl)†	565
Cholesterol (mg/dl)†	204

*To convert values for urea nitrogen to millimoles per liter, multiply by 0.357. To convert values for creatinine to micromoles per liter, multiply by 88.4. To convert values for triglyceride to millimoles per liter, multiply by 0.01129. To convert values for cholesterol to millimoles per liter, multiply by 0.02586.
†Measured in a blood specimen obtained while the patient was not fasting.

Table 2 Serum and Plasma Endocrine Values.

Variable*	Patient	Normal Range
Testosterone (mg/dl)	10	300–1100
Follicle-stimulating hormone (U/liter)	0.3	1.6–16.8
Luteinizing hormone (U/liter)	<0.1	3.3–25
Prolactin (μg/liter)	24	0–10
Thyroid-stimulating hormone (μU/ml)	0.88	0.5–5
Total triiodothyronine (ng/dl)	96	75–195
Thyroxine (ng/dl)	3	0.8–2.7
Thyroid hormone–binding index	0.83	0.83–1.17
Somatomedin C (ng/ml)	75.6	54–328.5

*To convert values for testosterone to nanomoles per liter, multiply by 3.467. To convert values for total triiodothyronine to nanomoles per liter, multiply by 0.01536. To convert values for thyroxine to picomoles per liter, multiply by 12.87.

deciliter (260 nmol per liter). An electrocardiogram was normal except for nonspecific ST-segment and T-wave abnormalities. A test for anti-HIV antibodies was negative.

A lumbar puncture was performed (Table 3). Cytologic examination of the fluid revealed polymorphous atypical lymphoid cells suggestive of lymphoma; the predominant cells were larger than small lymphocytes. Radiographs of the chest were normal. A radionuclide scan of the head, neck, and thorax, obtained after the intravenous injection of gallium citrate Ga 67, showed no hilar or mediastinal lymphadenopathy. CT scan images of the brain (Fig. 1 and 2), obtained before and after the intravenous administration of contrast material, revealed a hyperdense, contrast-enhancing mass, 2 by 2 cm, in the region of the suprasellar cistern, optic chiasm, and hypothalamus, with thickening and enhancement of the fornices; tissue loss in the left inferior frontal lobe was noted. An MRI scan demonstrated a hyperintense signal in the hypothalamus (Fig. 3); sagittal T_1-weighted images obtained after the intravenous administration of gadolinium revealed enhancement of a suprasellar mass with infiltration of contiguous structures (Fig. 4). A neuro-ophthalmologic consultant found that the best corrected visual acuity was 20/40 in the right eye and 20/20 in the left eye; color vision was normal. The anterior segments of both eyes were normal on slit-lamp examination. There was a temporal paracentral scotoma in the visual field of the right eye; a dilated-fundus examination revealed fibrous strands and acellular debris in the vitreous of the right eye. No optic atrophy, papilledema, or retinal or choroidal infiltrates were seen. The findings were considered inadequate to explain the extent of the impaired vision in the right eye.

During the first hospital day the fluid intake was 3900 ml, and the urinary volume 4000 ml. Desmopressin acetate was administered intranasally in the evening, without satisfactory control. On the second hospital day the dose was increased; the sodium concentration became normal on the third hospital day and remained normal thereafter. The patient was afebrile. The hemodynamic status was stable, and no corticosteroid replacement therapy was administered. Oxycodone–acetaminophen was

Table 3 Findings on Lumbar Puncture.

Variable*	Finding
Fluid characteristics	Clear, colorless
Initial pressure (mm H$_2$O)	180
White-cell count (per mm^3)	2
Differential count (%)	
Neutrophils	2
Lymphocytes	86
Atypical lymphocytes	4
Monocytes	4
Nonhematic cells	4
Glucose (mg/dl)	52
Protein (mg/dl)	59
Albumin	46
IgG (mg/dl)	5.9
Agarose-gel electrophoresis (in 80-fold concentrate)	No oligoclonal bands
Microorganisms	0
Alpha-fetoprotein (IU/ml)	<10 (normal, <12.8)
Chorionic gonadotropin, beta subunit (IU/liter)	<2.5 (normal, not defined)
Culture	Sterile

*To convert values for glucose to millimoles per liter, multiply by 0.05551.

prescribed for headaches, and prochlorperazine was given for intermittent nausea and vomiting.

A diagnostic procedure was performed.

DIFFERENTIAL DIAGNOSIS

DR. MARTIN A. SAMUELS[*]: In this 49-year-old man the onset of impotence and decreased libido, with an absence of morning erections, occurred six months before admission, suggesting a neurologic disease. When nocturnal thirst and nocturia developed four months later, one might have considered diabetes mellitus or diabetes insipidus. Even though no studies were performed at that time, diabetes insipidus was more likely, since impotence due to the neuropathy of diabetes mellitus is rarely seen at the time of presentation of the disease and would not cause a reduction in libido. Six weeks before admission the illness entered a subacute, clearly neurologic phase, with

---

[*] Chief of neurology, Brigham and Women's Hospital; director, Harvard–Longwood Neurology Training Program; professor of neurology, Harvard Medical School. Currently Chair, Department of Neurology, Brigham and Women's Hospital.

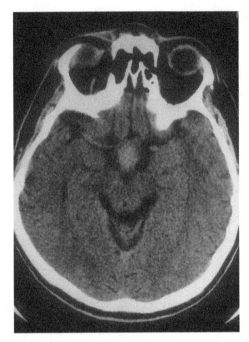

FIG 1 Axial CT Image of the Brain before the Intravenous Administration of Iodinated Contrast Material, Demonstrating a Hyperdense Mass Centered in the Suprasellar Cistem.

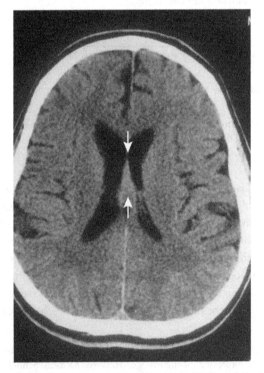

FIG 2 Axial CT Image before the Intravenous Administration of Iodinated Contrast Material, Showing Thickening and Hyperdensity of the Fomix (Arrows).

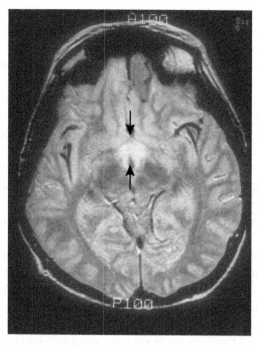

FIG 3 Proton-Density–Weighted MRI Image, Demonstrating an Abnormal, Hyperintense Signal Infiltrating the Hypothalamus (Arrows).

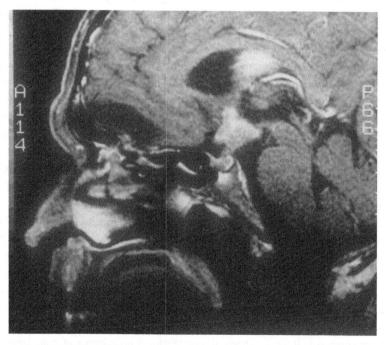

FIG 4 Sagittal T_1-Weighted MRI Image after the Intravenous Administration of Gadolinium–Pentetic Acid Contrast Material, Revealing an Enhanced Suprasellar Mass Infiltrating Contiguous Structures, Including the Pituitary Infundibulum, Mamillary Bodies, Tuber Cinereum, Optic Chiasm, and Fornix.

headache, gait difficulty, and visual blurring. The assumed diabetes insipidus worsened, and the patient lost 10 kg in weight. Although he had experienced chronic gait instability and anosmia since a severe head injury 10 years earlier, his gait became more unsteady than usual during this more aggressive phase of the illness. The hearing loss provides an important clue, indicating that the disease was not due to a single localized process involving the pituitary gland or hypothalamus, or both. The marked asymmetry of the hearing loss suggests a malfunction of the cochlear nerve rather than the central nervous system auditory pathways. That observation, combined with the evidence that the brunt of the disease occurred in the pituitary gland or hypothalamus, or both, suggests that the cochlear nerve dysfunction was caused by infiltration of right cranial nerve VIII by cells that reached it by way of the spinal fluid. The dysarthria may also have been related to a similar process involving cranial nerves IX, X, and XII, although that hypothesis is less certain since the precise nature of the dysarthria is not described.

After a brief evaluation at another hospital revealed the expected hypothalamic lesion, the patient was transferred to this hospital. It is important that there was no definite evidence of an immunocompromised state. In particular, HIV testing was negative. Of interest is the history of severe infectious mononucleosis. I shall mention later the possible role of the Epstein—Barr virus in this patient's illness. His history of heavy smoking is a source of concern, but an extensive search for a lung tumor was negative. The remote history of severe head trauma is important only in that the recent illness worsened some of his chronic deficits, such as his unsteady gait. The remnants of that earlier injury were visible on neuroimaging but ought to have been easily distinguishable from the new disease.

The neurologic and neuro-ophthalmologic examination at this hospital served only to reinforce what was already known from the history—namely, that there was involvement of the hypothalamic–pituitary axis and neighboring structures, in particular the optic nerves. The endocrine values (Table 2) documented the presence of diabetes insipidus and hypothalamic failure. On stimulation with 1–24 corticotropin, a synthetic subunit of adrenocorticotropic hormone, the adrenal glands responded with the release of cortisol. The slightly elevated prolactin level, however, suggests that the pituitary gland was capable of releasing prolactin and perhaps too much, presumably because of inadequate delivery of the prolactin-inhibitory hormone (dopamine) from the diseased hypothalamus.

Another spinal fluid analysis again showed an elevated protein level, and cytologic examination revealed abnormal lymphocytes. There is no mention of whether they were B or T lymphocytes or whether they were monoclonal. It is now possible to use the polymerase chain reaction to amplify B-cell immunoglobulin gene rearrangements and distinguish monoclonal neoplastic lymphoid proliferation from a reactive spinal fluid pleocytosis, but that test apparently was not done in this case. There were no abnormal immunoglobulin levels in the spinal fluid or blood.

An extensive search for a systemic disease disclosed no evidence of granulomatous, infectious, or neoplastic disease. However, repeated neuroimaging studies with CT and MRI scans showed a lesion in the expected location. May we review the imaging studies?

DR. BRADLEY R. BUCHBINDER: An axial CT image of the brain before the administration of contrast material demonstrates a round, hyperdense mass centered in the suprasellar region (Fig. 1). A more superior slice at the level of the lateral ventricles shows thickening and slight hyperdensity of the fornices (Fig. 2). After the intravenous administration of iodinated contrast material, both the suprasellar mass and the forniceal thickening were enhanced homogeneously. Axial proton-density–weighted MRI demonstrates hyperintensity within the suprasellar mass and the hypothalamus (Fig. 3). Signal abnormalities are present in the inferior frontal lobes, a finding consistent with remote post-traumatic tissue loss and gliosis. In contrast to the proton-density–weighted hyperintensity, the suprasellar mass is slightly hypointense on T_2-weighted images. T_1-weighted imaging in the sagittal plane after the intravenous administration of gadolinium paramagnetic contrast material (Fig. 4) demonstrates that the suprasellar mass involved many contiguous structures, including the mamillary bodies, tuber cinereum, pituitary infundibulum, optic chiasm, and hypothalamus, with apparent spread along the columns and bodies of the fornices. The pituitary gland is normal. Other images show involvement of the prechiasmatic right optic nerve.

DR. SAMUELS: Having seen the imaging studies, I am reminded of the perhaps apocryphal story of the famous neurologist who was asked to give a differential diagnosis in a particularly complicated case and responded, "I don't know what you mean by a differential diagnosis. If you wish, I can give the right diagnosis and a list of wrong diagnoses." It appears obvious to me that this patient had a central nervous system lymphoma occurring in the context of an immunocompetent host. What, then, are the "wrong" diagnoses?

The diagnosis is *not* an intracranial germ-cell tumor, such as a germinoma, teratoma, embryonal carcinoma, yolk-sac tumor, or choriocarcinoma,[1] which could involve the hypothalamus, although the posterior third ventricle is a more common location. Tumors in this category could spread by spinal fluid pathways and seed cranial nerves. However, the age of this patient argues powerfully against a germ-cell tumor, and the absence of production of either alpha-fetoprotein or the beta subunit of chorionic gonadotropin is evidence against a yolk-sac tumor and choriocarcinoma, respectively.

This was also *not* a metastatic tumor. There was no evidence of a primary tumor elsewhere despite extensive efforts to find one. In addition, the pattern of growth and spread of this lesion along the fornices and diffusely into the corpus callosum, as well as the occurrence of drop metastases by way of the cerebrospinal fluid to cranial nerves, would be extremely atypical for any form of metastatic tumor.

This was *not* infundibulohypophysitis, a cryptogenic inflammatory disease with infiltration of the neurohypophysis by T lymphocytes.[2] This rare disorder can cause diabetes insipidus and perhaps even minor additional neuroendocrine disturbances as well as loss of the normal hyperintense signal of the neurohypophysis seen on T_1-weighted MRI. However, infundibulohypophysitis never acts as aggressively as this patient's lesion did and would not infiltrate the fornix or produce nerve deafness.

This was *not* a form of granulomatous disease. Infectious granulomatous disease of the leptomeninges, such as tuberculosis, syphilis, and fungal diseases, could involve the infundibulum and infiltrate cranial nerves, but such involvement would produce a marked cerebrospinal fluid pleocytosis and a much higher spinal fluid protein level, and the patient would almost certainly have had a systemic illness probably involving the lungs.

Of all the illnesses that this patient's disorder was not, perhaps the most compelling is histiocytosis X, which usually involves multiple organs but may be limited to the nervous system, particularly in the Letterer–Siwe variety. When the nervous system is involved, the hypothalamus and neighboring structures are the principal sites, with the development of diabetes insipidus and other neuroendocrine abnormalities. The leptomeninges may be widely infiltrated by abnormal histiocytes, producing cranial-nerve and other nerve palsies. However, nearly all patients with histiocytosis are children, and the spinal fluid cytologic pattern in this case suggested that the abnormal cell was a medium-sized lymphocyte rather than a histiocyte or monocyte. Of most importance, the subacute course of this patient's illness, in contrast to the usual indolent course of histiocytosis X, suggests a rapidly proliferating tumor. Nonetheless, the distinction between histiocytosis X and lymphoma may be difficult, and some observers believe that histiocytosis X is a proliferative disease in the monocyte line that may transform into a neoplasm such as monocytic leukemia.

Lastly, this patient's disease was *not* sarcoidosis, even though the serum angiotensin-converting–enzyme level was slightly elevated. Sarcoidosis is nearly always mentioned in the differential diagnosis of a mysterious disorder of the nervous system and is nearly always the wrong diagnosis, particularly when there is no evidence of systemic involvement, as was true in this case. The prevalence of neurologic symptoms in sarcoidosis is about 5 percent, but the neurologic effects are the presenting feature of the illness in only half this small number.[3] When sarcoidosis affects the nervous system, it involves the leptomeninges, with a predilection for the area of the infundibulum. It can produce hypothalamic failure and various cranial-nerve palsies, including nerve-VIII palsy, although involvement of nerve VII is far more common. However, sarcoidosis would not spread aggressively into the fornices and corpus callosum. Furthermore, extensive studies to uncover hilar lymphadenopathy, even with use of a gallium scan, were negative in this patient. The angiotensin-converting–enzyme level may be elevated for many reasons other than sarcoidosis, including various tumors. A very elevated spinal fluid level of angiotensin-converting enzyme would have been more suggestive of sarcoidosis, but a test for it was not done.

Unfortunately, there is no escape from the "right" diagnosis of central nervous system lymphoma. Both the hyperintensity of the lesion demonstrated on CT scanning with enhancement and the isointensity with brain substance of the center of the lesion on T_2-weighted MRI suggest a highly cellular lesion, typical of lymphoma. The pattern of diffuse spread along the fornix into the corpus callosum and the probable drop metastases along cerebrospinal fluid pathways also are characteristic.

The cell of origin of primary central nervous system lymphoma is a lymphocyte, usually a B cell, but up to a third of primary central nervous system lymphomas are T-cell lymphomas, a much higher proportion than is seen in cases of systemic lymphoma. Primary central nervous system lymphoma has been increasing markedly in frequency, from about 1 percent to 3 percent of all intracranial neoplasms. Part of this increased frequency is attributable to the increase in HIV infections, but for unknown reasons the disease is also increasing greatly among HIV-negative people.[4–7]

Among immunocompromised patients primary central nervous system lymphoma is a major problem. Such patients include those with congenital immunodeficiencies, immunoglobulin A deficiency, combined immunodeficiency syndrome, and immunodeficiency associated with systemic lupus erythematosus and rheumatoid arthritis; organ-transplant recipients; and patients with the acquired immunodeficiency syndrome (AIDS). The tumor cells in lymphomas that arise in immunocompromised patients are usually polyclonal, tend to have high-grade histologic characteristics (i.e., immunoblastic and small, noncleaved cells), and contain Epstein–Barr virus genomic material.

Treatment for primary central nervous system lymphoma depends on whether it arises in a normal or immunocompromised host.[8] Treatment of immunocompromised patients is aimed at reversing the immunosuppression. If it is reversed, the tumor may regress. In patients with AIDS-associated primary central nervous system lymphoma, therapy of this type is not possible and the prognosis is very poor, with an average survival of only 2½ months despite the use of corticosteroids followed by cranial irradiation. In immunocompetent patients the tumors are usually monoclonal, large-cell lymphomas of B-cell origin with a low-grade histologic appearance and no evidence of Epstein–Barr virus infection. Chemotherapy, most often with high-dose intravenous, intrathecal, or intraventricular methotrexate, followed by radiotherapy, with about 4000 cGy to the whole brain plus a boost of about 1500 cGy to the mass, has resulted in a mean survival of about 3½ years, a substantial improvement over the mean survival of about 1½ years in patients treated with radiation therapy alone. Other agents, such as high-dose cytarabine and cyclophosphamide, have also been used either alone or in combination.

In conclusion, I believe that the diagnostic test was a stereotactic brain biopsy and the diagnosis is primary central nervous system large-cell lymphoma, B-cell type.

CLINICAL DIAGNOSIS

Probable lymphoma of the brain.

DR. MARTIN A. SAMUELS'S DIAGNOSIS

Primary central nervous system large-cell lymphoma, B-cell type.

PATHOLOGICAL DISCUSSION

DR. SUZANNE DE LA MONTE: The cerebrospinal fluid specimen received for cytologic examination was markedly cellular and contained a pleomorphic population of lymphomononuclear cells composed of mature lymphocytes, monocytes, and scattered atypical lymphocytes. The atypical lymphocytes were characterized by striking nuclear folding and irregularity, with tulip-like silhouettes, large prominent nucleoli, and hyperchromasia. These features suggested the diagnosis of a malignant lymphoma, but immunocytochemical staining failed to demonstrate a predominance of expression of either kappa- or lambda-light-chain immunoglobulin in the atypical lymphoid cells.

The diagnostic procedure was a stereotactic biopsy of the hypothalamus. Histologic sections of the 3-mm³ specimen revealed a diffuse infiltrate of neoplastic mononuclear cells with irregular nuclei and scanty cytoplasm (Fig. 5). The neoplastic cells were distributed throughout the neuropil, without a clear vasculocentric arrangement. The tumor cells were admixed with small mature lymphocytes. Immunohistochemical staining demonstrated leukocyte–common antigen immunoreactivity in all the infiltrating cells. Virtually all the neoplastic cells were also immunoreactive with the B-1, pan–B-lymphocyte marker, CD20 (Fig. 6); immunoreactive, small mature T cells accounted for a very small proportion of the infiltrating mononuclear-cell population. Most of the neoplastic cells had immunoreactivity for kappa-light-chain immunoglobulin (Fig. 7), whereas immunoreactivity for lambda immunoglobulin was detected only in small lymphocytes scattered throughout the tumor or associated with blood vessels. Immunostaining for glial fibrillary acidic protein (GFAP) revealed reactive glial fibers distributed among the neoplastic cells, but none of the neoplastic cells had positive staining for GFAP. The diagnosis was primary diffuse large-cell malignant lymphoma of the central nervous system, B-cell type, with expression of kappa-light-chain immunoglobulin.

Most primary central nervous system lymphomas are of the high-grade immunoblastic or diffuse large-cell type with a B-cell immunophenotype.[9–12] Despite the high-grade histopathologic features, many primary central nervous system lymphomas are arrested at relatively mature stages of differentiation, as evidenced by immunoreactivity for FMC7 and the presence of light-chain and heavy-chain immunoreactivity.[12] Primary

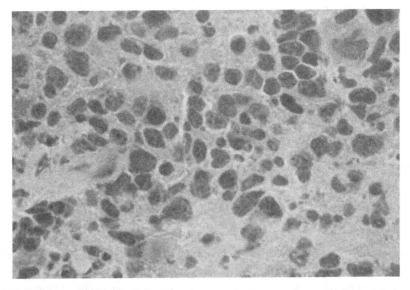

FIG 5 Brain-Biopsy Specimen (×355).
There is a diffuse infiltrate of malignant neoplastic mononuclear cells with dense chromatin, mixed with occasional small mature lymphocytes.

FIG 6 B-1, Pan–B-Lymphocyte Immunoreactivity (CD20) in Most of the Neoplastic Cells (Immunoperoxidase, ×225).

central nervous system lymphomas are largely clonal on the basis of their monotypic expression of either kappa- or lambda-light-chain immunoglobulin,[12] as demonstrated in the case under discussion. Molecular studies have also demonstrated consistent profiles of light-chain and heavy-chain immunoglobulin gene rearrangements in primary, recurrent, and metastatic central nervous system lymphomas.[12–14] Interpretation of biopsy and cerebrospinal fluid cytologic specimens should therefore include evaluation

FIG 7 Intense Immunoreactivity for Kappa Light Chain Throughout the Tumor (Immunoperoxidase, ×225).

of immunohistochemical markers to demonstrate the largely monomorphous and probably clonal nature of the neoplastic lymphomononuclear-cell infiltrates. Molecular analysis of the immunoglobulin gene rearrangement is being used with increasing regularity to aid in the diagnosis. However, molecular techniques alone are diagnostically unreliable because of the frequent admixture of non-neoplastic mononuclear cells. In addition, Epstein–Barr virus–associated polyclonal lymphoproliferative lesions, which may be clinically and histopathologically indistinguishable from malignant lymphoma, frequently develop in immunosuppressed patients.[15,16] Another potential adjunctive marker of central nervous system lymphoma is an elevated beta$_2$-microglobulin concentration (> 160 nmol per liter) in cerebrospinal fluid.[17]

DR. LAWRENCE CHER: After the diagnosis the patient received intravenously administered high-dose methotrexate, which is our current treatment for primary central nervous system lymphoma. His hearing loss, gait abnormality, and headaches have resolved, and his subjective visual impairment has improved. An MRI scan after six cycles of therapy showed complete resolution of the enhancing tumor, with an area of T$_2$-weighted bright signal within the hypothalamus. The patient continues to require replacement therapy for hypothyroidism, adrenocortical insufficiency, and hypogonadism.

The therapy for primary central nervous system lymphoma has changed substantially in the past decade. The median survival has been only about 13 months after radiation therapy alone.[18] Recently, the use of chemotherapy has been highlighted, but standard protocols for non-Hodgkin's lymphoma are not of benefit,[19] probably because of poor penetration of the central nervous system by the drugs. Regimens that involve agents known to enter the central nervous system prolong the median survival or disease-free interval to between 40 and 45 months. Almost all these regimens have been used in conjunction with radiation therapy. Morbidity from radiation encephalopathy can occur in long-term survivors.

At this hospital, experience with methotrexate treatment before radiotherapy has shown the benefit of this approach in the treatment of primary central nervous system lymphoma.[20–22] Neuwelt et al.,[23] however, achieved similarly beneficial results using intravenous and intraarterial chemotherapy with intraarterial blood–brain barrier modification and without radiation therapy. Our initial experience has suggested that high-dose methotrexate-based regimens with leucovorin rescue may produce a similar disease-free interval with minimal toxicity.[24] This treatment achieves uniform central nervous system and cerebrospinal fluid levels throughout the neuraxis and when given without radiation is only rarely associated with methotrexate leukoencephalopathy.

In this patient the methotrexate therapy was complicated by diabetes insipidus, creating a challenge in management. To prevent crystallization of methotrexate within the renal tubules and to promote its renal excretion, aggressive hydration with intravenously administered fluids and sodium bicarbonate and alkalinization of the urine are mandatory. The sodium load, however, can induce polyuria and hyperosmolality. Desmopressin acetate can reduce urine flow and methotrexate excretion, but it increases the likelihood of toxicity. We plan to continue maintenance therapy at three-month intervals and administer radiation treatment only if the tumor recurs.

ANATOMICAL DIAGNOSIS

Primary malignant lymphoma of the central nervous system, diffuse large-cell B-cell type, with kappa-light-chain immunoglobulin.

REFERENCES

1. Jennings MT, Gelman R, Hochberg F. Intracranial germ-cell tumors: natural history and pathogenesis. J Neurosurg 1985;63:155–67.
2. Imura H, Nakao K, Shimatsu A, et al. Lymphocytic infundibuloneurohypophysitis as a cause of central diabetes insipidus. N Engl J Med 1993;329: 683–9.
3. Stern BJ. Neurosarcoidosis. Neurol Chron 1992;2:1–6.
4. De Angelis LM. Primary central nervous system lymphoma. In: DeVita VT, Hellman S, Rosenberg SA, eds. Cancer: principles and practice of oncology. Update, Vol. 6, No. 11, Philadelphia: J.B. Lippincott, 1992:6–13.
5. Fine HA, Mayer RJ. Primary central nervous system lymphoma. Ann Intern Med 1993;119:1093–104.
6. Hochberg FH, Miller DC. Primary central nervous system lymphoma. J Neurosurg 1988;68:835–53.
7. O'Neill BP, Illig JJ. Primary central nervous system lymphoma. Mayo Clin Proc 1989;64:1005–20.
8. Hochberg FH, Loeffler JS, Prados M. The therapy of primary brain lymphoma. J Neurooncol 1991;10:191–201.
9. Kanavaros P, Mikol J, Nemeth J, et al. Stereotactic biopsy diagnosis of primary non-Hodgkin's lymphoma of the central nervous system: a histological and immunohistochemical study. Pathol Res Pract 1990;186:459–66.
10. Murphy JK, O'Brien CJ, Ironside JW. Morphologic and immunophenotypic characterization of primary brain lymphomas using paraffin-embedded tissue. Histopathology 1989;15:449–60.
11. Chang KL, Flaris N, Hickey WF, Johnson RM, Meyer JS, Weiss LM. Brain lymphomas of immunocompetent and immunocompromised patients: study of the association with Epstein-Barr virus. Mod Pathol 1993;6:427–32.
12. Smith WJ, Garson JA, Bourne SP, Kemshead JT, Coakham HB. Immunoglobulin gene rearrangement and antigenic profile confirm B cell origin of primary cerebral lymphoma and indicate a mature phenotype. J Clin Pathol 1988;41:128–32.
13. Kumanishi T, Washiyama K, Nishiyama A, Abe S, Saito T, Ichikawa T. Primary malignant lymphoma of the brain: demonstration of immunoglobulin gene rearrangements in four cases by the Southern blot hybridization technique. Acta Neuropathol (Berl) 1989;79:23–6.
14. Shibata D, Nichols P, Sherrod A, Rabinowitz A, Bernstein-Singer L, Hu E. Detection of occult CNS involvement of follicular small cleaved lymphoma by the polymerase chain reaction. Mod Pathol 1990;3:71–5.
15. Joshi VV, Kauffman S, Oleske JM, et al. Polyclonal polymorphic B-cell lymphoproliferative disorder with prominent pulmonary involvement in children with acquired immune deficiency syndrome. Cancer 1987;59:1455–62.
16. Cinque P, Brytting M, Vago L, et al. Epstein-Barr virus DNA in cerebrospinal fluid from patients with AIDS-related primary lymphoma of the central nervous system. Lancet 1993;342:398–401.

17. Hansen PB, Kjeldsen L, Dalhoff K, Olesen B. Cerebrospinal fluid beta-2-microglobulin in adult patients with acute leukemia or lymphoma: a useful marker of early diagnosis and monitoring of CNS-involvement. Acta Neurol Scand 1992;85:224–7.

18. Nelson DF, Martz KL, Bonner H, et al. Non-Hodgkin's lymphoma of the brain: can high dose, large volume radiation therapy improve survival? Report on a prospective trial by the Radiation Therapy Oncology Group (RTOG): RTOG 8315. Int J Radiol Oncol Biol Phys 1992;23:9–17.

19. Lachance DH, Gockerman J, Halperin E, et al. Cyclophosphamide, doxorubicin, vincristine, and prednisone (CHOP) for primary central nervous system lymphoma (PCNSL): short-duration response, multi-focal intracerebral recurrence preceding radiotherapy. Neurology 1992;42:Suppl 3:343, abstract.

20. Gabbai AA, Hochberg FH, Linggood RM, Bashir R, Hotleman K. Highdose methotrexate for non-AIDS primary central nervous system lymphoma: report of 13 cases. J Neurosurg 1989;70:190–4.

21. Glass J. Pre-irradiation-methotrexate chemotherapy of primary central nervous system: long-term outcome. J Neurosurg 1994; 81: 188–95.

22. Glass J, Gruber ML, Hochberg FH. Chemotherapy of primary central nervous system lymphoma (PCNSL) with MCHOD (methotrexate [MTX], cyclophosphamide, adriamycin, vincristine, dexamethasone) prior to radiation therapy (RT). Neurology 1993;43:Suppl 2:A209. abstract.

23. Neuwelt EA, Goldman DL, Dahlborg SA, et al. Primary CNS lymphoma treated with osmotic blood-brain barrier disruption: prolonged survival and preservation of cognitive function. J Clin Oncol 1991;9:1580–90.

24. Cher L, Glass J, Hochberg FH. Therapy of primary central nervous system lymphoma (PCNSL) with methotrexate (MTX)-based intravenous chemotherapy (MBISC) and deferred whole-brain radiation therapy (WBRT). Neurology 1994;44:Suppl 2:A378–A379, abstract.

The Massachusetts General Hospital wishes to acknowledge the generous support of Glaxo Inc., whose sponsorship makes possible the continued preparation of the Case Records.

Perspectives and Updates

What was obvious to me when I was 17 years younger seems somewhat more nuanced to me today. Looking at this unusual case in retrospect, I wonder whether both I and the pathologists were unable to make the correct diagnosis.

The neuroendocrine aspect of the presentation was and is rather straightforward, though its initial presentation was certainly not an easy one to recognize. A man in his late 40s develops erectile dysfunction with decreased libido. As an aside, it is interesting that what was called impotence then is now called erectile dysfunction, presumably as a manifestation of political correctness ("impotence" sounds vaguely characterologic whereas "erectile dysfunction" sounds medical). In any case, decreased libido in a 49-year-old man would hardly cause the primary care doctor to raise the question of a brain tumor. In fact, only an infinitesimal number of men with this complaint will ever be found to have any diagnosable medical illness. Depression is commonly considered likely, but simple aging, anxiety, and distraction by other matters (e.g., finances, work, and satisfaction with partner) are probably the most common causes of this complaint. Another common phenomenon is what I call the "failed athlete syndrome," by which I mean the exaggerated memory of one's formal prowess as compared with the realities of the moment. Sexual prowess is perhaps the most common capacity that men exaggerate in memory. In this case, it was only when unequivocal neuroendocrine symptoms developed (nocturnal thirst, asymmetrical hearing loss, and visual blurring) that a pathological process in the hypothalamus and meninges became obvious. The MRI, electrolytes, and endocrine studies confirmed this suspicion.

I confidently discarded the history of Epstein-Barr virus infection, arguing that EBV-positive lymphomas were seen only in the context of HIV infection, which did not apply to this patient. I did not acknowledge that a primary CNS lymphoma presenting with a hypothalamic syndrome would be very rare. Most lymphomas of the CNS are periventricular, not infundicular.

What I did not mention was that an EBV infection that produced such a picture, now known as lymphomatous granulomatosis (Liebow disease), was described in 1972.[1] This is a lymphoproliferative disorder that most commonly affects the lung, but primary CNS forms of the disease exist.[2] It shares many of the characteristics of post-transplantation lymphoproliferative disease and is one of the angiocentric lymphoproliferative processes. Care must be taken not to confuse this illness with Castleman disease, which is caused by human herpesvirus 8, the Kaposi sarcoma–associated virus. Castleman disease is probably caused by overproduction of the cytokine IL-6; as such, it usually presents with a systemic syndrome of microcytic anemia, fevers, and weight loss. It can be unicentric or polycentric and can affect the nervous system, but a hypothalamic syndrome of this type would be highly atypical.

There continues to be a disconcerting increase in prim ary CNS lymphoma, which is not completely explained by lymphomas caused by HIV. Could EBV and other viral infections account for this increase in incidence? Subtle immune deficiencies have been demonstrated in some HIV-negative patients with lymphoproliferative disease of this type. This patient's history of infection with EBV raises the question of whether his was indeed such a case.

Martin A. Samuels

REFERENCES

1. Liebow AA, Carrington CR, Friedman PJ. Lymphomatoid granulomatoisis. Hum Pathol 1972; 3:457–558.
2. Patsalides AD, Atac, G, Hedge U, Janik J, Grand N, Jaffe ES, Dwyer A, Patrones NJ, Wilson WH. Lymphomatous granulomatosis: abnormalities of the brain at MR imaging. Radiology 2005; 237;266–73.

An 18-Year-Old Man with Headache, Ataxia and Slurred Speech

Q FEVER CEREBELLITIS
CPC 38-1996

PRESENTATION OF CASE

An 18-year-old right-handed man was admitted to the hospital because of severe, persistent headache and the development of ataxia and slurred speech.

The patient had been in good health until one week earlier, when he awoke with severe retro-orbital pain, bilateral frontal headache, and pain at the base of the skull, with photophobia. His pains were similar to those he had experienced during repeated bouts of sinusitis and occasional ear infections since the age of 12 years but were much more severe. Thereafter, the headache and retro-orbital pain awakened him from sleep, and he received minor relief from the use of ibuprofen. Four days before admission, his physician prescribed the patient's customary treatment of amoxicillin and an antihistamine, but on the next day his headache worsened. He vomited once and felt weak. He began to have slightly slurred speech, with unsteadiness on walking and shaking on reaching for objects. One day before admission, he had coryza, nasal stuffiness, and a dry cough. He was referred to this hospital.

The patient was a high-school student who worked as a volunteer providing meals to children and cleaning public parks in Boston during the summer. He had received measles vaccine one year earlier. There was no history of insect bites, exposure to animals, meningitis, trauma, pharyngitis, stiff neck, vertigo, fever, chills, sweats, diplopia or other visual symptoms, dysarthria, dysphagia, paresthesias, focal weakness, use of tobacco, use of alcohol or illicit drugs, recent travel, risk factors for human immunodeficiency virus (HIV) infection, or contact with ill persons.

The temperature was 36.7°C, the pulse was 67, and the respirations were 16. The blood pressure was 115/65 mm Hg.

Examination disclosed bilateral mild conjunctival injection, with edema of the eyelids and a clear, mucoid nasal discharge. No rash or lymphadenopathy was found. The neck was supple. The lungs, heart, abdomen, and arms and legs were normal.

On neurologic examination the patient was alert and oriented; he remembered two of three objects at five minutes. His speech was fluent, with mild dysarthria but no aphasia. Cranial-nerve functions were preserved. There was mild left pronator drift, with a slight increase in tone in both arms and both legs; muscle power was 5/5 throughout. Sensation was intact on testing with light touch, pinprick, and vibration. Slight dysmetria was noted on finger-to-nose testing bilaterally, with a slight overshoot on the evaluation of coordination. Movements of the left fingers were rapid and normal, but those of the right fingers were slightly slower and less accurate. There was slight ataxia on heel–shin testing bilaterally, and rapid alternating movements were slightly clumsy on both sides. The deep-tendon reflexes were ++ and equal; the plantar reflexes were flexor. His gait was wide-based, with a decreased arm swing; he performed tandem walking with minimal unsteadiness and walked in tandem backward. Romberg's test was negative.

The urine was normal. The hematocrit was 43.7 percent; the white-cell count was 7600 per cubic millimeter, with 67 percent neutrophils, 18 percent lymphocytes, 12 percent monocytes, and 3 percent eosinophils. The platelet count was 211,000 per cubic millimeter.

The glucose level was 113 mg per deciliter (6.27 mmol per liter); the values for urea nitrogen, creatinine, total bilirubin, total protein, albumin, globulin, electrolytes, amylase, aspartate aminotransferase, and lactate dehydrogenase were normal. Radiographs of the chest were normal. A computed tomographic scan of the head revealed slight mucosal thickening of the right maxillary sinus; evaluation of the posterior fossa was limited by a beam-hardening artifact. A lumbar puncture was performed (Table 1).

Table 1. Findings on Lumbar Puncture

Variable	Finding
Appearance of cerebrospinal fluid	Clear, colorless
Initial pressure (cm of water)	12
Cells (per mm^3)*	
Red	8
White	168
Differential count (%)	
Neutrophils	1
Lymphocytes	84
Monocytes	15
Total protein (mg/dl)	260
Glucose (mg/dl)†	62
Latex-agglutination tests for antigens	
Cryptococcus neoformans	Negative
Haemophilus influenzae	Negative
Streptococcus pneumoniae	Negative
Neisseria meningitidis	Negative

*Cells were measured in the fourth tube.

†To convert the value for glucose to millimoles per liter, multiply by 0.05551.

A cranial magnetic resonance imaging (MRI) scan showed a focal area of increased signal on an axial image obtained after the administration of gadolinium, which was interpreted as a contrast-enhanced vein. Mucosal thickening was noted in the maxillary antra and ethmoid air cells.

Specimens of cerebrospinal fluid and blood were obtained for culture and other studies, and ceftriaxone was administered by vein.

A diagnostic report was received.

DIFFERENTIAL DIAGNOSIS

DR. ALLAN H. ROPPER*: This one-week illness in a previously healthy young man involved sequentially a severe headache and lymphocytic or aseptic meningitis, an acute but mild cerebellar syndrome, and a nondescript upper respiratory tract infection, with coryza, a stuffy nose, and a dry cough. The singular finding was ataxia, which provides the clue to the diagnosis. I shall not discuss the interpretation of the neurologic signs, because the ataxia of gait and limbs, coupled with dysarthria, is a straightforward manifestation of a cerebellar syndrome. It is difficult to assess the slightly increased limb tone in the absence of corroborating signs of corticospinal disease, such as Babinski's sign.

The most common form of postinfectious ataxia is probably Guillain–Barré polyneuropathy, either the sensory-ataxic variant or Fisher's syndrome (ataxia with ophthalmoplegia). The absence of reduced reflexes, Romberg's sign, and paresthesias and the presence of dysarthria rule out ataxia originating in the peripheral nervous system.

The challenge in this case is to identify one factor that explains the cerebellar ataxia and the infectious manifestations. The first consideration on the basis of cerebellar signs, increased limb tone, and a severe headache is an abscess or septic infarct of the cerebellum. Cerebellar abscesses are usually otogenous, but the scans showed no mass or hydrocephalus from obstruction of the fourth ventricle. Also, abscesses tend to be located in one cerebellar hemisphere and generally cause asymmetric limb dysmetria, increased cerebrospinal fluid pressure, and if they have been present for several days, papilledema. Another possible but unlikely diagnosis is a partially treated bacterial meningitis resulting in a deceptive lymphocytosis in the cerebrospinal fluid. Occasionally, *Haemophilus influenzae* meningitis in children is accompanied by ataxia,[1] and listeria infection may cause ataxia as a manifestation of a brain-stem encephalitis. However, there were no features of bacterial meningitis, such as meningismus, an increased cerebrospinal fluid pressure, or a reduced cerebrospinal fluid glucose level. Multiple sclerosis often affects the cerebellum in young people and occasionally becomes apparent during an infection. None of the usual features of that disease were present in this case, however, and the cerebrospinal fluid findings do not support that diagnosis. Finally, numerous drugs and toxins produce ataxia, in addition to sedatives

---

* Chief, Neurology Department, St. Elizabeth's Hospital; professor of neurology, Tufts University School of Medicine. Currently Executive Vice Chair of Neurology, Brigham and Women's Hospital.

and anticonvulsant agents, which are common culprits. In 10 years of experience with 40 children at the University of South Florida, drug ingestion was one of the most frequent causes of ataxia, even in youngsters under the age of six years.[2] None of the medications administered in this case cause ataxia.

In this patient, who had headache, brain dysfunction, and inflammation in the cerebrospinal fluid in the context of a respiratory tract infection, there are only two possible causes of ataxia: meningoencephalitis and postinfectious immune encephalitis. As I shall explain, these two diseases are intertwined, and despite distinctly different pathological features, they can have almost identical clinical manifestations.

Sporadic cases of viral encephalitis have been reported in young adults, and the cerebellum may be involved as part of a more widespread infection. More noteworthy, in regard to this patient, are the few cases of viral encephalitis in which the cerebellum has been the sole site of involvement. Almost all the viruses that cause aseptic meningitis and a few bacteria have produced an ataxic illness of this nature. The viruses that are most often implicated are those in the enterovirus group (coxsackievirus, echoviruses, and poliovirus)[3,4] and those that cause childhood exanthems. The enteroviruses are neurotropic and should receive diagnostic consideration not only because they cause cerebellar encephalitis but also because they are the most common agents of aseptic meningitis. The Epstein–Barr virus and *Mycoplasma pneumoniae* have also been reported to cause cerebellitis. Ataxia has occurred with HIV seroconversion,[5] and cerebellitis due to Epstein–Barr virus has been reported in a patient with HIV infection.[6] A few cases of cerebellar encephalitis have occurred in patients with Lyme disease, Q fever, rabies, legionellosis, herpes zoster, or herpes simplex. In all these cases, including those of bacterial origin, the cause of the cerebellar dysfunction was assumed to be infectious.

The alternative diagnosis to infectious cerebellitis in this case is cerebellar inflammation caused by a postinfectious immune process. The most generalized form of postinfectious disease of the nervous system is postinfectious encephalomyelitis, which is characterized by multifocal or disseminated demyelination of the brain and spinal cord. It is thought to be caused by an immune reaction to the systemic infection. Microscopical examination reveals perivenous inflammation and adjacent streaky demyelination, in contrast to the zones of tissue damage with neuronophagia and microglial infiltration that are seen in cases of infectious encephalitis.

Whether infectious or postinfectious, acute ataxia caused by encephalitis is most closely linked with the childhood exanthems, especially chickenpox. In many textbooks this disorder has been designated "acute cerebellar ataxia." Our understanding of acute ataxia after childhood exanthems is limited because of the benign nature of the illness, which precludes autopsy studies. The results of experimental studies of measles encephalitis in animals have led to the prevalent opinion that cerebellitis in children is a form of postinfectious encephalomyelitis. In cases of varicella cerebellitis in humans, however, the mechanism is not clear, and viral antigen has been found in the cerebrospinal fluid in some cases.[7] With techniques of molecular amplification that allow the detection of minuscule quantities of organisms in the cerebrospinal fluid and nervous tissue, many types of meningoencephalitis that were previously thought to be immune-mediated now seem more likely to be infectious. This change in interpretation applies especially to mycoplasma, which has often been reported to cause a postinfectious encephalitis, but in such cases, fragments of the organism's DNA have been found in the cerebrospinal fluid.[8] These modern bacteriologic findings have led to the recognition of a new category of disease: bacterial encephalitis.

Reflecting the lack of clarity in the distinction between postinfectious and infectious meningoencephalitis, authoritative textbooks, such as the *Handbook of Clinical Neurology*,[9] regard the ataxia that follows infection with most of the common viruses, Epstein–Barr virus, and mycoplasma as a manifestation of infectious encephalitis but classify the ataxia that follows the childhood exanthems as postinfectious. The designations are based largely on the infectious agent and its putative interaction with the immune system, but they are supported by very limited pathological evidence. It may be preferable to use the term "acute parainfectious cerebellitis" unless the organism or its genetic material is isolated from nervous system tissue or cerebrospinal fluid.

Batten[10] is usually credited with the first description of parainfectious ataxia, in 1905, but similar cases had been reported more than 30 years earlier by Westphal,[11] who identified ataxia in adults after smallpox and typhoid fever. Batten associated the cerebellitis with measles, pertussis, and scarlet fever. Under the title "A Case of Acute Ataxia (Encephalitis Cerebelli)," Batten[12] presented before the London Clinical Society the case of a three-year-old patient who had had measles in March and in April "got dazed, vomited and was unconscious." Several days later, "he was quite conscious, but his arms and legs shook.... He spoke in a hesitating manner. He was unable to sit up in bed without support and when put on his legs walked in the most incoordinate manner. There was marked incoordination of both hands, but the grasp was fairly good. There was no facial weakness, no ocular palsies or nystagmus, and the optic disks were normal." Batten noted that "since his illness the boy has become most untruthful. Not only does he tell lies to obtain his purpose, but he invents stories which can obtain him no possible advantage. His moral sense is perverted."

The typical case of parainfectious cerebellitis has clinical features similar to those seen in the patient under discussion. Ataxia develops within days after the onset of the infection and sometimes before it. The cerebellar signs can be mild; the presence of nystagmus and dysarthria varies. Recovery is usually complete. Often there is evidence of corticospinal tract dysfunction, as in this patient, indicating more widespread involvement of the central nervous system.

I could reasonably end the neurologic discussion at this point with a diagnosis of parainfectious cerebellitis. The severity of the aseptic meningitis (over 100 white cells) and the degree of protein elevation in the cerebrospinal fluid, however, are out of proportion to this patient's mild neurologic dysfunction and suggest a direct infection of the cerebellum and meninges. An intense cerebrospinal fluid reaction would be unusual in a case of ataxia associated with measles or varicella, which is usually characterized by fewer than several dozen mononuclear cells in the cerebrospinal fluid or, in some cases, none. Moreover, in my experience, when aseptic meningitis is the first indication of a cerebral illness, the entire process is likely to be infectious rather than postinfectious, and the normal findings on MRI are inconsistent with the presence of demyelination, which is the main pathological feature of postinfectious encephalomy-elitis. For these reasons, an infectious cerebellitis is most likely.

I assume that the diagnostic report identified an organism by DNA amplification or enzyme-linked immunosorbent assay or indirectly through a serologic test or detection of some other marker. In the absence of overt chickenpox or a characteristic syndrome of some type of infection, however, it is practically impossible to ascertain on clinical grounds alone the organism that caused the cerebellitis and meningitis in this case.

Table 2 lists the organisms that have been associated with acute cerebellar ataxia. The division into infectious and postinfectious causes is tentative for the reasons I have mentioned.

In the largest recent series of children with acute ataxia (73 consecutive cases), 26 percent had had chickenpox, 52 percent had had a presumably viral illness that could not be identified specifically, and 3 percent had recently been vaccinated.[13] In contrast, in a prospective series of 11 adults with cerebellitis, 4 had evidence of Epstein–Barr virus infection, and 2 had serologic evidence of reactivated varicella–zoster virus infection in the absence of chickenpox.[14] The most frequent nonexanthematous causes of an acute cerebellar syndrome in a patient of this age are Epstein–Barr virus[15] and *M. pneumoniae*.[16,17]

Although this patient had no fever, his headache, coryza, injected conjunctiva, and dry cough could have been caused by any number of respiratory tract pathogens. The common adenovirus and related denizens of the upper respiratory tract may cause aseptic meningitis but rarely of this intensity, and they have not been associated with cerebellitis. The enteroviruses, especially coxsackievirus, can also cause cerebellitis, but the absence of fever and the prominent respiratory symptoms are not consistent with infection by these agents. Antibodies to varicella–zoster virus have been found in adults with cerebellitis, but in the absence of chickenpox, the meaning of these antibodies is uncertain. Reactivated or preeruptive varicella would be unlikely, but varicella is so specifically and frequently associated with pure cerebellitis that it must always be con-sidered in the differential diagnosis. Listeria rhombencephalitis would be associated with signs of cranial-nerve or brain-stem involvement and abnormalities on the MRI scan. There is no clinical evidence of Epstein–Barr virus infection, such as pharyngitis or lymphadenopathy, to support this diagnosis.

Among the respiratory infectious agents associated with cerebellitis, *M. pneumoniae* or a similar organism is most consistent with the dry cough of a tracheobronchitis. Influenzavirus is also a possible cause. The other agent of atypical pneumonia that produces meningitis and ataxic encephalitis is Q fever.[18] According to some textbooks, monocytosis as described in the patient under discussion occurs with this rickettsial infection. It must also be considered because of the characteristic extreme prodromal headache in the absence of a stiff neck, a symptom noted in this case.[19] However, there was no fever and nothing obvious in the history to suggest this type of infection. The same severe prodromal headache with minimal or no meningismus also occurs with influenza and mycoplasma infections.

In summary, this is a case of acute infectious or postinfectious ataxia, probably an infectious cerebellar encephalitis caused by a bacterial or, less likely, a viral respiratory pathogen, possibly one of the agents that causes atypical pneumonia. If this patient's

Table 2. Causes of Postinfectious and Infectious Acute Cerebellar Ataxia[*]

Exanthematous viruses

Varicellavirus

Measles virus

Rubella virus

Mumps virus

Vaccinia virus

Other viruses

Epstein–Barr virus

HIV

Influenzavirus

Enteroviruses (echoviruses, poliovirus, and coxsackievirus)

Cytomegalovirus

Rabies virus

Herpesvirus

Bacteria and other organisms

Mycoplasma pneumoniae

Typhoid bacilli

Coxiella burnetii (Q fever)

β-Hemolytic streptococci (scarlet fever)

Leptospira

Legionella

Borrelia burgdorferi (Lyme disease)

Listeria monocytogenes

Bacteria causing abscesses

Tubercle bacilli

Cryptococcus

Plasmodia (malaria)

Previous vaccination

Against hepatitis B

Against smallpox

Against measles

---

[*]Acute cerebellitis caused by infection with varicella, measles, rubella, mumps, vaccinia, or Epstein–Barr viruses; HIV; β-hemolytic streptococci; or previous vaccination against hepatitis B, smallpox, or measles is presumably postinfectious. All the other causes are infectious or of uncertain type. Varicella, measles, and Epstein–Barr viruses and *M. pneumoniae* are the organisms most commonly associated with ataxia.

illness, with its mild neurologic manifestations, was typical of others with infectious cerebellitis, he should have recovered in several weeks.

Dr. Vincent B. Young: Our initial impression was that the patient had aseptic (viral) meningitis, but given his history of cleaning public parks, we assumed that he could have been exposed to rat urine and feces. That possible exposure and his conjunctival injection strongly suggested leptospirosis.

CLINICAL DIAGNOSES

? Aseptic (viral) meningitis.
  ? Leptospirosis.

DR. ALLAN H. ROPPER'S DIAGNOSIS

Infectious cerebellitis due to an atypical pneumonia agent.

PATHOLOGICAL DISCUSSION

DR. ANGELA M. CALIENDO: The diagnostic report presented the results of rickettsial serologic testing by the Centers for Disease Control and Prevention. The IgG titer for Q fever phase II antigen rose from less than 16 in the serum sample obtained during the acute infection to more than 512 in the sample obtained during convalescence, indicating recent Q fever. In addition, *Ehrlichia chaffeensis* antigen titers rose from less than 16 to 64, a finding interpreted as due to a cross reaction with the Q fever antigen. The leptospirosis titer rose from an undetectable value to 100, and the reaction occurred with only one serovar. Titers over 400 develop in most cases of leptospirosis, with reactions to multiple serovars. Low-level leptospirosis titers can be seen in acutely ill patients and in this case may represent cross reactivity. The serologic results were consistent with the diagnosis of acute Q fever.

Rocky Mountain spotted fever and typhus fever antigens were undetectable in serum samples obtained during both the acute and the convalescent phases of the illness. The results of serologic tests for *M. pneumoniae* and adenovirus during the acute and convalescent phases were not consistent with acute infection. Heterophile tests and serologic tests for cryptococcal and Lyme disease antigens were negative. General viral cultures of throat washings and cerebrospinal fluid and tests for HIV infection and syphilis were also negative. Routine bacterial, mycobacterial, and fungal cultures of the blood and cerebrospinal fluid were all negative.

Coxiella burnetii, the cause of Q fever, displays an antigenic-phase variation that is unique among the rickettsiae. It has two antigenic phases (I and II), which are analogous to the smooth and rough forms of some species of bacteria. *C. burnetii* exists in antigenic phase I in nature, but it changes to phase II after continuous passage in tissue culture. The phase I antigen is a polysaccharide component of the coxiella lipopolysaccharide, and the transition from phase I to phase II occurs when one or more carbohydrate components are deleted from the lipopolysaccharide moiety.[20] In acute Q fever, antibodies to *C. burnetii* phase II antigen dominate the immune response, whereas in chronic Q fever, phase I antigen levels become elevated. The phase II IgG titers, which were measured with the use of an indirect immunofluorescence assay, usually peak four to eight weeks after the onset of the disease.[21]

Acute *C. burnetii* infection causes a variety of clinical syndromes, the most common of which are a self-limited febrile illness and a mild-to-moderate atypical pneumonia. Unlike other rickettsial diseases, Q fever is not associated with a rash. Years after the initial infection with *C. burnetii*, chronic Q fever can occur in the form of endocarditis, usually involving abnormal or prosthetic cardiac valves.[22] Headache is the most common neurologic manifestation of *C. burnetii* infection. Rickettsial lymphocytic meningitis and encephalitis are well recognized.[23] Both meningoencephalitis and abnormal cerebrospinal fluid findings are much less frequent in Q fever than in other rickettsial diseases.[24] Meningoencephalitis due to acute infection with *C. burnetii* was reported in a soldier returning from the Persian Gulf War who had a headache and a crescendo pattern of transient ischemic attacks.[25] Lymphocytic meningitis has also been described as the sole manifestation of Q fever.[26] A recent review of 21 cases of Q fever meningoencephalitis reported a variety of symptoms, including aphasia, ataxia, seizures, and confusional states, as well as ocular symptoms such as diplopia and decreased visual acuity. Most of the cases of meningoencephalitis occurred in the absence of pneumonia, but antecedent influenza-like symptoms were common, as in this case. Most patients had a lymphocytic pleocytosis, with a normal or elevated protein concentration and a normal glucose concentration in the cerebrospinal fluid. Recovery was usually complete, although permanent neurologic deficits did occur.[25]

The primary reservoirs of *C. burnetii* are cattle, sheep, and goats, but many other species, including rodents and cats, are known to be infected.[24] The infection in animals is usually not clinically apparent, but *C. burnetii* may be excreted in milk, urine, feces, and amniotic fluid.[27] Large numbers of *C. burnetii* can be present in the parturient fluids of sheep, cattle, and cats.[28] Humans usually acquire the disease by inhaling aerosolized particles, but transmission can occur through the ingestion of unpasteurized milk. A single organism may be sufficient to cause the disease.[24] This patient had no history of known exposure to animals, although it is possible that while he was working in the public parks, he acquired *C. burnetii* infection from exposure to infected feces or urine from rodents or cats.

Most acute Q fever infections resolve spontaneously. Treatment is often given to prevent the development of chronic infection and to shorten the duration of fever. Tetracycline and its analogues are the recommended therapy.[29]

MR. LUIS MORENO: Leptospirosis is a biphasic illness. During the second phase, leptospires cannot be found in the blood or the cerebrospinal fluid, despite the presence of meningitis. Can serologic testing detect leptospirosis during the second phase?

DR. CALIENDO: Leptospires can be isolated from the blood and cerebrospinal fluid only during the first 10 days of illness. Organisms usually appear in the urine during the second week. However, the laboratory diagnosis of leptospirosis is usually made by serologic testing. Agglutinins appear by the end of the first week of illness and peak in the third or fourth week. The antibody titer may be suppressed or delayed by antibiotic therapy.[30]

DR. YOUNG: The patient was discharged after the second hospital day, when the initial cerebrospinal fluid cultures were negative for routine bacterial pathogens. A week after discharge, when the followup sample for serologic testing was obtained, he was almost asymptomatic. A day later, the neurologist performed another lumbar puncture, which revealed persistent pleocytosis (52 white cells, of which 79 percent were polymorphonuclear leukocytes and 21 percent were monocytes).

DR. ELIZABETH C. DOOLING: Was he treated with antibiotics?

DR. YOUNG: He received ceftriaxone initially for 48 hours. It was discontinued when the cerebrospinal fluid cultures remained negative for routine bacterial pathogens. He was given doxycycline for four days because of a presumptive diagnosis of leptospirosis.

Both leptospirosis and Q fever are generally self-limited illnesses. In patients with leptospirosis who are not severely ill, a five- to seven-day course of doxycycline may shorten the duration of symptoms. Although coxiella endocarditis is usually treated with extended courses of antibiotics, there is no evidence that they affect the neurologic manifestations of coxiella infections.

DR. ROPPER: This case is unusual. The question arises whether there have been other cases of cerebellitis with Q fever. Generalized meningoencephalitis is well recognized. The cerebellum is special in regard to both its proclivity for infection by certain organisms and the tendency for its white matter to be involved by postinfectious encephalomyelitis.

LABORATORY DIAGNOSIS

Q fever, acute (with cerebellar and meningeal involvement).

REFERENCES

1. Schwartz JF. Ataxia in bacterial meningitis. Neurology 1972;22:1071–4.
2. Gieron-Korthals MA, Westberry KR, Emmanuel PJ. Acute childhood ataxia: 10-year experience. J Child Neurol 1994;9:381–4.
3. Feldman W, Larke RPB. Acute cerebellar ataxia associated with the isolation of coxsackievirus type A9. Can Med Assoc J 1972;106:1104–7.
4. McAllister RM, Hummeler K, Coriell LL. Acute cerebellar ataxia: report of a case with isolation of type 9 ECHO virus from the cerebrospinal fluid. N Engl J Med 1959;261:1159–62.
5. Scarpini E, Sacilotto G, Lazzarin A, Gereinia L, Doronzo R, Scarlato G. Acute ataxia coincident with seroconversion for anti-HIV. J Neurol 1991;238:356–7.
6. Pulik M, Lionnet F, Genet P, Petitdidier C, Rosenberg F. Cérébellite à virus Epstein-Barr chez un patient infecté par le virus de l'immunodéficience humaine: mise en évidence du génome viral par amplification génome (PCR). Presse Med 1995;24:417.
7. Peters ACB, Versteeg J, Lindeman J, Bots GTAM. Varicella and acute cerebellar ataxia. Arch Neurol 1978;35:769–71.
8. Narita M, Matsuzono Y, Togashi T, Kajii N. DNA diagnosis of central nervous system infection by *Mycoplasma pneumoniae*. Pediatrics 1992;90:250–3.
9. Weiss S, Guberman A. Acute cerebellar ataxia in infectious disease. In: Vinken PJ, Bruyn GW, eds. Infections of the nervous system. Vol. 34 of Handbook of clinical neurology. Amsterdam: North-Holland Publishing, 1978:619–39.
10. Batten FE. Ataxia in childhood. Brain 1905;28:484–505.

11. Westphal C. Ueber eine Affection des Nervensystems nach Pocken and Typhus. Arch Psychiatr Nervenkr 1872;3:376–406.
12. Batten FE. A case of acute ataxia (encephalitis cerebelli). Trans Clin Soc Lond 1905;38:193.
13. Connolly AM, Dodson WE, Prensky AL, Rust RS. Course and prognosis of acute cerebellar ataxia. Ann Neurol 1994;35:673–9.
14. Klockgether T, Doller G, Wullner U, Petersen D, Dichgans J. Cerebellar encephalitis in adults. J Neurol 1993;240:17–20.
15. Cleary TG, Henle W, Pickering LK. Acute cerebellar ataxia associated with Epstein-Barr virus infection. JAMA 1980;243:148–9.
16. Steele JC, Gladstone RM, Thanasophon S, Fleming PC. Acute cerebellar ataxia and concomitant infection with Mycoplasma pneumoniae. J Pediatr 1972;80:467–9.
17. Endtz LJ, Hers JFP. Ataxie cérébelluese aiguë causée par *Mycoplasma pneumoniae*. Rev Neurol 1970;122:52–4.
18. Kohler J, Mergner T, Bohl E, Neumann-Haefelin D. Neurologische Komplikationen bei Q-Fieber (Coxiella burnetii). Fortschr Neurol Psychiatr 1992;60:110–13.
19. Marrie TJ, Raoult D. Rickettsial infections of the central nervous system. Semin Neurol 1992;12:213–24.
20. Hackstadt T, Peacock MG, Hitchcock PJ, Cole RL. Lipopolysaccharide variation in Coxiella burnetii: intrastrain heterogeneity in structure and antigenicity. Infect Immun 1985;48:359–65.
21. Dupuis G, Peter O, Peacock M, Burgdorfer W, Haller E. Immunoglobulin responses in acute Q fever. J Clin Microbiol 1985;22:484–7.
22. Tellez A, Sainz C, Echevarria C, et al. Q fever in Spain: acute and chronic cases, 1981–1985. Rev Infect Dis 1988;10:198–202.
23. Silpapojakul K, Ukkachoke C, Krisanapan S, Silpapojakul K. Rickettsial meningitis and encephalitis. Arch Intern Med 1991;151:1753–7.
24. Sawyer LA, Fishbein DB, McDade JE. Q fever: current concepts. Rev Infect Dis 1987;9:935–46.
25. Ferrante MA, Dolan MJ. Q fever meningoencephalitis in a soldier returning from the Persian Gulf War. Clin Infect Dis 1993;16:489–96.
26. Schattner A, Kushnir M, Zhornicky T, Fenakel G. Lymphocytic meningitis as the sole manifestation of Q fever. Postgrad Med J 1993;69:636–7.
27. Aitken ID. Clinical aspects and prevention of Q fever in animals. Eur J Epidemiol 1989;5:420–4.
28. Leedom JM. Q fever: an update. Curr Clin Top Infect Dis 1980;1:304–31.
29. Holtom PD, Leedom JM. Coxiella burnetii (Q fever). In: Gorbach SL, Bartlett JG, Blacklow NR, eds. Infectious diseases. 4th ed. Philadelphia: W.B. Saunders, 1992:1657–9.
30. Farrar WE. Leptospira species (leptospirosis). In: Mandell GL, Bennett JE, Dolin R, eds. Mandell, Douglas and Bennett's principles and practice of infectious diseases. 4th ed. Vol. 2. New York: Churchill Livingstone, 1995:2137–41.

Perspectives and Updates

This was one of the most peculiar and diagnostically unsatisfying cases I have discussed in a CPC. The problem presented was one of a young man with ataxia and dysarthria with essentially no other findings but with severe retro-orbital pain and frontal headache, symptoms for which I ultimately had only a feeble explanation. The CSF was intensely inflammatory with mononuclear cells, and the glucose was normal. The final surprising diagnosis, based on serologic evidence, was an immune or infectious cerebellitis from Q fever.

Curiously, the timing and progression of the ataxia were not described in the case report; I presumed that it was acute or subacute over days. It was this temporal profile that made the case distinctive and offered the chance of at least a generic diagnosis for the acute cerebellar syndrome. The best-characterized acute cerebellitis with an inflammatory CSF is that following chickenpox in children and young adults. My discussion pointed out the important and unanswered question of whether this varicella-cerebellar disorder is a direct viral neurotropic infection or a form of postinfectious disorder akin to Guillain-Barré syndrome. For the latter, I have used the term "parainfectious" to indicate uncertainty about the mechanism. From time to time there are reports in cases of myelitis or cerebellitis of positive PCR in the spinal fluid for an organism such as *Mycoplasma pneumoniae*. In the case of Q fever— the imputed diagnosis in this CPC—as well as of *Mycoplasma* and *Legionella*, it is difficult to comprehend that there is a true bacterial infection of neurons, even with the inflammatory CSF formula, but we cannot be certain of the biology of these conditions. A similar ambiguity pertains to Lyme infections that implicate the nervous system. The presence of mononuclear cells in the spinal fluid does not help to differentiate the two mechanisms, but their absence might hint at a postinfectious cause in a particular case.

The rickettsial disease Q fever, caused by *Coxiella burnetti*, is unusual enough, but to then attribute a rare neurologic syndrome to the organism seems to be multiplying low probabilities, to the point of skepticism. I was told at the time of this CPC that a rise in the titer of the serologies in seum from less than 1:16 to more than 1:512 during convalescence was specific for recent infection with the organism, so I take the case on face value, but I do not anticipate seeing another case in my career. What led the clinicians even to send this test remains a puzzle.

Since the publication of this CPC, many chapters and articles have included Q fever in the lists of the postinfectious causes of cerebellitis. However, as far as I have been able to determine, there have been exceedingly few well documented cases.[1] There is a better-characterized generalized encephalitis from this organism, again, with lack of clarity regarding a direct infections versus a post-infectious process.[2]

Allan H. Ropper

REFERENCES

1. Sawaishi Y, Takahashi I, Hirayama Y, et al. Acute cerebellitis caused by *Coxiella burnetii*. Ann Neurol 1999; 45:124–7.
2. Brooks RG, Licitra CM, Peacock MG. Encephalitis caused by *Coxiella burnetii*. Ann Neurol 1986; 20:91–3.

A 43-Year-Old Woman with Adult Respiratory Distress Syndrome

ROCKY MOUNTAIN SPOTTED FEVER

CPC 32-1997

PRESENTATION OF CASE

A 43-year-old woman was admitted to the hospital in early June because of possible adult respiratory distress syndrome.

The patient had been in excellent health until nine days earlier, when she began to have low-grade fever, chilliness, and headache. On the next day, she slept excessively. One week before admission to this hospital, she vomited and lost consciousness for 15 seconds while kneeling. Later that day, an examination at another hospital revealed tender postoccipital lymph nodes; the white-cell count was 7600 per cubic millimeter. Her husband recalled that he had removed a tick from her neck about nine days earlier. Amoxicillin was prescribed. The next day, the occipital headache persisted, with myalgia and a temperature of 38.2°C. Amoxicillin was discontinued. A nurse who saw the patient at about this time recalled having observed a very fine rash, with papular lesions, sprinkled over the body except for the palms.

Five days before admission to this hospital, the patient returned to the other hospital with a persistent headache, a prominent dry cough, and severe dyspnea and was admitted. The temperature was 40.3°C. Examination showed no rash or lymphadenopathy. Crackles were present over the anterior aspect of the right hemithorax. Laboratory tests were performed (Tables 1 and 2). A radiograph of the chest (Fig. 1) showed diffuse bilateral air-space opacification with air bronchograms. Erythromycin, cefuroxime, and methylprednisolone were administered. The headache and respiratory distress worsened. Arterial-blood gases were measured (Table 3) four days before admission to this hospital. The trachea was intubated, and ventilatory assistance was begun with 100 percent oxygen, which was soon reduced to 40 percent. The results of a bronchoscopic examination were normal, and an examination of bronchial washings revealed no acid-fast bacilli, fungi, *Pneumocystis carinii*, or other microorganisms; cultures of the washings were negative, as were six blood-culture specimens.

Table 1 Hematologic Laboratory Values

Variable	Five Days before Admission	One Day before Admission	On Admission
Hematocrit (%)	39.6	27.2	25.4
Mean corpuscular volume (μm^3)			90
White-cell count (per mm^3)	6,200	13,200	
Differential count (%)			
Neutrophils	79	84	
Band forms	15		
Lymphocytes	5		
Monocytes	1		
Platelet count (per mm^3)	72,000	168,000	197,000

On the fourth hospital day, the temperature was 39.7°C. Another radiograph of the chest (Fig. 2) showed resolution of the consolidation in the right lung, with residual interstitial opacification and persistent consolidation in the left lower lobe.

On the fifth hospital day, the administration of furosemide was followed by a negative fluid balance of 4 liters, and the trachea was extubated. The patient opened her eyes in response to verbal and tactile stimuli but did not speak. She moved her arms and legs slowly. Laboratory tests and a lumbar puncture were performed (Tables 1 and 4). Later in the day, the temperature was 39.6°C; respiratory distress recurred and worsened despite the administration of furosemide, and the trachea was again intubated.

Table 2 Blood Chemical Findings*

Variable	Five Days before Admission	On Admission
Sodium (mmol/liter)	126	153
Potassium (mmol/liter)		3.8
Chloride (mmol/liter)		116
Carbon dioxide (mmol/liter)		29.7
Protein (g/dl)		4.2
Albumin		1.8
Globulin		2.4
Glucose (mg/dl)		158
Calcium (mg/dl)		6.8
Aspartate aminotransferase (U/liter)	118	
Alanine aminotransferase (U/liter)	138	

*To convert the value for glucose to millimoles per liter, multiply by 0.05551. To convert the value for calcium to millimoles per liter, multiply by 0.250.

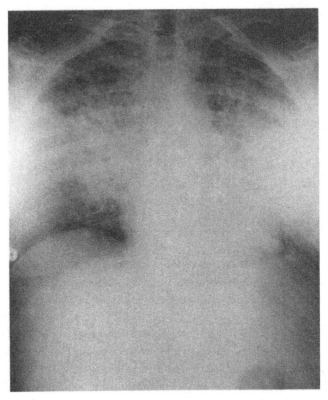

FIG 1 Anteroposterior Chest Radiograph Obtained with the Patient in a Supine Position, Showing Diffuse Bilateral Air-Space Opacification with Air Bronchograms.

The heart is of normal size, and there are no pleural effusions.

On the sixth hospital day, another chest radiograph was unchanged. A cardiac ultra-sonographic examination showed moderate global hypokinesis, severe anteroseptal hypokinesis, and an estimated left ventricular ejection fraction of 30 to 40 percent. A Swan–Ganz catheter was inserted, and the pulmonary–capillary wedge pressure was 14 mm Hg. One dose of doxycycline was administered, and the patient was transferred to this hospital on a respirator.

The patient resided on the Rhode Island coast in a wooded area with many deer present. She lived with her husband, one cat, and one dog; both animals were healthy.

Table 3 Arterial-Blood Gases

Variable	Four Days before Admission*	On Admission†
Partial pressure of oxygen (mm Hg)	53	187
Partial pressure of carbon dioxide (mm Hg)	30	37
pH	7.3	7.54

*Measurements were performed while the patient was receiving 50 percent oxygen by mask.
†Measurements were performed while the patient was receiving 60 percent oxygen.

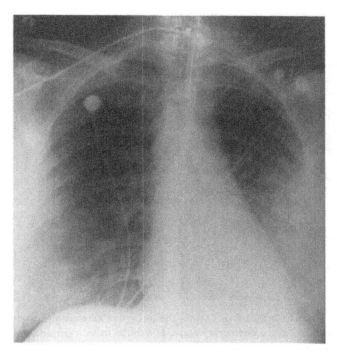

FIG 2 Anteroposterior Chest Radiograph Obtained with the Patient in a Supine Position, Showing Resolution of the Consolidation in the Right Lung, with Residual Interstitial Opacification.
There is persistent consolidation in the left lower lobe.

There was no history of exposure to toxic chemicals or medications, risk factors for human immunodeficiency virus infection, or recent travel.

The temperature was 38.2°C, and the pulse was 74. The blood pressure was 90/50 mm Hg.

On examination, the patient was pharmacologically paralyzed and could not be aroused. No rash, petechiae, or lymphadenopathy was found. The lungs were clear, with diminished breath sounds at the bases. A cardiac examination revealed a hyperdynamic

Table 4 Results of Lumbar Puncture One Day before Admission*

Variable	Value
Red cells (per mm³)	190
White cells (per mm³)	11
Differential count (%)	
Neutrophils	66
Lymphocytes	34
Total protein (mg/dl)	190
Glucose (mg/dl)	74
Culture	Negative

*The procedure yielded 2 ml of fluid. To convert the value for glucose to millimoles per liter, multiply by 0.05551.

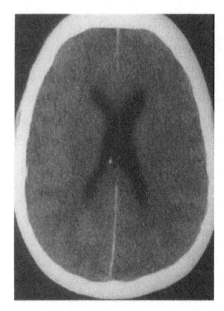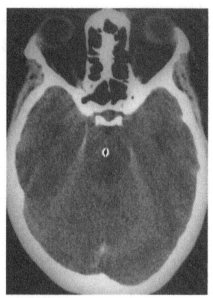

FIG 3 Nonenhanced Cranial CT Scans Showing Diffuse Cerebral Edema, with Effacement of the Sulci and Basal Cisterns and Evidence of Uncal and Cerebellar Tonsillar Herniation. No focal lesion is present.

precordium. A neurologic examination showed that the pupils were 7 mm in diameter and unreactive to light; no extraocular movement was detected. The corneal and gag reflexes were absent. No spontaneous movement of the arms or legs was seen. The deep-tendon reflexes were ++ and equal, except that the knee and ankle jerks were +; the plantar responses were absent. There was no response to the doll's-head maneuver, noxious stimuli, or cold caloric stimulation.

The urea nitrogen, creatinine, bilirubin, phosphorus, magnesium, creatine kinase, and alkaline phosphatase levels were normal, as were the prothrombin and partial-thromboplastin times. The results of other laboratory tests and measurements of arterial-blood gases are shown in Tables 1, 2, and 3. Serum tests for toxic drugs were negative except for the presence of carbamazepine. An electrocardiogram revealed a normal rhythm at a rate of 79 and a QT interval, corrected for rate, of 498 msec; inverted T waves were present in leads V_2 through V_5. A computed tomographic (CT) cranial scan (Fig. 3), obtained without the administration of contrast material, revealed diffuse cerebral edema, with effacement of the sulci and basal cisterns and uncal and cerebellar tonsillar herniation.

Mannitol, doxycycline, ceftriaxone, and acyclovir were administered intravenously, with an infusion of norepinephrine as needed to maintain an adequate blood pressure. A right frontal intracranial-pressure monitor was inserted. The intracranial pressure was 71 mm Hg, with a contemporaneous mean arterial pressure of 55 to 60 mm Hg, and was generally 10 to 15 mm Hg higher than the mean arterial pressure. A transcranial Doppler examination showed no cerebral perfusion. An apnea test showed no movement of the chest wall as the partial pressure of carbon dioxide rose from 37 to 63 mm Hg, with a fall in pH from 7.57 to 7.28. Treatment was continued until the next morning, when an electroencephalographic study showed no electrical activity.

The patient was declared brain dead. She died after life support measures were terminated.

DIFFERENTIAL DIAGNOSIS

DR. MARTIN A. SAMUELS[*]: This previously healthy 43-year-old woman died in less than two weeks from massively increased intracranial pressure that occurred as part of a systemic illness characterized by progressive encephalopathy. May we see the imaging studies?

DR. BEATRICE TROTMAN-DICKENSON: The radiograph of the chest obtained five days before admission to this hospital (Fig. 1) shows extensive bilateral, predominantly peri-hilar consolidation with air bronchograms in the upper lobes. The radiograph obtained three days later (Fig. 2) shows that the consolidation in the right lung has resolved, with residual interstitial opacification, but the consolidation in the left lower lobe persists. The radiograph obtained on the day of admission shows no change. The cranial CT scan (Fig. 3) obtained on the same day without the administration of intravenous contrast material shows extensive edema, with effacement of the sulci, loss of differentiation between gray and white matter, and effacement of the basal cisterns. There is also evidence of uncal and tonsillar herniation, but no focal abnormality is present.

DR. SAMUELS: Between 1873 and 1910, 295 cases of a multisystem disease, 190 of them fatal, were reported in the Bitterroot Valley of western Montana. Howard Ricketts investigated this disease and found it was caused by a microorganism transmitted by the wood tick, *Dermacentor andersoni*. In 1909, Ricketts died of the disease he was studying at that time, epidemic typhus (known in Mexico as tabardillo). In 1916, the microbiologist da Rocha-Lima (after whom the closely related rochalimaea have been named) designated the agent of epidemic typhus *Rickettsia prowazekii*, in honor of Ricketts and Stanislaw Prowazek, who died in Europe while trying to isolate the organism responsible for this important disease. Typhus fever has dwarfed influenza, tuberculosis, and the acquired immunodeficiency syndrome as a cause of death in the past two centuries.[1]

The family Rickettsiaceae includes the genus rickettsia as well as ehrlichia, coxiella, wolbachia, and rochalimaea. These organisms are small, gram-negative, pleomorphic, coccobacillary bacteria that contain both DNA and RNA and with two exceptions, rochalimaea and wolbachia, are obligate intracellular parasites. The phylogeny and taxonomy of these organisms are undergoing some revision on the basis of nucleic-acid sequencing, but it is convenient to divide them into three groups: the spotted fevers, the typhus group, and others.[2] Almost all the organisms are maintained in an arthropod-animal cycle in which human infection is incidental. Only *R. prowazekii* is

---

[*] Neurologist-in-chief, Brigham and Women's Hospital, Boston; cochairman, Partners Neurology, Boston; professor of neurology, Harvard Medical School. Currently Chair, Department of Neurology, Brigham and Women's Hospital.

maintained in a louse-human cycle. One organism, *Coxiella burnetii*, the cause of Q fever, is transmitted by inhalation, but all the other organisms require human contact with the arthropod vector. That vector is the louse for epidemic typhus and trench fever, the mite for rickettsial pox and scrub typhus, the flea for murine typhus, and the tick for Rocky Mountain spotted fever, boutonneuse fever, and Queensland tick typhus. Of the three tick-borne rickettsial diseases, only Rocky Mountain spotted fever is seen in North America. The disease is transmitted by the dog tick, *D. variabilis*, in the eastern United States, the Lone Star tick, *Amblyomma americanum*, in the Southwest, and the wood tick, *D. andersoni*, in the Rocky Mountains, where the disease was first reported. The ticks acquire the causative organism, now known as *R. rickettsii*, by feeding on infected animals or by transovarial transmission.[3]

The largest number of cases of Rocky Mountain spotted fever are reported in the southeastern United States, mostly from May to September, when the ticks are active. About 650 cases were reported in 1990. North Carolina had the highest density of cases, and Oklahoma the largest number. The initial fatality rate of 70 percent, reported by Ricketts, has been reduced to roughly 5 percent by the use of tetracycline and chloramphenicol. The chance of becoming infected appears to increase with the length of time the tick remains in place. Use of tick repellents and inspection of the skin and clothing several times daily and before going to bed are probably effective methods of prevention.[4]

After an incubation period of two to seven days, fever, chills, and headache, often associated with gastro-intestinal symptoms, develop. The rash, for which the disease is named, appears on approximately the second day of illness, beginning in the cooler areas of the body, affecting the palms and soles, and migrating in a centripetal fashion. The rash may be severe, becoming purpuric and even necrotic, or it may be evanescent. In about 10 percent of cases, there is no rash. In severe or untreated cases, a noncardiac pulmonary edema, cardiomyopathy, renal and hepatic failure, and coma develop. The pathologic process is virtually the same in all organs, reflecting the propensity of the organism to infect endothelial cells and lead to capillary leakage, intravascular volume depletion, and cerebral and pulmonary edema. The pulmonary edema may be due in part to capillary leakage caused by direct pulmonary involvement and in part to the cerebral lesion, which results in "neurogenic" pulmonary edema. In addition, there may be a component of cardiac pulmonary edema resulting from the cardiomyopathy caused by rickettsial vasculitis of the coronary vessels. Cardiac pulmonary edema is due to the movement of fluid from pulmonary capillaries into the air spaces as a result of increased pressure rather than the incompetency of the capillary tight junctions.[5] In this patient, all three mechanisms of pulmonary edema were probably present. The partial improvement of the pulmonary radiologic abnormalities caused by fluid diuresis and ventilation probably reflects successful treatment of the cardiac component of the pulmonary edema, whereas the residual abnormality was most likely due to the noncardiac components. Consumption of coagulation factors results in thrombocytopenia and anemia, as noted in this patient. Sometimes a full-blown thrombotic thrombocytopenic purpura develops or, more commonly, disseminated intravascular coagulation.[3]

It may be difficult to establish an early diagnosis, which depends on recognizing the characteristic clinical picture and epidemiologic background. Serologic testing, including complement fixation, indirect hemagglutination, and indirect fluorescence antibody studies, are now possible but are generally not useful in establishing an early diagnosis. The Weil-Felix reaction is an older technique that depends on cross-reactivity with proteus strains OX-19, OX-K, and OX-2. It is not a specific test, however, and may be positive in cases of infections with other organisms—in particular, leptospira, borrelia, and proteus itself. Organisms in the endothelial cells can be identified in a biopsy specimen of the skin rash by immunofluorescence staining,[3] but the study is rarely performed because of the length of time required. Treatment involves the administration of tetracycline or chloramphenicol. Once a serious neurologic syndrome has developed, the prognosis is very grave, even with appropriate treatment.[6]

A neuropathological examination shows a widespread vasculitis caused by rickettsial organisms in the endothelial cells, resulting in the generalized cerebral edema that is visible on the CT scan. So-called typhus (microglial) nodules are found but are nonspecific. Thrombosis, vessel-wall destruction, and perivascular inflammation, sometimes with neuronophagia, are seen. The location of the most severe lesions probably corresponds to the clinical syndrome observed. The description of the patient as awake but unresponsive leads me to believe that one of the important lesions may have been in the top of the reticular formation near the mesencephalic—diencephalic junction. It is clear from the CT scan, however, that the disease became widespread and diffuse, and at the time of the postmortem examination, it may have been impossible to determine where the illness began in the brain. In some rickettsial diseases, there may be a predilection for certain parts of the nervous system for unknown reasons. For example, the brain stem is said to be affected more frequently than other parts of the brain in patients with epidemic or scrub typhus, but that does not appear to be true in patients with Rocky Mountain spotted fever, according to most postmortem evaluations.[7-9] Imaging studies in cases of encephalopathy associated with Rocky Mountain spotted fever have been limited. The CT scan usually shows only generalized cerebral edema, as in this case. In one patient, magnetic resonance imaging showed increased signal intensity in an apparent perivascular-space distribution on T_2-weighted images. The authors believed that these findings were due to perivascular inflammation, although this conclusion was not confirmed, since the patient recovered and the finding disappeared.[10]

Other tick-borne illnesses are relatively unlikely in this patient. Ehrlichiosis, which has been increasing lately in the northeastern United States, is the best match. There are two forms of ehrlichiosis: human monocytic ehrlichiosis, caused by *Ehrlichia chaffeensis*, and human granulocytic ehrlichiosis, caused by *E. phagocytophila*, which is probably identical to the organism *E. equi*. Ehrlichiosis in humans differs slightly from the disease that veterinarians see. *E. canis* causes a similar illness in dogs and is a major problem in veterinary practice. Both *E. chaffeensis* and *E. phagocytophila* may cause severe illness, but there have been only a few reported deaths, all in older, debilitated people. According to Dr. John S. Bakken, an expert on ehrlichiosis, only four deaths have been caused by ehrlichia to date. When death does occur, it is due to superinfection with other organisms, since ehrlichia causes immunosuppression. Ehrlichiosis can cause thrombocytopenia, elevated values on liver-function tests, and cardiomyopathy, but the degree of cerebral edema seen in this case has not been reported in association with ehrlichiosis. The ehrlichia organism may be visible in white cells on a buffy-coat examination of a peripheral-blood specimen, but the organism has to be sought specifically, and even when sought, it is often not seen. A rash is also rare but can develop in patients with ehrlichiosis.[11–14]

Acute Lyme disease due to infection with *Borrelia burgdorferi* can be severe, with pulmonary and cardiac involvement, but this woman did not have the characteristic erythema migrans or joint symptoms, and her very severe cerebral edema would be exceedingly unusual, even in the most aggressive cases of Lyme disease. Babesiosis is also prevalent in the Northeast and may be cotransmitted with Lyme disease by the same *Ixodes dammini* ticks, but it is a malaria-like illness with prominent hemolysis, reticulocytosis, depressed haptoglobin levels, elevated bilirubin levels, and excess urobilinogen in the urine, none of which were noted in this patient. Although some central nervous system symptoms are common in babesiosis, the severity of cerebral involvement seen in this case would be distinctly unusual except in asplenic patients.[15] In fact, asplenic persons should probably be immunized against this disease or take prophylactic antibiotics if they travel to areas where babesiosis occurs, which includes southeastern New England.

Tularemia is also prevalent along the New England coast. The infection is caused by the arthropodborne *Francisella tularensis*, a small, gram-negative, aerobic coccobacillus that is nonmotile and pleomorphic. The most common form of infection, known as ulceroglandular tularemia, is characterized by a skin lesion at the site of the tick bite, with localized tender lymphadenopathy. This patient was said to have tender, palpable lymph nodes, but no localized lesion was seen in the region. A typhoidal form of the disease is associated with a worse prognosis and is often accompanied by severe pneumonia. Although this patient's illness is in many ways compatible with typhoidal tularemia, the severe nature of the central nervous system involvement and the noncardiac pulmonary edema make it a very unlikely diagnosis.

In retrospect, the presence of multisystem involvement makes a primary encephalitic illness (e.g., eastern equine encephalitis, herpes simplex encephalitis, Powassan virus encephalitis, or meningococcal or viral meningitis) very unlikely. The overall clinical picture in this epidemiologic context makes the diagnosis of Rocky Mountain spotted fever virtually certain. As part of my research into this case, I asked Dr. Utpala Bandy, of the Department of Public Health of Rhode Island, for a map showing the distribution of the disease in that state. She spontaneously told me that a patient with Rocky Mountain spotted fever had been transported by helicopter to the Massachusetts General Hospital this past summer, and the diagnosis was not made until postmortem examination. This information, obviously not available to the treating physicians in this case, helped me a great deal.

CLINICAL DIAGNOSIS

Encephalitis, ? viral, ? rickettsial.

DR. MARTIN A. SAMUELS'S DIAGNOSIS

Rocky Mountain spotted fever.

PATHOLOGICAL DISCUSSION

DR. KATHY L. NEWELL: At postmortem examination, the heart was grossly normal, but histologic examination showed scattered foci of mixed chronic inflammatory cells within the myocardium (Fig. 4). The lungs were congested, with a combined weight of 1131 g and bilateral pleural effusions of 50 ml each. Microscopical examination revealed a focal vasculitis with patchy collections of fibrin, proteinaceous fluid, and macrophages in alveolar spaces. The spleen was congested, and the liver had scattered areas of mild, chronic periportal inflammation. No organisms were identified with the use of special stains.

Removal of the calvaria revealed diffuse swelling of the brain, with flattening of gyri. There was mild uncal grooving. The cerebellar tonsils were tightly apposed to the medulla, although no necrosis was seen. Coronal sectioning of the brain revealed a mild right-to-left hemispheric shift with softening and slight compression of the left cerebral peduncle. No focal lesions were seen. Microscopical examination showed a subarachnoid infiltration of lymphocytes, monocytes, plasma cells, and macrophages, with extension along Virchow–Robin spaces and infiltration of vessel walls. These findings were prominent within the cerebral white matter and the spinal cord (Fig. 5). The walls of some vessels were destroyed focally, with extravasation of proteins and inflammatory cells into the adjacent tissue (Fig. 6). Only rare foci of fibrinoid change were seen in the vessel walls. Microglia, microglial nodules, and chronic inflammatory cells were present throughout the parenchyma of the brain and spinal cord (Fig. 7). Periodic acid–Schiff, Brown and Hopps, Gomori's methenamine-silver, and Steiner stains for organisms were all negative.

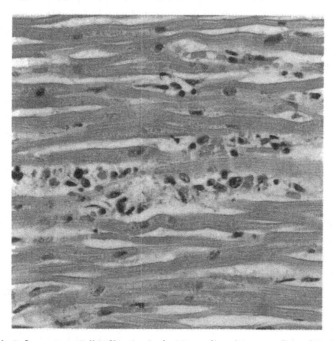

FIG 4 Patchy Inflammatory-Cell Infiltration in the Myocardium (Hematoxylin and Eosin, ×220).

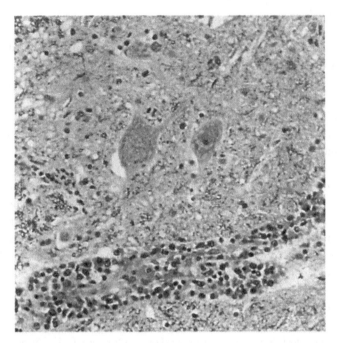

FIG 5 Perivascular and Vascular Inflammation in the Spinal Cord (Luxol Fast Blue–Hematoxylin and Eosin, ×150).

Serologic tests performed by the state laboratory on a specimen of blood obtained before death revealed elevated titers of IgG for *R. typhi* (1:256) and *R. rickettsii* (>1:256). To interpret the results of serologic studies, it is desirable to compare titers in specimens obtained during the acute and convalescent stages of infection. A four-fold increase in the titer during the convalescent stage provides confirmation of recent infection. In this case, we have only one value, for a specimen obtained on the day of death. Serum was sent to the Centers for Disease Control and Prevention (CDC) for additional testing, which revealed an IgM titer of 1:2048 for *R. rickettsii* and 1:64 for *R. typhi;* repeated IgG titers revealed values of 1:512 and <64, respectively. Antibodies for human granulocytic ehrlichiosis, hantavirus, and *B. burgdorferi* were not detected. There was evidence of probable past infection with *E. chaffeensis.*

Since serologic cross-reactivity within a particular rickettsial group is common, a specimen from a person infected with *R. rickettsii* may show antibody cross-reactivity with another species in the spotted-fever group. Less commonly, there is cross-reactivity between groups. When a person has a robust serologic response, such as an IgM titer of 1:2048, however, nonspecific cross-reactivity between groups is possible. Therefore, the IgM response for *R. typhi* in this case is probably spurious, according to Dr. Jacqueline Dawson, at the CDC.

After receiving this information, we carefully screened Giemsa-stained sections of the brain for rickettsiae and identified rare structures in endothelial cells that were suggestive of these organisms. Dr. Sherif Zaki, at the CDC's Laboratory of Molecular Pathology and Ultrastructure Activity, Viral, and Rickettsial Diseases Division,

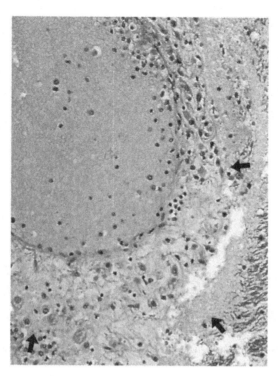

FIG 6 Inflamed Wall of Blood Vessel with Focal Destruction (Arrows) and Leakage of Proteins into Adjacent White Matter (Luxol Fast Blue–Hematoxylin and Eosin, ×190).

performed immuno histochemical staining for *R. rickettsii* on paraffin-embedded sections of brain, liver, lung, bone marrow, and spleen. There was high reactivity in and around endothelial cells in the brain and rare focal staining in the spleen and lung. On the basis of the pathological and serologic findings, we concluded that the meningoencephalitis was due to Rocky Mountain spotted fever.

Rickettsial species infect endothelial cells resulting in vasculitis, typically with necrosis, thrombosis, and hemorrhage. The lesions may occur in virtually any organ. Only 0.3 to 2 μm in length, the organisms are difficult to identify in tissue sections by routine methods and are best visualized with Giemsa, Macchiavello's, or Giménez stains or immunohisto chemical techniques.[16]

Pneumonitis due to infection of the pulmonary microcirculation occurs in severe cases. Retrospective studies have shown evidence of lower respiratory tract involvement in up to 42 percent of cases.[17] Neurologic manifestations are common,[7,8,18,19] with encephalitis apparent in 27 percent of cases.[20] The reason for the severity of the infection in the central nervous system in this patient is unknown. Similar findings were reported by Katz et al.[21] in a 40-year-old man with Rocky Mountain spotted fever who died after a brief respiratory illness had progressed to severe pulmonary edema. At autopsy, the inflammatory changes were limited to the central nervous system. The authors suggest that an autopsy in similar cases in which Rocky Mountain spotted fever is unsuspected may fail to establish that diagnosis if the central nervous

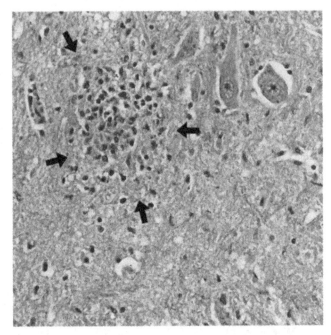

FIG 7 Microglial Nodule (Arrows) in the Medulla (Luxol Fast Blue–Hematoxylin and Eosin, ×150).

system has not been examined. Because of the vasculitis, it has been proposed that aggressive corticosteroid therapy may be useful and potentially more effective than antibiotics in treating the later stages of the infection.[22] The absence of more extensive vascular necrosis and thrombosis in this case may be related to the administration of methylprednisolone.

There is currently no commercially available laboratory test to detect Rocky Mountain spotted fever early in the clinical course, when treatment must be initiated. The standard serologic method for detecting rickettsiae is indirect immunofluorescence, which was used in testing serum from this patient. The polymerase chain reaction may have a future role in the detection of rickettsial infections.[23] Culture of the organisms, which is dangerous and difficult, is performed only in reference laboratories.

ANATOMICAL DIAGNOSIS

Rocky Mountain spotted fever with meningoencephalomyelitis, vasculitis, and focal myocarditis.

REFERENCES

1. Marrie TJ, Raoult D. Rickettsial infections of the central nervous system. Semin Neurol 1992;12:213–24.
2. Weisburg WG, Dobson ME, Samuel JE, et al. Phylogenetic diversity of the rickettsiae. J Bacteriol 1989;171:4202–6.

3. Relman DA, Swartz MN. Rickettsial diseases. Part 17 of Infectious disease. In: Rubenstein E, Federman DD, eds. Scientific American medicine Vol. 2. New York: Scientific American, 1994:XVII-1–XVII-11.

4. Kirk JL, Fine DP, Sexton DJ, Muchmore HG. Rocky Mountain spotted fever: a clinical review based on 48 confirmed cases, 1943–1986. Medicine (Baltimore) 1990;69:35–45.

5. Malik AB. Mechanisms of neurogenic pulmonary edema. Circ Res 1985;57:1–18.

6. Shaked Y. Rickettsial infection of the central nervous system: the role of prompt antimicrobial therapy. QJM 1991;79:301–6.

7. Miller JQ, Price TR. The nervous system in Rocky Mountain spotted fever. Neurology 1972;22:561–6.

8. Bell WE, Lascari AD. Rocky Mountain spotted fever: neurological symptoms in the acute phase. Neurology 1970;20:841–7.

9. Miller JQ, Price TR. Tick-borne typhus including Rocky Mountain spotted fever. In: Vinken PJ, Bruyn GW, eds. Infections of the nervous system. Part 2. Vol. 34 of Handbook of clinical neurology. Amsterdam: Elsevier North-Holland Biomedical Press, 1978:651–8.

10. Baganz MD, Dross PE, Reinhardt JA. Rocky Mountain spotted fever encephalitis: MR findings. AJNR Am J Neuroradiol 1995;16:Suppl:919–22.

11. Fishbein DB, Dawson JE, Robinson LE. Human ehrlichiosis in the United States, 1985 to 1990. Ann Intern Med 1994;120:736–43.

12. Standaert SM, Dawson JE, Schaffner W, et al. Ehrlichiosis in a golf-oriented retirement community. N Engl J Med 1995;333:420–5.

13. Bakken JS, Krueth J, Wilson-Nordskog C, Tilden RL, Asanovich K, Dumler JS. Clinical and laboratory characteristics of human granulocytic ehrlichiosis. JAMA 1996;275:199–205.

14. Fishbein DB, Dennis DT. Tick-borne diseases—a growing risk. N Engl J Med 1995;333:452–3.

15. Case Records of the Massachusetts General Hospital (Case 28-1993). N Engl J Med 1993;329:194–9.

16. White WL, Patrick JD, Miller LR. Evaluation of immunoperoxidase techniques to detect Rickettsia rickettsii in fixed tissue sections. Am J Clin Pathol 1994;101:747–52. [Erratum, Am J Clin Pathol 1994;102:559.]

17. Donohue JF. Lower respiratory tract involvement in Rocky Mountain spotted fever. Arch Intern Med 1980;140:223–7.

18. Horney LF, Walker DH. Meningoencephalitis as a major manifestation of Rocky Mountain spotted fever. South Med J 1988;81:915–8.

19. Massey EW, Thames T, Coffey CE, Gallis HA. Neurologic complications of Rocky Mountain spotted fever. South Med J 1985;78:1288–90.

20. Walker DH. Rocky Mountain spotted fever: a seasonal alert. Clin Infect Dis 1995;20:1111–17.

21. Katz DA, Dworzack DL, Horowitz EA, Bogard PJ. Encephalitis associated with Rocky Mountain spotted fever. Arch Pathol Lab Med 1985; 109:771–3.

22. Woodward TE. Remember Rocky Mountain spotted fever—a lesson in ethical principles. Clin Infect Dis 1996;23:165–6.

23. Tzianabos T, Anderson BE, McDade JE. Detection of Rickettsia rickettsii DNA in clinical specimens by using polymerase chain reaction technology. J Clin Microbiol 1989;27:2866–8.

Perspectives and Updates

There is very little update on the recognition and management of tick-borne rick-ettsial diseases (TBRD). Human granuloctytic ehrlichiosis (HE) is now known as human granulocytic anaplasmosis (HGA), and a few new diagnostic tests are available. For example in the CPC, the pathologist predicts that the polymerase chain reaction (PCR) will probably become available. It has, indeed, become available, but it is disappointing in its sensitivity in early infection (i.e., no better than about 75 percent). Its usefulness is highly laboratory-dependent and its sensitivity falls off with exposure to doxycycline. The major principles of management of TBRD involve a high index of suspicion in people at risk and early treatment with doxyclycline if any of the TBRDs are suspected. The definite diagnosis is usually made after the fact using acute and convalescent sera sent to the state laboratory. Immunofluorescent assays (IFAs) and enzyme-linked immunosorbent assays (ELISAs) are available, but the results are too slow in coming to allow the clinician to intervene successfully in the seriously ill patient.

One of the amusing aspects of this CPC was my accidental learning of the correct diagnosis as part of my research into the case. I was hoping to show a map of New England indicating the reported cases of TBRDs, so I called the Department of Public Health in a neighboring state and reached Dr. Utpala Bandy. As I mentioned in the last line of my discussion, she innocently told me that she had become aware of a case of Rocky Mountain spotted fever. The patient had been transferred to the Massachusetts General Hospital the summer before my discussion. She told me that the correct diagnosis was made only on postmortem examination. It was obvious to me that she was talking about this very case.

It is remarkable how many people contacted me after the discussion, complimenting me on my honesty in admitting that I knew the diagnosis. I even received a framed "award" for unusual candor. This outpouring of support was heartwarming, but it implied that the readers of the CPC don't actually believe that the discussers are blind to the diagnosis. Certainly the seemingly uncanny correct percentage obtained by the medical students can give one the impression that some people are in on the secret. Let me assure the reader that in most cases the discusser is actually in the dark. It is not true, however, that these discussions are off-the-cuff analyses, presented as one would imagine the usual case would be handled in a teaching conference. In fact, the discusser receives the case several weeks before the discussion, thus giving him a long time to ruminate about the various possibilities and to make an erudite discussion. In my own personal experience of 12 CPCs, I was aware of the diagnosis in advance only twice: in the case of this patient and the one whom I had also seen as an attending physician. In both cases I made it clear that I was aware of the diagnosis.[1]

Martin A. Samuels

REFERENCE

1. Chapman AS and the Tickborne Rickettsial Diseases Working Group. Diagnosis and management of tickborne rickettsial diseases: Rocky Mountain spotted fever, ehrlichioses and anaplasmosis. MMWR. 2006; 55:1–29.

A 74-Year-Old Woman with Diarrhea and Fever Followed By Multiple Cranial Nerve Palsies

CAMPYLOBACTER RELATED

GUILLAIN-BARRE SYNDROME

CPC 39-1999

PRESENTATION OF CASE

A 74-year-old woman was admitted to the hospital because of diarrhea and fever followed by multiple cranial-nerve palsies.

She had a one-week history of fever (temperature, 40°C), watery diarrhea, nausea, abdominal pain, weakness, and fatigue. Her physician prescribed diphenoxylate hydrochloride–atropine sulfate. At 9 p.m. on the day before admission, the patient was speaking normally. She later applied a benzocaine–eugenol preparation to her gingiva because of several hours of dental pain. At 3 a.m. on the next day, her speech became severely slurred.

The patient was taken to another hospital. She was able to drink water and to walk satisfactorily. She was oriented and, although unable to speak, wrote complete, coherent sentences. She reported perioral numbness and dysphagia. Bilateral ptosis, greater on the right side, and left skew deviation were present. She could not move either eye in any direction. Corneal reflexes were absent. There was bilateral facial weakness. The gag reflex was intact; the tongue deviated to the left. Muscle strength was normal, and the deep-tendon reflexes were intact, with plantar flexor responses. The vocal cords were normal.

The results of laboratory tests throughout the course of the patient's illness are shown in Tables 1 through 3. A computed tomographic (CT) scan of the head, obtained without the intravenous injection of contrast material, showed moderate cerebral atrophy and a lacunar infarct in the right internal capsule. Specimens of blood and urine were obtained for culture. Methylprednisolone, ceftriaxone, and heparin were administered intravenously. The patient was transferred to this hospital, where her trachea was intubated on arrival.

Table 1 Hematologic Laboratory Values

| | Day 1 | | |
Variable	Before Admission	On Admission	Day 3
Hematocrit (%)	37.1	38.8	34.5
Mean corpuscular volume (μm^3)			90
Erythrocyte sedimentation rate (mm/hr)		91	
White-cell count (per mm^3)	20,000	27,700	21,800
Differential count (%)			
Neutrophils	68		85
Band forms	5		0
Metamyelocytes	3		1
Lymphocytes	14		7
Atypical lymphocytes	6		1
Monocytes	4		5
Eosinophils	0		1
Platelet count (per mm^3)	474,000	445,000	469,000
Prothrombin time	Normal	Normal	
Partial-thromboplastin time	Normal	Normal	
Fibrinogen (mg/dl)			502*

*The normal range is 75 to 400 mg per deciliter.

The patient had a long history of hypertension and aortic stenosis; she had undergone aortic-valve replacement with a porcine bioprosthesis five years before admission. Lung cancer had been diagnosed six years before admission, with resection of the right upper lobe followed by radiation therapy. She had smoked and had chronic obstructive pulmonary disease. Herpes zoster had developed on the right side of her back four months before admission. Additional problems included gallstones, peptic ulcer, and gastroesophageal reflux disease. The patient's medications at the time of admission consisted of hydrochlorothiazide–triamterene, potassium chloride, and verapamil. There was no history of recent ingestion of chicken or unusual or canned foods, exposure to pets, recent foreign travel, use of alcohol or drugs, exposure to ticks, previous neurologic problems, chest pain, or loss of vision.

The temperature was 36.6°C, the pulse was 105, and the respirations were 25. The blood pressure was 210/150 mm Hg.

A general physical examination showed no abnormalities.

On neurologic examination, the patient was oriented and could read, write, and count fingers when her eyelids were held open. She understood complex commands and gave appropriate positive or negative responses by turning either thumb up or down. The pupils were unreactive. No extraocular movements were present, and the doll's-head maneuver elicited no movements. She felt a cotton swab on the corneas but did not blink. Facial sensation and hearing were intact, and the uvula was in the

Table 2 Results of Lumbar Puncture on Day 1 before Admission

Variable	Finding
Appearance of fluid	Clear, colorless
Cells (per mm³)*	1 lymphocyte
Glucose (mg/dl)†	65
Protein (mg/dl)	26
Stained smear	No microorganisms

*Cells were measured in the fourth tube of fluid.

†To convert the value for glucose to millimoles per liter, multiply by 0.05551.

midline position. She could not protrude her tongue. Sternocleidomastoid strength was 4/5 bilaterally. Left-sided strength was 2/5 in the deltoid, biceps, and triceps muscles; 4/5 in the dorsal and palmar interosseous muscles; and 5/5 in the iliopsoas, quadriceps, anterior tibial, extensor hallucis longus, gastrocnemius, and hamstring muscles. Right-sided strength was 2/5 in the deltoid, biceps, and triceps muscles; 4/5 in the dorsal and palmar interosseous muscles; and 5/5 in the iliopsoas, quadriceps, anterior tibial, extensor hallucis longus, gastrocnemius, and hamstring muscles. Vibratory sensation was slightly diminished in the distal arms and legs; the sensation of a pinprick,

Table 3 Blood Chemical Values*

Variable	On Admission	Day 3
Protein (g/dl)	7.0	
Albumin	2.8	
Globulin	4.2	
Uric acid (mg/dl)	7.2	
Glucose (mg/dl)	151	140
Sodium (mmol/liter)	138	142
Potassium (mmol/liter)	3.8	4.6
Chloride (mmol/liter)	103	110
Carbon dioxide (mmol/liter)	20.1	22.6
Lactate dehydrogenase (U/liter)	783	637
Alkaline phosphatase (U/liter)	253	217
Aspartate aminotransferase (U/liter)	56	37
Amylase (U/liter)		78
Lipase (U/liter)		23.9†
Creatine kinase (U/liter)	317	
Creatine kinase MB	Normal	

*Blood chemical values other than those shown were normal. To convert the value for uric acid to micromoles per liter, multiply by 59.48. To convert the values for glucose to millimoles per liter, multiply by 0.05551.

†The normal range is 3 to 19 U per liter.

light touch, joint position, and temperature was intact. The patient could not cooper-
ate during tests of coordination. The deeptendon reflexes were absent in the arms and
++ at the knees and ankles; the plantar responses were flexor.

The urine was positive (+) for protein; the sediment contained 50 to 100 red cells,
0 to 2 white cells, and a few bacteria per high-power field. A specimen of arterial
blood, drawn after tracheal intubation, while the patient was breathing an enriched
oxygen mixture, showed that the partial pressure of oxygen was 151 mm Hg, the partial pressure of carbon dioxide was 36 mm Hg, and the pH was 7.43. An electrocardiogram showed a normal rhythm, with a short PR interval (120 msec) and a prolonged
corrected QT interval (496 msec). A magnetic resonance imaging (MRI) study of the
brain revealed diffuse enlargement of the ventricles, sulci, and cisterns; prominent
Virchow–Robin spaces; and foci of hyperintensity in the periventricular white matter, right pons, and midbrain—findings consistent with the presence of small-vessel
ischemia.

A chest radiograph showed low lung volumes and patchy opacities in the right
lung—findings consistent with the presence of either atelectasis or pneumonia. A cranial CT angiographic study showed no occlusions of the major intracranial arteries.

Heparin therapy was changed to a minidose regimen, and thiamine was given intravenously. Tests of urine and blood specimens for toxins were negative. Specimens of
stool, serum, and urine were obtained for culture and other studies.

On the second hospital day, the blood pressure was 150/75 mm Hg. The temperature was 37.7°C and did not exceed 37.9°C thereafter. The patient was weaker.
Complete ophthalmoplegia persisted; pupillary reflexes were absent. Both arms
were flaccid, and she could not raise either arm from the bed. Bilateral muscle
strength was 1/5 in the wrist extensors, 2/5 in the fingers, 1/5 in the trapezius muscles, 4/5 in the iliopsoas muscles, and 5/5 in the distal muscles of the legs. The arms
remained areflexic. The knee and ankle jerks were ++ bilaterally, and the plantar
responses were flexor.

Motor conduction studies of the right median and tibial nerves showed a low-
amplitude compound response. The F responses were normal in the tibial nerve but
were inconsistently evoked in the median nerve (Table 4). The sensory-nerve action
potentials were normal in the arms and legs. Needle electromyographic studies showed
no spontaneous activity. Motor unit potentials were normal; recruitment patterns
were reduced. A blink reflex could not be elicited from the right orbicularis oculi muscle on ipsilateral and contralateral stimulation, but the muscles responded normally
to stimulation of the facial nerve at the stylomastoid foramen (Table 5); the left orbicularis oculi muscle responded normally (Table 5). Repetitive-stimulation studies of
the intrinsic hand muscles before and after exercise showed no decremental responses
or postexercise facilitation. Botulinum antitoxin A and B, penicillin (24 million units
daily), and ofloxacin (800 mg daily) were administered.

On the third day, the patient's mental status remained normal. The cranial-nerve
deficits were unchanged. She was able to move her right thumb only minimally. She
could not lift either leg, but she could wiggle her feet up and down. There was a marked
decrease in vibratory sensation in the hands, ankles, and knees; the sensation of light

Table 4 Motor Conduction of Right Median and Tibial Nerves

Variable	Day 2	Day 3	Day 11
Median nerve			
Wrist stimulation			
Latency (msec)	3.7	4.1	No response
Amplitude (mV)	10.1	7.0	No response
Elbow stimulation			
Amplitude (mV)	8.3	4.2	No response
Velocity (m/sec)	56.5	39.7	No response
F response	Inconsistent	Absent	
Tibial nerve			
Ankle stimulation			
Latency (msec)	9.1	9.7	10.4
Amplitude (mV)	2.1	1.3	0.4
Popliteal fossa stimulation			
Amplitude (mV)	1.6	1.1	
Velocity (m/sec)	42.5	35.8	
F response	Normal	Absent	Absent

touch was preserved. No deep-tendon reflexes could be elicited. The urea nitrogen and creatinine levels were normal. A chest radiograph showed patchy bibasilar opacities that were consistent with the presence of subsegmental atelectasis. Motor conduction studies were repeated (Table 4).

Two diagnostic procedures were performed.

Table 5 Blink Reflex and Facial Motor Conduction on Day 2

	*Response**		
Site of Stimulation	*ipsilateral R1*	*ipsilateral R2 msec*	*contralateral R1*
Supraorbital nerve			
Right	No response	No response	37.5
Left	13.8	37.8	No response
	LATENCY		AMPLITUDE
	msec		mV
Facial nerve			
Right	4.5		5
Left	4.1		4

*For the facial motor conduction studies, the stylomastoid foramen was stimulated, and the response of the orbicularis oculi muscle recorded. R1 is the first component of the blink reflex, relayed oligosynaptically through the pons. It is recorded only ipsilateral to the stimulus. R2 is the later bilateral blink response. It is delayed or absent on the involved side of a facial-nerve lesion.

DIFFERENTIAL DIAGNOSIS

DR. ALLAN H. ROPPER[*]: This patient had acute, bilateral cranial-nerve paralysis that worsened over a period of hours. At the time, her physicians did not know that generalized paralysis, distal sensory loss, and areflexia would ensue. I shall analyze this case from their perspective early in the course.

Muscle weakness must be explained by a lesion at one of four sites: the central motor neurons and their descending tracts, the nerves, the neuromuscular junctions, or the muscles themselves. When one evaluates each site in this case, the diagnosis becomes apparent.

Primary muscle disease can result in oropharyngeal weakness, and ptosis can occur in cases of primary muscle disease, but it would be exceptional for a myopathy to evolve over a period of two or three days. Furthermore, oculomotor paralysis is not a typical feature of muscle disease, except in cases of progressive external ophthalmoplegia (a type of mitochondrial myopathy), thyroid ophthalmopathy, and oculopharyngeal dystrophy, all of which are ingravescent processes. Muscle disease is therefore unlikely because of the rapid progression, distribution, and severity of the weakness in this case.

Disorders of the neuromuscular junction could explain this patient's illness, since they preferentially involve ocular and cranial muscles—the ones with the lowest threshold for synaptic failure. The most common neuromuscular disorder, myasthenia gravis, may progress rapidly, causing ptosis and oropharyngeal, oculomotor, and proximal-limb weakness. Until the reflex and sensory loss became evident later in the course of the disease, myasthenia gravis was a defensible diagnosis. However, the pupils are not overtly affected in patients with myasthenia gravis, as they were in this patient, and acute total ophthalmoplegia is uncommon with this disorder. Another disease of the neuromuscular junction that warrants consideration is botulism, which generally begins with a nasal quality of the voice, dysarthria, and dysphagia and causes strabismus, ptosis, and fixed pupils. In this case, the evolution of neurologic signs over a period of hours, and then days, after a gastrointestinal illness is also suggestive of botulism. The long interval between the gastrointestinal illness and the neurologic difficulty, however, is evidence against the diagnosis; the interval is typically less than 24 hours with botulism. Also, there is no mention of prominent dryness of the mouth and throat, which is typical of the early stage of botulism, and this patient had fever, whereas in the gastrointestinal phase of botulism, the patient is usually afebrile. I would have administered botulinum antitoxin, as the clinicians did in this case, but when sensory loss became apparent, botulism could be confidently ruled out.

Any acute weakness of the cranial musculature demands a consideration of diseases of the cranial-nerve nuclei in the brain stem, especially the common problem of infarction of the pons and midbrain from occlusion of the basilar artery. Can a structural brainstem lesion that abolishes eye movements and pupillary reactions, implicating the rostral midbrain tegmentum (the region around the aqueduct that

---

[*] Chief of neurology, St. Elizabeth's Medical Center; chairman and professor of neurology, Tufts University School of Medicine—both in Boston. Currently Vice-Chair, Department of Neurology, Brigham and Women's Hospital.

encompasses the cranial-nerve nuclei), spare the immediately adjacent upper reticular neurons, leaving the patient fully awake? I think not. It is also difficult to conceive of a process that affects the widely dispersed brain-stem nuclei innervating the ocular, facial, and oropharyngeal muscles but spares the adjacent corticospinal tracts. Involvement of the corticospinal tracts is almost essential for the diagnosis of occlusion of the midbasilar artery. Exceptions to these rules include Wernicke's disease that involves the brain-stem nuclei and causes ophthalmoplegia and syringobulbia, which may affect several cranial-nerve nuclei, but neither disease explains the other features of this patient's illness. A diagnosis of acute brain-stem multiple sclerosis is inconsistent with the absence of involvement of structures near the brain-stem nuclei. Bulbar poliomyelitis could account for the pattern of destruction of brain-stem motor neurons in this patient, but it rarely causes ophthalmoplegia and is unlikely because of the absence of fever during the early phase of the neurologic illness and the normal findings in the cerebrospinal fluid.

By ruling out these sites of disease, we must conclude that this patient had a cranial-nerve disorder—namely, cranial polyneuropathy. Among the polyneuropathies, the syndrome of acutely advancing ocular, facial, and oropharyngeal weakness coupled with limb weakness is familiar to all physicians as the Guillain–Barré syndrome. However, when only the cranial nerves are involved, the illness is not as easily recognizable as the typical syndrome. Other causes of cranial polyneuropathy do not satisfactorily explain acute symmetric paralysis involving cranial nerves III through XII. Neoplastic meningeal infiltration evolves more gradually, affects the nerves unilaterally or asymmetrically, and results in abnormalities in the cerebrospinal fluid. Infectious diseases and noninfectious granulomatous diseases, including tuberculosis, fungal infections, syphilis, Lyme disease, sarcoidosis, Wegener's granulomatosis, and idiopathic granulomatous disease, can cause cranial polyneuropathy, but not as acute and severe as in this case. Also, these diseases do not explain the limb weakness and sensory changes in this case. Ciguatera (poisoning from marine toxins) can be associated with perioral numbness and a gastrointestinal prodrome, but cranial-nerve weakness, present only rarely, is not as severe as in this case.

The cranial neuropathy associated with diphtheria is perhaps the closest clinical and electrophysiologic imitator of the cranial form of the Guillain–Barré syndrome, especially when palatal paralysis is the first symptom, as it was in this case. Paralysis of the extraocular muscles develops in about 15 percent of patients with diphtheria. It may be difficult to differentiate diphtheria from the Guillain–Barré syndrome if an exudative pharyngeal membrane is not detected, and it would not be seen by a neurologist consulted at this time, because both the generalized and oculomotor neuropathies appear weeks after the pharyngitis. Diphtheria is rare in developed countries. It is also unlikely in this case because of the simultaneous rather than sequential occurrence of pharyngeal and generalized cranial weakness and the absence of early paralysis of accommodation.

As often happens in neurology, the many normal and abnormal test results are not helpful in establishing a diagnosis in this case, and the diagnosis must be based on the clinical features. From a general perspective, acute total ophthalmoplegia as the sole clinical manifestation of a neurologic illness strongly suggests the diagnosis of the Guillain–Barré syndrome. In Keane's series of 60 cases of acute bilateral ophthalmoplegia, 25 cases were due to the Guillain–Barré syndrome; 15 to brain-stem diseases, mostly strokes; 8 to disorders with a neuromuscular origin; and 12 to various other causes.[1]

The processes I have discussed (Guillain–Barré syndrome, diphtheria, myasthenia gravis, and botulism), however, can be distinguished by their electrophysiologic features. There are characteristic electromyographic abnormalities in patients with the Guillain–Barré syndrome—mainly reduced compound muscle action potentials and slowed or blocked nerve conduction—but in patients with cranial variants of the Guillain–Barré syndrome, the results of these standard tests may initially be normal or almost normal. The greatest value of the electromyographic studies in this case is that they rule out the diagnosis of neuromuscular disease—specifically, myasthenia gravis—by demonstrating the absence of a decrement in muscle contraction with repetitive nerve stimulation, and botulism, by demonstrating the absence of an increment in muscle contraction.

Predominant weakness of the ocular and oropharyngeal muscles characterizes one of several variants of the Guillain–Barré syndrome in which weakness is purely or predominantly regional. Guillain et al. described afebrile generalized paralysis in 1916, and numerous refinements of the clinical picture were presented at a symposium in Brussels, Belgium, in 1937.[2] Several French neurologists described syndromes of multiple symmetric cranial-nerve palsies that were later redescribed in the English literature.[3] In 1956, Fisher identified a syndrome of ataxia, external (and sometimes internal) ophthalmoplegia, and areflexia.[4] Additional variants have subsequently been delineated (Table 6).[5] All these variants are linked to the typical form of the

Table 6 Regional and Functional Variants of the Guillain-Barré Syndrome

Variant	Associated Ganglioside Autoantibody*
Regional	
Oculomotor paralysis with ataxia (Fisher's syndrome) or without it	GQ1b
Pharyngeal–brachial–cervical weakness	GT1a (GQ1b, GD1a)
Lumbar–crural syndrome	
Bilateral facial or abducens paresis, with paresthesia	GM1
Pure motor syndrome	
Functional	
Pure sensory syndrome	GD1b
Ataxia (with or without ophthalmoplegia)	GD1b (GD3, GQ1b)
Pure dysautonomia	
Mixed types	GQ1b, GT1a

*Antibodies in parentheses are infrequent, subsidiary, or cross-reacting antibodies. Anti-GQ1b autoantibody is regularly associated with Fisher's syndrome. With all the other disorders, the association with the specified autoantibodies is variable.

Guillain–Barré syndrome by the presence of generalized areflexic weakness; shared electrophysiologic features, which may be abnormal only in weakened regions; and an elevated cerebrospinal fluid protein level in some cases. The variant forms of the Guillain–Barré syndrome are often combined with generalized paralysis. The oculomotor and lower-cranial-nerve variants have a particular proclivity to coalesce, as in the case under discussion.[6,7] This patient did not have Fisher's syndrome, a designation best reserved for cases with only ataxia and ophthalmoplegia.

Another interesting aspect of this case is the subtle meaning of the early neurologic signs in relation to the Guillain–Barré syndrome. The first symptom, perioral numbness, usually indicates the presence of basilar-artery occlusion, but I have seen that symptom in patients with the Guillain–Barré syndrome. Disconjugate skew deviation may be a symptom of a peripheral oculomotor palsy but always raises the possibility of brain-stem or cerebellar stroke. The absence of diplopia is common because of the complete ophthalmoplegia that is characteristic of the Guillain–Barré syndrome, in which the globes are kept in an orthotopic position. In this case, the deeptendon reflexes, which were initially normal, directed attention away from this syndrome, but areflexia may not appear for days, and then only in weak limbs. A loss of reflexes from one day to the next is almost diagnostic of the Guillain–Barré syndrome. Normal levels of protein in the cerebrospinal fluid are common in the initial days of the illness; 70 percent of patients have protein levels below 45 mg per deciliter in the first three days, and many variants of the Guillain–Barré syndrome are associated with normal levels even later in the illness.

Autoantibodies directed against peripheral-nerve antigens, particularly gangliosides, have been identified in patients with the Guillain–Barré syndrome. The most consistent association is that between anti-GQ1b autoantibody and Fisher's syndrome.[8] The putative explanation for the paralysis of the ocular muscles is the high concentration of GQ1b ganglioside in paranodal regions of the oculomotor nerves.

Furthermore, the enteric pathogen *Campylobacter jejuni* is the most common infectious trigger for the development of the Guillain–Barré syndrome, and the lipopolysaccharide coat of some strains of this organism shares epitopes with gangliosides of the peripheral nerve, specifically GQ1b and GM1. This finding validates the concept of cross-reacting antibodies, or "molecular mimicry," which has been postulated to explain the postinfectious, immunologic nature of the Guillain–Barré syndrome. In the process of evicting *C. jejuni*, the immune system purportedly produces antibodies that damage elements of the peripheral nerve. Concentrations of specific gangliosides in certain nerves may account for the regional and functional variants of the syndrome that I have listed.

The diagnostic procedure in this case was probably a serologic test for autoantibody to GQ1b ganglioside. Since an enteritis with fever preceded this patient's neurologic illness, she must have had *C. jejuni* infection, which may have been cultured from the stool specimen. There are effective treatments for the main causes of acute, multiple, symmetric cranial palsies (the Guillain–Barré syndrome, botulism, myasthenia gravis, diphtheria, and basilar-artery occlusion), and their distinction on the basis of clinical features and the results of electromyographic and antibody tests is therefore of great practical value.

CLINICAL DIAGNOSES

Guillain–Barré syndrome.
Campylobacter jejuni enteritis.

DR. ALLAN H. ROPPER'S DIAGNOSES

Mixed cranial-nerve variant of the Guillain–Barré syndrome (oculomotor–pharyngeal type) associated with anti-GQ1b autoantibody.
Campylobacter jejuni enteritis.

PATHOLOGICAL DISCUSSION

DR. DIDIER P. CROS: One of the diagnostic procedures was an extension of the initial neurophysiologic assessment, which continued during the patient's three-week hospital stay. The normal results of repetitive nerve stimulation on the initial examination, performed on the second hospital day, ruled out the diagnosis of a presynaptic or postsynaptic neuromuscular-junction disorder. On the next day, rapid changes in the neurophysiologic findings were consistent with the fulminant course of the patient's illness. There was a further decrease in the amplitude of the compound motor response of the right ulnar and tibial nerves. F responses were unobtainable in the right median, ulnar, and tibial nerves, and the sensory-nerve action potentials were all absent. In many of the weak muscles, no spontaneous or voluntary activity was seen. Eight days later, motor amplitudes were very low or unobtainable (Table 4). Widespread spontaneous activity was recorded in many muscles from which voluntary responses could not be elicited.

The neurophysiologic findings indicate a generalized polyneuropathy of recent onset. The conduction abnormalities indicate the presence of disease of the peripheral nerves, and the absence of voluntary electromyographic activity is correlated with the severity of the weakness. The criteria for the diagnosis of primary demyelination of the motor fibers, which include conduction block, marked prolongation of motor latencies, marked slowing of conduction velocities, and an absence of F responses (in nerves with normal compound muscle action potentials),[9] are not met in this case.

Can the findings and their rapid progression nonetheless provide clues to the nature of the neuropathy? In this regard, the neurophysiologic findings are mostly ambiguous. The rapidly decreasing amplitude of the compound motor responses could be due to distal conduction block or to degeneration of the motor fibers. Similarly, the disappearance of sensory-nerve action potentials over a 24-hour period is consistent with primary demyelination as the cause of conduction block or desynchronization in the large sensory fibers, but extensive fiber degeneration could also be the cause. The progression of abnormalities in the F responses from persistently low to absent responses is suggestive but not diagnostic of primary demyelination because of the low amplitude of the compound motor responses. The results of the studies of the blink reflex and facial motor conduction on the right side also suggest that primary demyelination caused conduction block of the motor fibers proximal to the stylomas-toid foramen. Extensive focal necrosis of these fibers in the same segment, however, could produce the same neurophysiologic pattern, since conduction persists for several days in axons distal to the site of focal axonal injury. The absence of spontaneous activ-ity on needle electromyography is similarly equivocal in a patient with acute paralysis. Spontaneous activity is not usually associated with a pure demyelinating lesion, but its development is delayed by at least several days in cases in which there is motor axonal degeneration.

The progression of the conduction abnormalities was so rapid that by the 11th hos-pital day all sensory potentials and blink reflexes were unobtainable, motor responses were of very low amplitude or were absent, and widespread fibrillation and positive wave activity were noted in muscles with no recorded voluntary activity. The sponta-neous activity unequivocally indicates the presence of motor axonal degeneration. Two questions remain. Was axonal degeneration or an inflammatory demyelinating lesion the primary pathophysiologic process?

The Guillain–Barré syndrome was for many years considered an acute, inflamma-tory demyelinating neuropathy.[10,11] The occurrence of axonal damage in the context of acute, overt demyelination has been noted in up to 64 percent of cases[12] and has gener-ally been attributed to nonspecific, severe endoneurial inflammation—the "bystander" effect. The question of an axonal variant of the Guillain–Barré syndrome was raised by a report on a small series of patients with inexcitable motor nerves and a poor outcome; limited pathological data failed to reveal the presence of primary demye-lination.[13] The importance of inexcitability of the nerves in the diagnosis of axonal Guillain–Barré syndrome was challenged,[14] and in several cases of acute paralysis, it was established that inexcitability of the nerves was due to the presence of demyeli-nating lesions rather than axonal disruption.[15–17] Acute motor axonal neuropathy was subsequently documented during epidemics in northern China, with detailed studies at autopsy.[18] At present, the Guillain–Barré syndrome should be considered patholog-ically heterogeneous, with a primary demyelinating variant, which is most common in North America and Europe,[11] a primary axonal motor variant, reported in northern China, and a rare, primary axonal sensory and motor variant. The distinction between the primary axonal and primary demyelinating forms of the disorder is important, because the efficacy of current treatments has been demonstrated mostly in patients with the primary demyelinating variant. The identification of reliable biologic mark-ers of each of these variants will be an important first step in developing improved treatments.

DR. DARRYL E. PALMER-TOY: The other diagnostic procedure was a stool cul-ture. Small, flat, mucoid colonies, which were positive for catalase, oxidase, and indoxyl acetate, grew on brucella–blood agar containing cefoperazone, vancomycin, and amphotericin B (Fig. 1) and were sensitive to nalidixic acid but resistant to cephalothin. Gram's staining revealed small, mostly curved or spiral gram-negative organisms (Fig. 2). The findings were consistent with the presence of *C. jejuni* infec-tion, although without a test of hippurate hydrolysis, *C. coli* infection could not be ruled out.

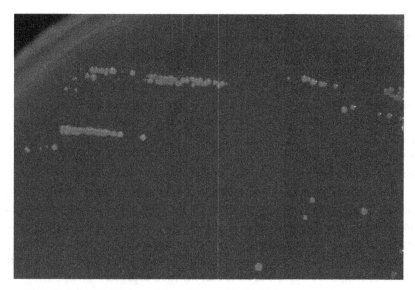

FIG 1 Small, Flat, Mucoid Colonies of *Campylobacter jejuni in Culture.*

C. jejuni is the most common bacterial cause of diarrhea in the United States, and about 1 percent of the U.S. population is infected by this organism each year.[19] The frequency of infection peaks in infancy, with a smaller peak between 15 and 30 years of age. Contaminated poultry has been implicated in 50 to 70 percent of cases that occur in areas where the infection is endemic.[20]

About 25 percent of patients with *C. jejuni* enteritis are asymptomatic.[19] Of symptomatic patients, 90 percent have fever, and most have severe diarrhea, abdominal pain,

FIG 2 Small, Curved or Spiral Gram-Negative *Campylobacter jejuni* Organisms (Gram's Stain, ×1200).

nausea, and malaise, all of which were present in this case. Symptoms usually resolve in one week, with or without treatment, but they persist from one to three weeks in about 20 percent of cases. The symptoms closely resemble those in patients with salmonella and shigella infections.

In patients who have *C. jejuni* infection in association with the Guillain–Barré syndrome, the weakness typically proceeds to maximal disability in less than a week, and sometimes in less than two days. Such patients are more likely to require ventilatory assistance and to have prolonged, severe disability than patients with the idiopathic form of the Guillain–Barré syndrome.[21] This patient had an elevated level of anti-GQ1b autoantibody but a normal level of anti-GM1 autoantibody.

DR. R. WESLEY FARRIS II: After the diagnosis was made, we began plasma-exchange therapy, with a total exchange of 21 liters. The patient's condition continued to deteriorate, and a five-day course of intravenously administered immune globulin was instituted. During this treatment, her weakness stopped progressing. After treating numerous medical complications, we discharged her to a rehabilitation facility. At the time of discharge, she was able to move only her right large toe.

DR. CROS: In the three months that have elapsed since the onset of the patient's illness, the cranial-nerve involvement has become less severe, and there has been a partial recovery from the ophthalmoplegia. The patient's arms have become stronger, and she uses them to communicate. She is still intubated.

DR. ROPPER: The Guillain–Barré disorder is indeed a syndrome, not a disease, encompassing a number of clinical and immune patterns. Many of the regional variants and some of the functional variants that have been mentioned have been associated with specific autoantibodies, and these associations may become diagnostically useful (Table 6). The anti-GQ1b autoantibody has the strongest association with a clinical feature—namely, ophthalmoplegia. Also, certain organisms have been associated with particular autoantibodies—*C. jejuni* with GM1 and cytomegalovirus with GM2. The humoral immune reactions to these organisms, particularly epitopes on campylobacter, demonstrate that the immune system can selectively attack both functional and regional components of the peripheral nervous system. This interesting point has not been widely appreciated. If there is a unifying feature of these variants, it is the relatively symmetric pattern of the clinical features.

ANATOMICAL DIAGNOSES

Guillain–Barré syndrome.
   Campylobacter jejuni enteritis.

REFERENCES

1. Keane JR. Acute bilateral ophthalmoplegia: 60 cases. Neurology 1986; 36:279–81.
2. Guillain G. Synthèse générale de la discussion. J Belg Neurol Psychiatry 1938;38:323–9.
3. Munsat TL, Barnes JE. Relation of multiple cranial nerve dysfunction to the Guillain-Barré syndrome. J Neurol Neurosurg Psychiatry 1965;28:115–20.

4. Fisher M. An unusual variant of acute idiopathic polyneuritis (syndrome of ophthalmoplegia, ataxia and areflexia). N Engl J Med 1956;255:57–65.

5. Ropper AH. Unusual clinical variants and signs in Guillain-Barré syndrome. Arch Neurol 1986;43:1150–2.

6. Shuaib A, Becker WJ. Variants of Guillain-Barré syndrome: Miller Fisher syndrome, facial diplegia and multiple cranial nerve palsies. Can J Neurol Sci 1987;14:611–16.

7. Ter Bruggen JP, van der Meche FG, de Jager AE, Polman CH. Ophthalmoplegic and lower cranial nerve variants merge into each other and into classical Guillain-Barré syndrome. Muscle Nerve 1998;21:239–42.

8. Chiba A, Kusunoki S, Obata H, Machinami R, Kanazawa I. Serum anti-GQ1b IgG antibody is associated with ophthalmoplegia in Miller Fisher syndrome and Guillain-Barré syndrome: clinical and immunohistochemical studies. Neurology 1993;43:1911–17.

9. Cornblath DR. Electrophysiology in Guillain-Barré syndrome. Ann Neurol 1990;27:Suppl:S17–20.

10. Asbury AK, Arnason BG, Adams RD. The inflammatory lesion in idiopathic polyneuritis: its role in pathogenesis. Medicine (Baltimore) 1969;48:173–215.

11. Albers JW, Donofrio PD, McGonagle TK. Sequential electrodiagnostic abnormalities in acute inflammatory demyelinating polyradiculoneuropathy. Muscle Nerve 1985;8:528–39.

12. Brown WF, Feasby TE. Conduction block and denervation in Guillain-Barré polyneuropathy. Brain 1984;107:219–39.

13. Feasby TE, Gilbert JJ, Brown WF, et al. An acute axonal form of Guillain-Barré polyneuropathy. Brain 1986;109:1115–26.

14. Triggs WJ, Cros D, Gominak SC, et al. Motor nerve inexcitability in Guillain-Barré syndrome: the spectrum of distal conduction block and axonal degeneration. Brain 1992;115:1291–302.

15. Hall SM, Hughes RAC, Atkinson PF, McColl I, Gale A. Motor nerve biopsy in severe Guillain-Barré syndrome. Ann Neurol 1992;31:441–4.

16. Berciano J, Figols J, Garcia A, et al. Fulminant Guillain-Barré syndrome with universal inexcitability of peripheral nerves: a clinicopathological study. Muscle Nerve 1997;20:846–57.

17. Berciano J, Coria F, Monton F, Calleja J, Figols J, Lafarga M. Axonal form of Guillain-Barré syndrome: evidence for macrophage-associated demyelination. Muscle Nerve 1993;16:744–51.

18. Griffin JW, Li CY, Ho TW, et al. Pathology of the motor-sensory axonal Guillain-Barré syndrome. Ann Neurol 1996;39:17–28.

19. Allos BM. Campylobacter jejuni infection as a cause of the Guillain-Barré syndrome. Infect Dis Clin North Am 1998;12:173–84.

20. Blaser MJ. Epidemiologic and clinical features of Campylobacter jejuni infections. J Infect Dis 1997;176:Suppl 2:S103–S105.

21. Hughes RAC, Rees JH. Clinical and epidemiologic features of Guillain-Barré syndrome. J Infect Dis 1997;176:Suppl 2:S92–S98.

Perspectives and Updates

Multiple cranial neuropathies present a vexing problem for neurologists and neuro-surgeons. After intrinsic brainstem disease has been excluded by determining that there are no long tract signs, the majority of cases are the result of inflammatory, infectious, invasive, or destructive processes. Cranial muscular weakness represents another category but is easier to detect clinically. The usual list of possibilities for multiple cranial neuropathies includes Guillain-Barré syndrome (GBS), sarcoidosis, viral infection including AIDS and CMV, carcinomatous meningitis, and the often cited but seldom seen diseases of botulism and diphtheria. When no diagnosis can be made with confidence, an inflammatory condition is often assigned as a default explanation.

As outlined in the discussion of this case, certain characteristic features of botulism, particularly dry mouth and a short interval between gastrointestinal illness and the neurologic features, assist in differentiating botulism from variants of GBS. Nonetheless, the two processes have many similarities and it is not unreasonable to administer anti–botulinum toxin in doubtful cases. Many textbooks give details of the pupillary features of botulism but few of these can be depended on with certainty for the diagnosis of the disease or in distinguishing its serotypes. However, light-fixed pupils in botulism are usually of mid-size, in contrast to the enlarged pupils of third nerve palsy in the GBS variants.

Diphtheria presents a similar diagnostic challenge when bulbar innervated muscles are affected. Many accounts of diphtheric cranial neuropathy in textbooks are somewhat muddled. First, a grayish diphtheric membrane in the oropharynx is helpful in the diagnosis, but it has usually disappeared by the time cranial polyneuropathy appears and a neurologist is called. The pharyngeal muscles weakness is due to direct diffusion of the bacterial toxin. Ocular motor palsies are infrequent. However, the polyneuropathy is usually (not always) delayed for days to weeks after the primary nasopharyngeal infection and cranial polyneuropathy. This polyneuropathy is predominantly motor; it is otherwise nondescript and may appear independently of the cranial palsies.

One of the most interesting causes of multiple cranial nerve palsies, not likely in this CPC, is retrograde local invasion of the fifth and seventh nerves by a cutaneous carcinoma on the face that had been resected up to several years previously. Squamous basal cell and a specific type of melanoma, lentigo maligna, are the usual causes in this category. The infiltrating dermal cancer cases I have seen began with numbness in the infraorbital nerve or forehead region. The neoplasm may eventually cause a small mass at the base of the skull.

There are, in addition, the "classic" syndromes of multiple palsies due to metastatic lesions at the base of the skull. Infiltration of the jugular foramen and posterior retroparotid and condylar regions are the commonest of these and give rise to the syndromes of Vernet (IX, X, XI), Collet-Siccard (IX, X, XI, and XII), and Villaret (the same as the previous one but with a Horner syndrome). These are usually due to prostate or breast cancer, or multiple myeloma.

With regard to GBS and its variants, I would caution against using the term "Fisher syndrome" for all forms of postinfectious cranial polyneuropathy. It is true that the ophthalmoplegic-ataxic-areflexic syndrome can blend into other more typical forms of GBS, but there is value in retaining the term for a pure or almost pure triad so that it remains distinguishable from other processes, such as the ophthalmoplegia of Wernicke disease.

Some of the most interesting work in peripheral neurology has come from Japanese laboratories, especially Yuki, who has studied the immunobiology of GBS.[1] As indicated in the table within the CPC, certain antibodies have a propensity to cause particular clinical syndromes. Aside from anti-GQ 1B and perhaps a motor syndrome associated with anti-GM1[2] these clinical and immunologic connections have been inconsistent. The most interesting result of these immunologic observations is that they suggest that different nerves express particular ganglioside epitopes, so that highly specific antibodies can tease apart the peripheral nervous system. Not only are certain regions of the nervous system, such as the cranial nerves, identified by particular antibodies (and therefore, presumably by different antigens) but functional features such as motor versus sensory, large fiber versus small fiber sensory as well as very specific components of the peripheral nerve such as the paranodal regions have autoantibody signatures that conform to clinical syndromes. Whether this also pertains to myelin, the axonal surface (most likely it does with anti-MAG), and components of the axon itself is not clear, but this question offers an exciting prospect for further elucidating in the biology of peripheral and cranial nerves.

The genesis of these anti-neural antibodies is not clear. Current thinking revolves around a "molecular mimicry" model in which viral or bacterial infection incites a panel of antibodies, one or more of which has antineural properties. The most compelling case for this mechanism is the connection between *Campylobacter jejuni* and anti-GM1 antibody. (*C. jejuni* is probably the most frequent identifiable predecessor to GBS, explaining 20 to 30 percent of typical cases and a similar proportion of cases of Fisher syndrome.). Yuki has also made the observation that *Haemophilus influenzae* precedes some cases of Fisher syndrome.[3]

At present there is no clear translation of these findings to the selection of specific treatment, such as informing the choice between IVIG infusion and plasma exchange. A current summary of the clinical syndrome of GBS and the autoantibodies that have been tentatively associated with them is given by Yuki and Hartung.[4]

Allan H. Ropper

REFERENCES

1. Yuki N: Ganglioside mimicry and peripheral nerve disease. Muscle Nerve 2007; 35:691–711.
2. Jacobs BC, Koga M, van Rijs W, et al. Subclass IgG to motor gangliosides related to infection and clinical course in Guillain-Barré syndrome Journal of neuroimmunology 2008; 194:1–90.
3. Koga M, Yuki N, Tai T, Hirata K. Miller Fisher syndrome and *Haemophilus influenzae* infection. Neurology. 2001; 57:686–91.
4. Yuki N, Hartung H-P. Guillain-Barré syndrome. N Engl J Med 2012; 366 :2294–2304.

A 31-Year-Old Man with an Apparent Seizure and A Cerebral Lesion

SCHISTOSOMIASIS

CPC 21-2001

PRESENTATION OF CASE

A 31-year-old man was admitted to the hospital because of an apparent seizure and radiologic evidence of a cerebral lesion.

The patient had been in excellent health until five days earlier, when he felt weak, was briefly unable to walk, and began to have mild headaches and dizzy spells, which lasted for several days. A computed tomographic (CT) scan of the head, obtained elsewhere, showed a hypodense lesion in the right parietal lobe. On the day of admission, uncontrollable flailing of the right arm and leg developed. The patient was referred to this hospital.

The patient was a research worker involved in a trial of a human immunodeficiency virus (HIV) vaccine; he had no contact with patients. Eighteen months before admission, he had participated in a field study in Uganda; a test for HIV antibodies had been negative on his arrival there. He had received vaccines against viral hepatitis A and B, typhoid fever, and yellow fever. During his stay in Africa, he also traveled to Kenya and Tanzania, rafted once on the Nile, and frequently swam in and sailed on Lake Victoria, five months before admission. He consumed a variety of meats, which included well-cooked pork. He had had a bout of diarrhea and fever one year before admission and again five months later; each bout lasted two days. His only medication was mefloquine (250 mg once a week). He had been accompanied in Africa by his wife, who remained well.

The temperature was 36.3°C, the pulse was 60, and the respirations were 18. The blood pressure was 140/80 mm Hg. Physical, neurologic, and ophthalmologic examinations revealed no abnormalities. The urine was normal. Laboratory tests were performed (Tables 1 and 2).

A magnetic resonance imaging (MRI) study of the brain (Fig. 1), performed after the administration of gadolinium, showed an ill-defined, irregular area of abnormal enhancement, 3.5 cm in maximal diameter, in the right parietal lobe, with increased

Table 1 Hematologic Laboratory Values

Variable	Value
Hematocrit (%)	42.6
Erythrocyte sedimentation rate (mm/hr)	11
White-cell count (per mm^3)	11,000
Differential count (%)	
Neutrophils	83
Lymphocytes	11
Monocytes	4
Eosinophils	2
Platelet count (per mm^3)	289,000
Prothrombin time	Normal
Partial-thromboplastin time	Normal

intensity of the signal on the T_1-weighted image; some of the enhancement within and posterior to the lesion appeared to indicate leptomeningeal involvement. This finding was consistent with a breakdown of the blood–brain barrier; the finding of a surrounding area of low attenuation was consistent with the presence of edema. Proton spectroscopy showed an elevation of choline resonance in relation to creatinine (1.66:1.0) and a decrease in N-acetyl aspartate; this finding is consistent with

Table 2 Blood Chemical Values

Variable	Value
Urea nitrogen	Normal
Creatinine	Normal
Protein (g/dl)	
Total	7.1
Albumin	4.4
Globulin	2.7
Calcium	Normal
Phosphorus	Normal
Bilirubin	
Total	Normal
Conjugated	Normal
Glucose	Normal
Sodium (mmol/liter)	134
Potassium (mmol/liter)	4.1
Chloride (mmol/liter)	103
Carbon dioxide (mmol/liter)	26.1

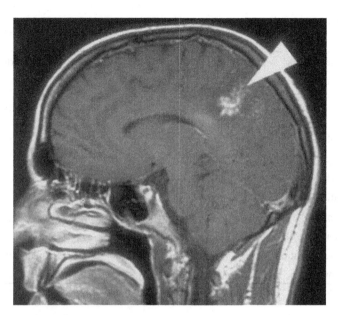

FIG 1 Sagittal T$_1$-Weighted Magnetic Resonance Image Obtained after the Administration of Contrast Material.
There is an area of increased enhancement in the right parietal lobe, with surrounding hypointensity (arrowhead).

inflammation. A small lactate doublet was present. Radiographs of the chest showed no abnormalities. Microscopical examination of urine and stool specimens disclosed no ova or parasites. A tuberculin skin test (5 TU), performed without controls, was negative at 72 hours. A lumbar puncture was performed (Table 3).

A diagnostic procedure was performed

DIFFERENTIAL DIAGNOSIS

Relation of the Main Neurologic Symptom to the Radiologic Lesion

Dr. ALLAN H. ROPPER[*]: Before discussing the causes of focal brain lesions in travelers who have returned from East Africa, I shall comment on this patient's main neurologic symptom, "uncontrollable flailing" of his right arm and leg. Flailing or flinging movements usually signify ballismus, an extraordinary type of movement disorder caused by a lesion in the contralateral subthalamic nucleus. Another possible interpretation is that the movements represent the rare choreoathetoid movement that originates from a seizure arising in the supplementary motor cortex. In a patient with a brain mass, however, a focal motor convulsion is the most likely interpretation of this symptom.

---

[*] Chief, Department of Neurology, St. Elizabeth's Medical Center; chairman and professor of neurology, Tufts University School of Medicine—both in Boston. Currently Vice-Chair, Department of Neurology, Brigham and Women's Hospital.

Table 3 Findings on Lumbar Puncture

Variable	Finding
Appearance of fluid	Clear, colorless
Cells (per mm^3)	
Red	136
White	2
Differential count (%)	
Lymphocytes	84
Monocytes	16
Unidentifiable cells	Rare
Glucose (mg/dl)*	71
Total protein (mg/dl)	75
Cytologic examination	No malignant cells
Microorganisms, including acid-fast bacilli and fungi	Absent

*To convert the value for glucos e to millimoles per liter, multiply by 0.05551..

With any of these explanations, the larger semiologic problem is the reconciliation of right-sided limb movements with the presence of a radiographically confirmed lesion on the right side of the brain. A convulsion ipsilateral to a cerebral lesion is most often explained by a generalized seizure discharge that is blocked from exciting the limbs of the opposite side because the causative lesion has produced a hemiplegia. Another explanation is the presence of a second, less apparent lesion in the contralateral hemisphere, as often happens in cases of metastatic and infectious diseases of the brain. The most intriguing possibility is that this patient had an uncrossed corticospinal system.[1,2] None of the possible explanations for this mismatch of sides is satisfactory in this case, however.

May we review the radiologic studies?

Dr. R. Gilberto Gonzalez (Neuroradiology): A sagittal T_1-weighted image in a right parasagittal plane from the MRI study performed at this hospital shows a hypointense lesion in the right parietal lobe. An image obtained after the administration of contrast material (Fig. 1) shows enhancement in the central portion of the lesion, indicating a breakdown of the blood–brain barrier.

Dr. Ropper: Neither the clinical appearance of a focal seizure nor the nonspecific appearance of this patient's small enhancing lesion even remotely permits a definite diagnosis. If we were to set aside his travel history, many relatively common processes, such as an incipient bacterial abscess (cerebritis), a granulomatous infection, or a tumor or tumor-like growth (particularly a tuberculoma, a glioma, or a metastatic tumor) would be prominent in the differential diagnosis. With the possibility of the acquired immunodeficiency syndrome (AIDS) suggested by this patient's history of involvement in an HIV-vaccine program, additional considerations are toxoplasmosis, cryptococcosis, and a brain lymphoma.

Table 4 Tropical Parasites That May Cause Focal Brain Lesions

Organisms	Diseases	Clinical Features	Radiographic Features
Cestodes (tapeworms)			
Taenia solium	Cysticercosis	Seizures with mature lesions, a mass, ventricular and subarachnoid implantation	Cyst with scolex, late calcification, often multiple cysts
Taen. multiceps	Coenurosis		
Spirometra	Sparganosis	Subcutaneous nodules, seizures	Migrating inflammation or mass
Echinococcus	Hydatid disease	Focal findings, raised intracranial pressure	Large fluid-filled cyst or solid chitinoma
Nematodes (roundworms)			
Trichinella	Trichinosis	Skin lesions, myositis, in rare cases brain granuloma	Granuloma
Angiostrongylus cantonensis	Angiostrongyliasis	Meningoen-cephalitis	Migrating lesions
Strongyloides stercoralis	Strongyloidiasis	Encephalitis, myelitis, seizures	Migrating lesions
Toxocara canis, Tox. cati	Visceral larva migrans	Eosinophilic meningoen-cephalitis	Irregular nodular enhancing lesions, migrating lesions
Trematodes (flukes)			
Schistosoma japonicum, S. mansoni, S. haematobium	Schistosomiasis	Myelopathy, brain lesions, seizures, tumorlike symptoms	Single granuloma
Paragonimus	Paragonimiasis	Seizures, meningoen-cephalitis	Single granuloma

(continued)

Table 4 (Continued)

Other tropical parasites			
Toxoplasma gondii	Toxoplasmosis	Seizures	Single enhancing lesion
Entamoeba histolytica, Balamuthia mandrillaris	Amebiasis	Hepatosplenic disease, granulomas, encephalopathy, meningoencephalitis, seizures	Abscess, meningoencephalitis
Mycobacterium tuberculosis, atypical forms	Tuberculoma	Seizures	Granuloma

Tropical Diseases

The salient feature of this patient's history is the onset of his illness on his return from East Africa, a factor that makes an exotic infectious cause of his brain lesion likely. I was taught by Dr. Benjamin H. Kean, former chief of tropical medicine at Cornell University Medical College, that the approach to diagnosing a tropical disease involves four questions: Where did the patient travel? What did he or she do there? What constellation of clinical features stands out? What would a local doctor think? The diseases I shall consider in detail are all common in East Africa and are known to cause single lesions in the brain.

In this case, there were no dermal, ocular, hepatosplenic, intestinal, hematologic, lymphatic, or other systemic findings characteristic of a specific tropical disease, and we are obliged instead to rely on epidemiologic and imaging features to establish the diagnosis. Two excellent sources of information for the differential diagnosis of tropical diseases, including parasitic diseases, involving the central nervous system are available.[3,4]

Diseases Due to Tapeworms

In a tropical or subtropical setting, a seizure associated with a focal lesion in the brain is most often due to cysticercosis caused by the pork tapeworm, *Taenia solium* (Table 4). Although this infection is one of the most common causes of acquired seizure disorders throughout the world, rivaled only by tuberculoma, it is easily overlooked by clinicians in the United States because of its rarity in this country. Cysticercosis occurs in East Africa but is not nearly as common there as it is in Latin America, including Mexico. This patient's lesion is probably not associated with cysticercosis, however, because the parasite larva in cysticercosis evokes little if any inflammatory response or edema in the early stages of brain infestation and therefore usually does not produce clinical manifestations or cause much radiologic change at that time. It takes approximately two months for the lesion to evolve into the highly recognizable, thin-walled, fluid-filled cavity containing a distinctive scolex. After about a year, the parasite dies, loses its distinctive internal structure, and incites an inflammatory response. Eventually, the lesion may calcify. It is in these later stages of evolution, as inflammation and gliosis become prominent, that seizures develop. The MRI study in this case does not reveal a scolex or a degenerating cyst. Conceivably, we are observing the early stage of larval invasion, but that phase is generally asymptomatic. I cannot dismiss cysticercosis because it is a common cause of seizures in the tropics, but I do not favor it.

Three other cestodes, besides *Taen. solium*, that may infect the brain and that characteristically encyst are echinococcus, *Taen. multiceps*, and spirometra (Table 4). Echinococcosis deserves consideration because it is endemic in the region where this patient traveled and, in particular, is hyperendemic in parts of Kenya. However, brain involvement is rare, and seizures are even rarer in echinococcosis. The tumor-like effects of a large, fluid-filled mass are more typical of this infection. The lesion in the current case does not have the radiologic appearance of a large hydatid cyst due to echinococcosis. Although there is a solid form of the echinococcal lesion, called a chitinoma, both the solid and the cystic forms enlarge very slowly, by approximately 1 to 2 cm per year. Thus the diagnosis of echinococcosis is very unlikely in this case. Coenurosis, due to *Taen. multiceps*, is almost identical to cysticercosis and causes single lesions in the brain more often than does cysticercosis, but it is extremely rare. Sparganosis, which is due to spirometra, should be considered because of its tendency to cause single granulomas of a configuration somewhat similar to the lesion in this case. However, the absence of the characteristic subcutaneous nodules of the disease in this patient and its relative infrequency in East Africa (as compared with the Far East, where most cases have been reported) help to rule out that diagnosis.

Diseases Due to Roundworms

Diseases due to roundworms typically cause meningoencephalitis, sometimes accompanied by a virtually diagnostic eosinophilia in the cerebrospinal fluid. Of the nematodes, toxocara, trichinella, strongyloides, and angiostrongylus cause focal lesions in the brain infrequently. *Toxocara canis* and *Tox. cati*, which cause visceral larva migrans, are acquired from dogs and cats, but the clinical disease almost always occurs in children and typically causes retinal lesions. Trichinosis is best known to neurologists for its involvement of muscle tissue; lesions in the brain are rare, occurring when there are large numbers of larvae; in such cases, eosinophilia in the peripheral blood is almost always present. The rarity of brain lesions caused by nematodes and the absence of eosinophilia and other characteristic systemic features of nematode infections make their presence unlikely in this case.

Diseases Due to Flukes

The flukes that may be implicated in brain disease are schistosomes and, very rarely, paragonimus (Table 4). Paragonimus causes a round, focal, granulomatous lesion in the brain, which is the most common extrapulmonary site of infestation, but in the absence of lung lesions, brain involvement is very rare. Furthermore, paragonimiasis, though reported in Uganda, is found predominantly in western Africa and the Far East.

Schistosomiasis is the probable diagnosis in this case because of the patient's history of rafting on the Nile and of frequent swimming in and sailing on Lake Victoria; both are warm, fresh-water locations where the snail hosts of schistosomes reside. Mention by the patient of either site would prompt a local doctor to make this diagnosis. Entry of the parasites from the water is transdermal, but their entry often goes unnoticed unless it causes so-called swimmer's itch. A pair of flukes mate and release eggs in the bloodstream; the eggs then spread to various parts of the body, occasionally including the nervous system.

According to authoritative textbooks, such as *Hunter's Tropical Medicine*,[5] brain lesions due to fluke infections are commonly caused by *Schistosoma japonicum*, which is native to the Far East, and only rarely by *S. mansoni* and *S. haematobium*, which are ubiquitous in Africa. The eggs of *S. mansoni* and *S. haematobium* usually spread to the lumbar spinal cord rather than the brain, but I have been unable to find corroboration of the statement that *S. mansoni* and *S. haematobium* only rarely affect the brain. One review[6] cites an autopsy study in Africa, in which over half the patients infected with *S. mansoni* or *S. haematobium* had brain lesions. In another study, *S. mansoni* eggs surrounded by granulomas were found in the brain in a quarter of infected patients at autopsy.[7] A review by Pittella[8] of published cases of *S. mansoni* infection up to 1991 reveals that 51 involved the brain and 60 involved the lumbar spinal cord. The author emphasizes the absence of evidence of systemic spread and the involvement of the central nervous system in the early stages of infestation.

The radiographic appearance of a schistosomal lesion in the brain is typically that of a moderately large granuloma with punctate enhancement and a heterogeneous internal structure. This appearance reflects the presence of a collection of eggs and is unlike the more homogeneous, nodular picture in this case.

Other Tropical Infections

Tuberculomas and amebic abscesses may form single lesions in the brain. *Entamoeba histolytica* must be contrasted with the so-called free-living amebas, such as *Naegleria fowleri*, which usually causes an aggressive meningitis, and acanthamoeba, which causes a multifocal, granulomatous reaction in the meninges and brain, usually in immuno-suppressed persons. At St. Elizabeth's Medical Center, my colleagues and I recently saw an infection caused by balamuthia,[9] an organism similar to acanthamoeba. Cerebral abscesses caused by entamoebas are very rare and are usually the result of dissemination from a heavily infested liver. Only the two bouts of diarrhea that this patient had 12 and 7 months before his admission even remotely support a diagnosis of entamoebic infection. Finally, African histoplasmosis (due to *Histoplasma capsulatum* var. *duboisii*) should be mentioned, since it occurs in baboons and monkeys that are used in AIDS vaccine research. *H. capsulatum*, the agent of typical histoplasmosis in the United States, can cause cerebral abscess. I was unable to find a case of involvement of the nervous system by the African variety.

CONCLUSIONS

In summary, an organism of East African origin, probably a parasite, was responsible for this patient's seizure and inflammatory brain lesion. The single, small, nonspecific enhancing lesion must have reflected an incipient phase of implantation. Schistosomiasis is the leading diagnosis because of its propensity to cause a solitary, irregular brain granuloma; the patient's history of exposure to the fresh water of Lake Victoria and the Nile; and the timing of the neurologic manifestations in relation to his travels. Tuberculoma cannot be completely ruled out, but the patient's negative tuberculin skin test is against that diagnosis. Surgical excision of the lesion is required for diagnosis and possibly for cure.

Dr. Howard M. Heller (Infectious Diseases): We were concerned about the possibility of schistosomiasis, especially in view of the patient's very-high-risk activities. The Centers for Disease Control and Prevention (CDC) have the most reliable serologic tests for schistosomiasis, but unfortunately, the turnaround time for these tests is relatively long. Because we were concerned that the patient had a tumor, we chose to do a brain biopsy before the results of serologic testing were received.

CLINICAL DIAGNOSIS

Neuroschistosomiasis.

DR. ALLAN H. ROPPER'S DIAGNOSIS

Parasitic cerebral lesion, probably schistosomiasis.

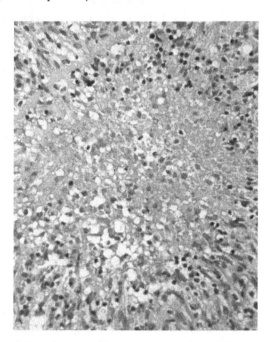

FIG 2 Granuloma with Central Necrosis (Hematoxylin and Eosin, ×250).

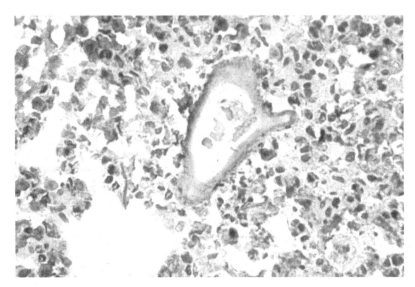

FIG 3 Ovum of *Schistosoma mansoni* with the Characteristic Broad Lateral Spine (Hematoxylin and Eosin, ×350).

PATHOLOGICAL DISCUSSION

DR. ANAT STEMMER-RACHAMIMOV (Neuropathology): The diagnostic procedure was a brain biopsy. Microscopical examination of the specimen (Fig. 2 and 3) revealed a necrotizing granuloma surrounding a refractile ovum of *S. mansoni*, identified by the presence of a prominent lateral spine. Chronic inflammatory cells, mostly lymphocytes and histiocytes with occasional plasma cells and eosinophils, clustered around adjacent blood vessels. The lateral spine of this ovum distinguishes it from the ova of *S. haematobium* and *S. japonicum*. It has been suggested that the large size of *S. mansoni* ova and their prominent lateral spines impede their progress along the vertebral venous plexus to the brain.

The pathologic response to ova in the central nervous system varies, depending on the intensity of the infection and the host's immunologic status. There may be no tissue reaction or only a scanty inflammatory reaction to scattered ova, localized vasculitis, or most commonly (as in this case), tissue necrosis with the formation of granulomas.[6] The distribution of the ova is also variable. The leptomeninges and cerebral cortex are the most common sites; the cerebellum, thalamus, hippocampus, midbrain, basal ganglia, choroid plexus, and white matter are less frequently involved.[10] The localized, tumor-like form of cerebral schistosomiasis is uncommon and is often not associated with severe visceral involvement.

DR. HELLER: The patient received two doses of corticosteroids and praziquantel, given eight hours apart. A week later, he was still having headaches, and subtle signs of dysmetria appeared on the right side. Because of the possibility that his neurologic status was worsening, we administered six doses of praziquantel over a two-day period. His headaches then subsided, and the findings on CT scanning improved. Three months after treatment, he was asymptomatic.

The serologic results from the CDC, which we received in four weeks, were positive for *S. mansoni*, and immunoblotting confirmed that result. The enzyme-linked immunosorbent assay has 97 to 100 percent sensitivity and 100 percent specificity for *S. mansoni*.

ANATOMICAL DIAGNOSIS

Schistosomiasis (*Schistosoma mansoni*), involving the cerebral cortex.

REFERENCES

1. Yakovlev PI, Rakic P. Patterns of decussation of bulbar pyramids and distribution of pyramidal tracts on two sides of the spinal cord. Trans Am Neurol Assoc 1966;91:366–7.
2. Terakawa H, Abe K, Nakamura M, Okazaki T, Obashi J, Yanagihara T. Ipsilateral hemiparesis after putaminal hemorrhage due to uncrossed pyramidal tract. Neurology 2000;54:1801–5.
3. Bia F, ed. Parasitic diseases of the nervous system. Semin Neurol 1993;13:1–239.
4. Maguire JH. Parasitic diseases of the central nervous system. Infect Dis Pract 1989;12:1–11.
5. Strickland GT, ed. Hunter's tropical medicine and emerging infectious diseases. 8th ed. Philadelphia: W.B. Saunders, 2000.
6. Scrimgeour EM, Gajdusek DC. Involvement of the central nervous system in *Schistosoma mansoni* and *S. haematobium* infection: a review. Brain 1985;108:1023–38.
7. Pittella JEH, Lana-Peixoto MA. Brain involvement in hepatosplenic Schistosomiasis mansoni. Brain 1981;104:621–32.
8. Pittella JEH. The relation between involvement of the central nervous system in Schistosomiasis mansoni and the clinical forms of the parasitosis: a review. J Trop Med Hyg 1991;94:15–21.
9. Katz JD, Ropper AH, Adelman LS, Worthington M, Wade P. A case of *Balamuthia mandrillaris* meningoencephalitis. Arch Neurol 2000;57:1210–2.
10. Alves W. The distribution of *Schistosoma* eggs in human tissues. Bull World Health Org 1958;18:1092–7.

Perspectives and Updates

In an endemic area, the diagnosis of schistosomiasis would not be so opaque. A young person with a single seizure would be identified by a local physician, one who dealt daily with tropical diseases, as almost always having a cerebral parasite or tuberculoma. The MRI in this case largely gives away the diagnosis, but there certainly are other parasites that could be considered in view of the patient's travel to East Africa.

Schistosomiasis is endemic in over 75 countries, with the highest proportion of infected people being in Africa. Both *Schistosoma hematobium* and *S. mansoni* are seen in sub-Saharan Africa and in the Nile Delta, but the first of these parasites is also endemic to Brazil and the southern Caribbean. Neurologic schistosomiasis, reflected by parasite deposition in the nervous system, is common in autopsy studies in the endemic areas. Travelers may be particularly susceptible to myelopathy and cerebral infections because they mount a more intense immune response than do chronically exposed hosts. One surprise in this case was the absence of eosinophilia in the peripheral blood. The diagnosis is otherwise made on a clinical basis unless there is hematuria, in which case inspection of the urine stool may be valuable. New PCR tests are being evaluated and seem to be most sensitive in infected persons who have traveled to an endemic area and not been previously exposed to the parasite.[1]

Treatment is with a brief course of albendazole or praziquantel, sometimes accompanied by steroids if there is marked brain edema. An interesting recent development is the observation that antimalarial drugs such as mefloquine and primaquine have activity against schistosomes, particularly if there are mature parasites.[2] So far these drugs, taken prophylactically by many travelers, have not been used to prevent or treat infections, but they may be altering the epidemiology of the disease.

Allan H. Ropper

REFERENCES

1. Wang C, Chen L, Yin X, Hua W. Application of DNA-based diagnostics in detection of schistosomal DNA in early infection and after drug treatment. Parasites Vectors 2011; 24;4:164.
2. Keiser J, N'Guessan NA, Adoubryn KD. Efficacy and safety of mefloquine, artesunate, mefloquine-artesunate, and praziquantel against *Schistosoma haematobium*: randomized, exploratory open-label trial. Clin Infect Dis 2010; 50:1205–13.

A 61-Year-Old Man with Headache and Multiple Infarcts

TROUSSEAU SYNDROME

CPC 31-2002

PRESENTATION OF CASE

A 61-year-old man was admitted to the hospital because of right hemiplegia, aphasia, and obtundation.

According to the patient's family, he had been well at his home in Haiti until about one month earlier, when pain developed in his right leg. Two days later, an ultrasonographic examination of the leg revealed no abnormalities, and a physician advised him to take aspirin. The pain resolved, but three weeks before admission, headache, nausea, and vomiting developed and shortly thereafter disappeared; two days later, the patient had a problem with balance. An ultrasonographic study of the liver raised the possibility of a tumor, and a stool specimen was found to contain *Entamoeba histolytica*; metronidazole was given for one week. Two weeks before admission, the patient's problem with balance resolved and a computed tomographic (CT) examination of the brain showed no abnormalities. One week before admission, abdominal pain and intermittent headaches developed, and he made plans to travel to the United States. On the morning of departure, a brother who accompanied him on the flight noted that the patient had difficulty signing his name. During the flight he spoke with increasing difficulty and had recurrent headache and weakness of the right leg. Weakness soon developed in the right arm, and he became aphasic. He was brought to this hospital awake and mute, but he quickly became obtunded. The trachea was intubated.

The patient, who resided in a rural area of Haiti, had stopped smoking 18 years earlier and drank a moderate amount of alcohol. There was a history of type 2 diabetes mellitus, for which he took an unknown oral medication. There was a history of diabetes mellitus in several relatives, and a sister had had three later-term spontaneous abortions, without further evaluation. The patient's family reported that to their knowledge he had not had chest pain, dyspnea, fever, chills, night sweats, weight loss, sickle cell disease, recent dental procedures, or exposure to animals or tuberculosis. There was no family history of stroke or clotting disorders.

Table 1 Hematologic Laboratory Data on the Day of Admission

Variable	Value
Hematocrit (%)	35.3
White cells (per mm3)	27,900
Differential count (%)	
Neutrophils	74
Band forms	3
Lymphocytes	17
Atypical lymphocytes	1
Monocytes	4
Metamyelocytes	1
Platelets (per mm3)	193,000
Erythrocyte sedimentation rate (mm/hr)	39
Mean corpuscular volume (μm3)	81
Prothrombin time (sec)*	14.1
Partial-thromboplastin time (sec)	Normal

*The normal range is 11.1 to 13.1 seconds.

The temperature was 36.4°C, the pulse was 137, and the respirations were 20. The blood pressure was 165/75 mm Hg.

On physical examination, the patient was obtunded and responded minimally to stimulation. No rash, petechiae, septic lesions, or lymphadenopathy was detected. Scleral icterus was noted. The lungs were clear. A grade 2 systolic apical murmur was present; a third heart sound was not heard. The liver was hard and descended 4 to 5 cm below the right costal margin; the spleen was not felt, and no fluid wave was detected. No bruit was heard. The left carotid pulse was absent; the right carotid, radial, femoral, and popliteal pulses were ++ bilaterally. The lower left leg was pale and cold below the middle of the calf, and the left posterior tibial and dorsalis pedis pulses were absent. The right foot was warm; the right posterior tibial and dorsalis pedis pulses were identified on Doppler examination but were not palpable. No peripheral edema was present.

On neurologic examination, the patient responded to sternal pressure with minimal movement of the left arm and leg; there was infrequent spontaneous movement of the left arm. The pupils were 4 mm in diameter, symmetric, and reactive. No gaze preference was detected. The right arm was flaccid. The deep-tendon reflexes were present bilaterally. The plantar responses were absent.

The urine was orange and was positive for protein (++) and bilirubin (+) and trace-positive for urobilinogen; the sediment contained three to five red cells, up to two white cells, and a few bacteria per high-power field. Hematologic tests and blood chemical studies were performed (Tables 1 and 2). The levels of calcium, amylase, and creatine kinase were normal. While the patient was breathing supplemental oxygen, the partial pressure of oxygen was 189 mm Hg, the partial pressure of carbon dioxide 37 mm Hg,

Table 2 Blood Chemical Values*

Variable	First Hospital Day	Second Hospital Day
Glucose (mg/dl)	188	142
Conjugated bilirubin (mg/dl)	3.5	
Haptoglobin (mg/dl)[†]		227
Total bilirubin (mg/dl)	4.9	
Phosphorus (mg/dl)	5.1	
Protein (g/dl)	7.7	
Albumin	2.4	
Globulin	5.3	
Sodium (mmol/liter)	134	
Potassium (mmol/liter)	5.7	
Chloride (mmol/liter)	102	
Carbon dioxide (mmol/liter)	19.9	
Magnesium (mmol/liter)	1.2	
Urea nitrogen (mg/dl)	66	70
Creatinine (mg/dl)	3.9	4.1
Iron (μg/dl)		27
Iron-binding capacity (μg/dl)		124
Creatine kinase (U/liter)		435
Creatine kinase isoenzyme (ng)[‡]	37.1	12.1
Creatine kinase isoenzyme index (%)[§]	13.1	3.0
Troponin T (ng/ml)[¶]	1.27	2.19
Alkaline phosphatase (U/liter)	415	
Aspartate aminotransferase (U/liter)	158	
Alanine aminotransferase (U/liter)	143	
Lactate dehydrogenase (U/liter)		1923
Ferritin (ng/ml)[‖]		7705
Lipase (U/liter)[**]	7.5	

*To convert the values for glucose to millimoles per liter, multiply by 0.05551. To convert the value for total bilirubin to micromoles per liter, multiply by 17.1. To convert the value for phosphorus to millimoles per liter, multiply by 0.3229. To convert the value for magnesium to milliequivalents per liter, divide by 0.5. To convert the values for urea nitrogen to millimoles per liter, multiply by 0.357. To convert the values for creatinine to micromoles per liter, multiply by 88.4. To convert the values for iron and iron-binding capacity to micromoles per liter, multiply by 0.1791.

[†]The normal range is 16 to 199 mg per deciliter.

[‡]The normal range is 0 to 6.9 ng per milliliter.

[§]The normal range is 0 to 3.5 percent.

[¶]The normal range is 0 to 0.09 ng per milliliter.

[‖]The normal range is 30 to 300 ng per milliliter.

[**]The normal range is 1.3 to 6.0 U per liter.

and the pH 7.33. An electrocardiogram showed a sinus tachycardia at a rate of 140, with occasional premature ventricular complexes; there was a pattern of inferior and probably lateral myocardial infarction, which may have been acute. A chest radiograph revealed that the endotracheal tube was in the appropriate position; there was patchy atelectasis at the base of the left lung; the other regions of the lungs and the cardiac silhouette were normal. CT and magnetic resonance imaging (MRI) of the brain, which showed multiple infarcts, and CT studies of the liver, kidneys, and lower abdomen were performed (Fig. 1, 2, 3, 4, and 5).

The patient was admitted to the intensive care unit. A urine specimen and two blood specimens were obtained for culture. Single doses of ceftriaxone and vancomycin were administered; treatment with aspirin (325 mg daily), minidose heparin, regular insulin, and metoprolol was begun. A transesophageal echocardiogram was obtained (Fig. 6).

On the second hospital day, the patient's temperature did not exceed 37.7°C, and the findings on examination were little changed. Blood chemical studies were performed (Table 2). A test for viral hepatitis B surface antibody was positive; tests for hepatitis B surface antigen, hepatitis C antibody, antibodies to human immunodeficiency virus (HIV) types 1 and 2, antinuclear antibodies, and rheumatoid factor were negative. Another chest radiograph revealed probable atelectasis at both lung bases and a small, linear opacity in the middle zone of the left lung, probably also atelectasis. A renal radioangiographic examination showed that there was virtually no perfusion of the left kidney, except for a small region at the lower pole, and minimal uptake of tracer material, predominantly in the lower pole on delayed images. There was normal perfusion of the right kidney on the initial images, with prompt concentration of tracer material, although clearance of

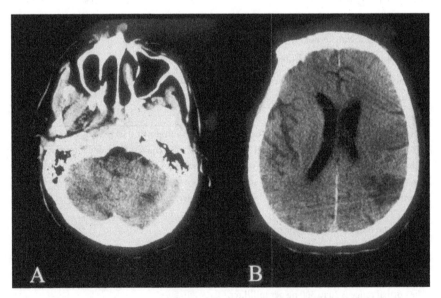

FIG 1 Axial CT Images of the Brain Obtained without the Use of Contrast Material, Showing Bilateral Cerebellar Infarctions (Panel A) and Left Frontal and Parietal Infarctions (Panel B).

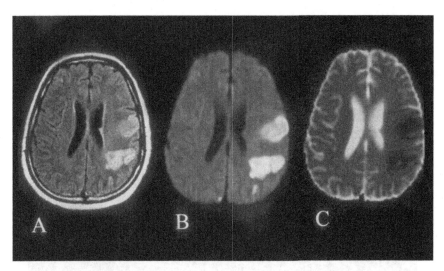

FIG 2 Axial MRI Scans of the Brain.

the material was delayed. Another CT study of the brain, performed without the use of intravenous contrast material, revealed no notable change in the multiple infarcts and no new infarcts, midline shift, mass effect, bleeding, or hydrocephalus.

An image obtained with fluid-attenuated inversion recovery (Panel A) shows infarctions in the left frontal and parietal lobes. The infarcts are hyperintense on diffusion-weighted images (Panel B) and hypointense on apparent-diffusion-coefficient images (Panel C), suggesting that they are acute.

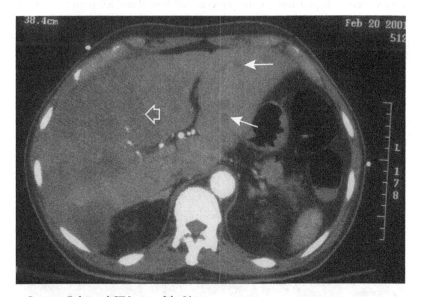

FIG 3 Contrast-Enhanced CT Image of the Liver.
Multiple focal, low-attenuation lesions with ill-defined borders (solid arrows) are present. A geographic pattern of low attenuation (open arrow) suggests abnormal perfusion. There is a more discrete, wedge-shaped area of low attenuation that was not enhanced, which indicates that the tissue is infarcted (arrowhead).

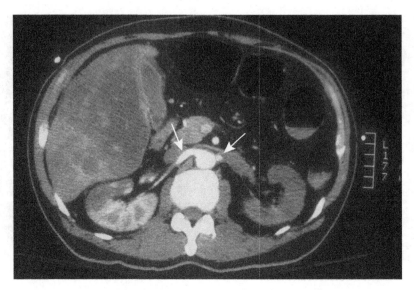

FIG 4 Contrast-Enhanced CT Image of the Liver and Kidneys.
There is abnormal perfusion of all three organs. There is minimal uptake of contrast material in the left kidney.
Contrast material is present in the renal arteries at their origins (arrows).

All culture specimens were negative, and the results of numerous other laboratory studies were still pending.

DR. PAMELA W. SCHAEFER (Neuroradiology): On the first hospital day, a CT examination of the brain (Fig. 1) was performed without the administration of contrast material. There are areas of hypodensity in the posterior left frontal and left parietal lobes; there

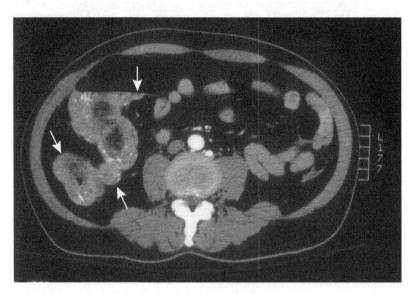

FIG 5 Contrast-Enhanced CT Image of the Lower Abdomen.
There is thickening, without dilatation, of the ascending colonic wall (arrows), with an abrupt transition to colonic wall of normal thickness (arrowhead).

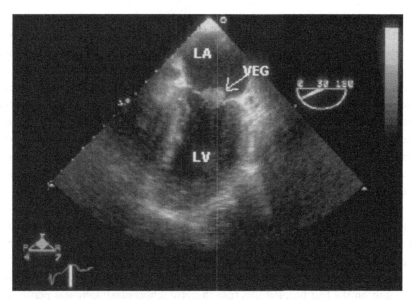

FIG 6 Transesophageal Echocardiogram.
A large vegetation is present on the mitral valve. LA denotes left atrium, LV left ventricle, and VEG vegetation.

is also loss of the normal distinction between gray matter and white matter and a local mass effect, as evidenced by effacement of the sulci. These changes are consistent with the presence of acute infarcts in the distribution of the left middle cerebral artery. Bilateral cerebellar infarcts are also present. There was no midline shift or hydrocephalus.

MRI of the brain (Fig. 2), with angiographic examination of the head and neck, showed multiple acute infarcts in several vascular territories. The largest infarcts were in the left middle cerebral artery in the posterior left frontal and left parietal lobes, with extension into the left temporal operculum; smaller, focal infarcts were seen elsewhere in the left and right middle cerebral arteries. Small, acute infarcts characterized by hyperintensity on diffusion-weighted imaging and by hypointensity on apparent-diffusion-coefficient imaging were present in both occipital lobes and extended into the temporo-occipital regions. Small, acute infarcts were also present bilaterally within the cerebellum, in the posteroinferior cerebellar arteries. Additional acute infarcts were present bilaterally along the border zones of the middle and posterior cerebral arteries and the middle and anterior cerebral arteries. Subacute infarcts (which were hypointense on diffusion-weighted imaging and hyperintense on apparent-diffusion-coefficient imaging) were seen in the right superior and right posteroinferior cerebellar arteries. Magnetic resonance angiograms of the neck and the circle of Willis showed no abnormalities.

DR. BRIAN C. LUCEY (Radiology): CT examination of the thorax, abdomen, and pelvis, performed after the intravenous administration of contrast material, disclosed minimal bibasilar atelectasis without pleural effusions, pulmonary masses or nodules, intrathoracic lymphadenopathy, or abnormalities of the thoracic or abdominal aorta or mesenteric vessels. The liver was enlarged, and both lobes contained multiple focal low-attenuation lesions with ill-defined borders, ranging from 2 to 20 mm in diameter. The lesions were so numerous in the right lobe that they appeared to be confluent. After the administration of contrast material, these areas showed heterogeneous enhancement during the portal venous phase. Thus, a diagnosis of hepatic abscess is unlikely. In addition, there were large irregular areas of decreased enhancement in the liver parenchyma, suggesting vascular insufficiency, and a wedge-shaped nonenhancing area, suggesting the presence of infarction (Fig. 3). No dilatation of the intrahepatic or extrahepatic ducts was observed; the hepatic arteries and portal vein were patent. In both kidneys, there were areas of hypoperfusion consistent with the presence of infarcts; the left kidney was more severely affected than the right. The renal arteries were patent at their origins (Fig. 4); the wall of the cecum and ascending colon was thickened, without dilatation, with a pattern of normal enhancement. In the wall of the ascending colon, there was an abrupt transition to normal thickness (Fig. 5)—a finding that is nonspecific but consistent with the presence of colitis. There were nonspecific inflammatory changes in the fat surrounding the ascending colon and inferior aspect of the right hepatic lobe. The findings suggested a focal ischemic colitis.

DR. MARY ETTA KING (Cardiology): After the patient's admission to the intensive care unit on the first hospital day, transthoracic echocardiography was performed because of his history of myocardial infarction and stroke. In the parasternal long-axis view, the anterior mitral leaflet was diffusely thickened. The mitral leaflets showed incomplete coaptation in a pattern consistent with the presence of papillary-muscle dysfunction. There was an eccentrically directed jet of mitral regurgitation. The aortic leaflets were slightly thickened but did not show obvious vegetations. In the parasternal short-axis view, the left ventricular chamber size, wall thickness, and systolic function were normal at the base and at the midventricular level. Apical views of the heart showed segmental dysfunction of the apex and diffuse thickening of the mitral valve, with a moderate degree of mitral regurgitation visible on color Doppler examination. The estimated left ventricular ejection fraction was 52 percent. Mild aortic insufficiency was also present. After the intravenous injection of agitated saline, both while the patient was at rest and while the Valsalva maneuver was being performed, there was dense opacification of the right atrium and right ventricle, with no contrast effect in the left atrium or left ventricle. Contrast material was administered to rule out the possibility that a paradoxical embolus had moved through an interatrial communication; no right-to-left intracardiac shunt was found. Although no discrete vegetations were seen, they could not be ruled out by the transthoracic study.

A diagnostic procedure was performed.

DIFFERENTIAL DIAGNOSIS

DR. MARTIN A. SAMUELS[*]: Armand Trousseau (1801–1867), professor of clinical medicine at the Faculty of Medicine, Paris, had an enormous impact on 19th-century

[*] Neurologist-in-chief and chair, Department of Neurology, Brigham and Women's Hospital; co-chief, Partners Neurology; professor of neurology, Harvard Medical School—all in Currently Chair, Department of Neurology, Brigham and Women's Hospital.

medicine. His lectures on clinical medicine, which he delivered as physician to the Hotel-Dieu, covered nearly every aspect of internal medicine, including neurology. Two of his most important contributions are the diagnoses in this case.

In a series of landmark articles published in the 1860s,[1-5] Paul Broca (of the Bicêtre Hospital, Paris) proposed the term "aphemia" for the language disorder that results from a lesion in an area of the left inferior frontal lobe. The observation was important because it suggested that different regions of the cerebral cortex have discrete functions and because it posited the concept of lateralization. Before this time, debate had raged over whether the brain functioned by means of specialized regions (the phrenology of Franz Gall)[6] or as a homogeneous whole (the argument put forth by Marie-Jean-Pierre Flourens, who refuted phrenology).[7] In 1864, Trousseau criticized Broca's term "aphemia" and suggested "aphasia" instead.[8] A debate ensued in the Academy of Medicine in which these terms, as well as "alalia" and "aphrasia," vied for dominance.[9] Trousseau was correct in that he favored the localization of language disorders (in the frontal lobes) but incorrect in that he did not recognize lateralization, since the left frontal lobe usually controls language. According to Henderson,[9] "aphasia" ultimately won, mostly because of Trousseau's power and influence. In the case under discussion, the aphasia, which was due to a left-frontal-lobe infarction, was the first of the patient's two Trousseau's syndromes.

In 1865, in lecture 95 of Trousseau's lecture series on clinical medicine, he described phlegmasia alba dolens (painful white inflammation) due to venous thrombosis in multiple circumstances, including the period after parturition, and in various cachectic diseases, such as tuberculosis and cancer.[10] This lecture included numerous clinical case presentations, autopsy results, and hypotheses concerning hypercoagulability. The physical findings and probable causes of death included pulmonary embolism, global cerebral ischemia (syncope), and stroke. In this lecture he said the following:

> I have long been struck with the frequency with which cancerous patients are affected with painful oedema of the superior or inferior extremities, whether or not either was the seat of cancer. The frequent concurrence of phlegmasia alba dolens with an appreciable cancerous tumor, led me to the inquiry whether a relationship of cause and effect did not exist between the two, and whether the phlegmasia was not the consequence of the cancerous cachexia. I have since that period had an opportunity of observing other cases of painful oedema in which, at autopsy, I found visceral cancer, but in which, during life, there was no appreciable cancerous tumor.[10]

About a year and a half after delivering this lecture, Trousseau himself had phlegmasia alba dolens affecting the left leg and predicted, correctly, that he had an occult stomach cancer.[11] His friend and colleague, Peter, later recorded the following: "It was on January 1, 1867 when I went to give him my best wishes for the new year that Trousseau told me with resigned sadness—'I am lost; a phlegmasia which showed itself that night leaves me no doubt about the nature of my affliction.'"[12] This paraneoplastic syndrome, characterized by phlebothrombosis related to a visceral cancer, is one of the few eponymous syndromes that deserves an apostrophe (i.e., the possessive form) because the discoverer both described the disorder and died of it.

In the 137 years since Trousseau's lecture on the subject, many studies have documented the association between venous thromboembolism and cancer.[13–20] Interestingly, treatment of recurrent deep venous thrombosis with warfarin may be associated with a reduced risk of cancer, raising the question of whether warfarin could be acting as an antineoplastic agent.[21] When cancer is diagnosed within one year after an episode of venous thrombosis, the likelihood of metastatic disease is greatly increased and the survival rate at one year is greatly reduced.[22]

Nearly every type of cancer (including gynecologic and urogenital neoplasms, lymphomas, and primary brain tumors) has been reported in association with a hypercoagulable state, but cancer of the gastrointestinal and hepatobiliary tracts, particularly mucinsecreting adenocarcinomas, predominate in this regard. The clinical maxim that pancreatic cancer is especially likely to result in Trousseau's syndrome is probably incorrect, but some patients with Trousseau's syndrome do have this cancer.[23]

The precise reason for the hypercoagulable state in some patients with cancer remains unknown, but it is likely that such a state, which resembles chronic disseminated intravascular coagulation, is due to a disruption in the delicate balance between fibrinolysis and inhibition of fibrinolysis. Tumors release substances that interfere with this balance, such as thromboplastin, factor X activator, prothrombinase, plasminogen-activator inhibitor, and plasmin inhibitor. The chronic state of disseminated intravascular coagulation in some patients with cancer has various causes, including genetic predisposition, such as that due to the presence of the factor V Leiden mutation or a mutation in the prothrombin gene. The fact that this patient's sister had had three spontaneous abortions raises the question of whether this family was prone to thrombosis as a result of the primary antiphospholipid-antibody syndrome or some other hypercoagulable state.

Trousseau's syndrome is characterized by microangiopathic changes on peripheral-blood smears and very friable vegetations, often invisible on echocardiograms, on the cardiac valves (nonbacterial thrombotic endocarditis). Visceral organs, including the brain, may thus be damaged by multiple interlocking mechanisms—mainly, venous thrombosis, arterial thrombosis, and cardiac source emboli.

There is little doubt that this patient had Trousseau's syndrome. Infarctions of the kidneys, bowel, heart, and brain followed an episode of pain in the right leg. The multiple small lesions in the liver probably represented metastases from a cancer of the stomach or colon or a cancer of the hepatobiliary system. The diagnostic test was probably a biopsy of the liver. One of the cerebral infarctions involved the left frontal lobe, resulting in a right hemiplegia and aphasia.

DR. ROBERT B. COLVIN (Pathology): Dr. Singhal, what were your thoughts?

DR. ANEESH B. SINGHAL (Neurology): When we first saw this patient, we knew his medical history and the findings on his cranial MRI scans. We considered hypercoagulable states such as the antiphospholipid-antibody syndrome, and we thought that vegetations, if present, could be secondarily infected. Since the levels of cardiac enzymes were abnormal, we considered the possibility of a left ventricular thrombus due to a recent myocardial infarction. However, because of the topography of the lesions on diffusion-weighted imaging, we favored a diagnosis of Trousseau's syndrome, with multiple strokes.

CLINICAL DIAGNOSIS

Multiple ischemic strokes, resulting from nonbacterial thrombotic endocarditis due to an underlying cancer (Trousseau's syndrome).

DR. MARTIN A. SAMUELS'S DIAGNOSES

Trousseau's syndrome (phlegmasia alba dolens as a manifestation of a hypercoagulable paraneoplastic syndrome).

Aphasia due to a frontal-lobe infarction as described by Trousseau.

PATHOLOGICAL DISCUSSION

DR. COLVIN: Two diagnostic procedures, transesophageal echocardiography and a biopsy of the liver (with a CT-guided core-biopsy needle), were performed.

DR. KING: Since valvular vegetations could not be ruled out by the transthoracic study, a transesophageal echocardiogram was obtained. The midesophageal views revealed a shaggy mass, 1 by 1 cm, attached to the posterior mitral-valve leafler; in addition, there was a small lesion on the tip of the anterior leaflet (Fig. 6). A video of the transesophageal echocardiogram is available as Supplementary Appendix 1 with the full text of this article at http://www.nejm.org. The aortic-valve cusps were diffusely thickened, and there were small, irregular lesions on both aspects of the cusps. On color Doppler examination, eccentrically directed mitral regurgitation was estimated to be moderately severe. Mild aortic insufficiency was present. The tricuspid and pulmonic valves were normal, and the interatrial septum was intact. On the transgastric views, there was segmental dysfunction of the cardiac apex, but no apical thrombus. The valvular findings are consistent with the presence of vegetations, which are due either to infection or to marasmus.

DR. ULYSSES BALIS (Pathology): Specimens from the hepatic biopsy, sectioned and stained with hematoxylin and eosin, reveal an infiltrative cancer with a focal microglandular pattern, consistent with the presence of a poorly differentiated adenocarcinoma (Fig. 7). The presence of pleomorphic nuclei and numerous mitoses indicate a high-grade cancer. There is focal mucin production (Fig. 8). Immunohistochemical studies were positive for cytokeratin 7, suggesting that the neoplasm is of pancreaticobiliary origin.

The hepatic architecture is almost totally effaced and has been replaced by a loosely cohesive, malignant-cell population with focal architectural features suggestive of microglandular formation.

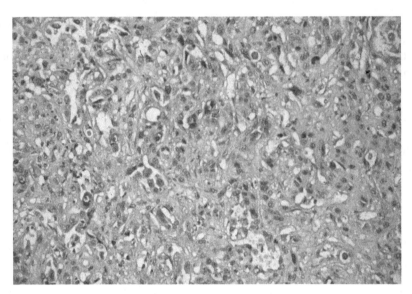

FIG 7 Biopsy Specimen of the Liver, Showing Metastatic Carcinoma (Hematoxylin and Eosin, ×250).

The findings are consistent with the presence of metastatic, poorly differentiated adenocarcinoma of probable pancreaticobiliary origin. The tumor cells have large, bizarre nuclei (Panel A; hematoxylin and eosin, ×500). Mucicarmine staining confirms the presence of focal areas of mucin production (Panel B; ×500).

DR. SINGHAL: The patient died after a cardiac arrest on the seventh hospital day.

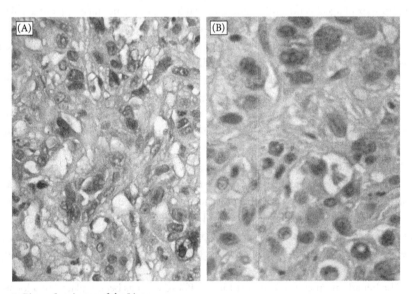

FIG 8 Biopsy Specimens of the Liver.

ANATOMICAL DIAGNOSIS

Adenocarcinoma, probably of pancreaticobiliary origin and metastatic to the liver, with a hypercoagulable state resulting in thrombophlebitis and nonbacterial thrombotic endocarditis, with multiple embolic infarcts (Trousseau's syndrome).

REFERENCES

1. Broca PP. Perte de la parole, ramollissement chronique et destruction partielle du lobe antérieur gauche du cerveau. Bull Soc Anthropol 1861;2:235–8.

2. *Idem.* Remarques sur le siège de la faculté du langage articulé, suivies d'une observation d'aphémie (perte de la parole). Bull Soc Anat 1861;36:330–57.

3. *Idem.* Nouvelle observation d'aphémie produite par une lésion de la moirtié postérieure des deuxième et troisième circonvolution frontales gauches. Bull Soc Anat 1861;36:398–407.

4. *Idem.* Localisation des fonctions cérébralis: siège de la faculté du langage articulé. Bull Soc Anthropol 1863;4:200–4.

5. *Idem.* Du siège de la faculté du langage articulé dans l'hémisphère gauche du cerveau. Bull Soc Anthropol 1865;6:377–93.

6. Gall FJ. Sur les fonctions du cerveau et sur celles de chacune de ses parties. Paris: J.-B. Baillière, 1825.

7. Flourens P. Recherches expérimentales sur les propriétés et les fonctions du système nerveux dans les animaux vertébrés. 2nd ed. Paris: J.-B. Baillière, 1842.

8. Trousseau A. De L'aphasie, maladie décrite recémment sous le nom impropre d'aphemie. Gaz Hop Civ Mil 1864;37:13–4, 25–6, 37–9, 49–50.

9. Henderson V. Alalia, aphemia, and aphasia. Arch Neurol 1990;47:85–8.

10. Trousseau A. Phlegmasia alba dolens (lecture XCV). In: Cormack JR, Bazire PV, trans. Lectures on clinical medicine. Philadelphia: Lindsay & Blakiston, 1873.

11. Aron E. Le centième aniversaire de la mort de A. Trousseau. Presse Med 1967;75:1429–30.

12. Soubiran A. Est-il roi dans quelque ile? Ou le demier Noël de Trousseau. Presse Med 1967;75:2807–10.

13. Monreal M, Lafoz E, Casals A, et al. Occult cancer in patients with deep venous thrombosis: a systematic approach. Cancer 1991;67:541–5.

14. Goldberg RJ, Seneff M, Gore JM, et al. Occult malignant neoplasm in patients with deep venous thrombosis. Arch Intern Med 1987;147:251–3.

15. Nordstrom M, Lindblad B, Anderson H, Bergqvist D, Kjellstrom T. Deep venous thrombosis and occult malignancy: an epidemiological study. BMJ 1994;308:891–4.

16. Prandoni P, Lensing AWA, Büller HR, et al. Deep-vein thrombosis and the incidence of subsequent symptomatic cancer. N Engl J Med 1992;327:1128–33.

17. Hettiarachchi RJ, Lok J, Prins MH, Buller HR, Prandoni P. Undiagnosed malignancy in patients with deep vein thrombosis: incidence, risk indicators and diagnosis. Cancer 1998;83:180–5.

18. Baron JA, Gridley G, Weiderpass E, Nyren O, Linet M. Venous thromboembolism and cancer. Lancet 1998;351:1077–80. [Erratum, Lancet 2000;355:758.]

19. Sørensen HT, Mellemkjær L, Steffensen FH, Olsen JH, Nielsen GL. The risk of a diagnosis of cancer after primary deep venous thrombosis or pulmonary embolism. N Engl J Med 1998;338:1169–73.

20. Gore JM, Appelbaum JS, Greene HL, Dexter L, Dalen JE. Occult cancer in patients with acute pulmonary embolism. Ann Intern Med 1982;96:556–60.
21. Schulman S, Lindmarker P. Incidence of cancer after prophylaxis with warfarin against recurrent venous thromboembolism. N Engl J Med 2000;342:1953–8.
22. Sørensen HT, Mellemkjær L, Olsen JH, Baron JA. Prognosis of cancers associated with venous thromboembolism. N Engl J Med 2000;343:1846–50.
23. Pinzon R, Drewinko B, Trujillo M, Guinee V, Giacco G. Pancreatic carcinoma and Trousseau's syndrome: experience at a large cancer center. J Clin Oncol 1986;4:509–14.

Perspectives and Updates

Many people believe that neurologists are particularly attracted to taxonomy. I prefer to think of the issue as one of precision rather than pointless obsessiveness. This discussion is a case in point. In preparing the case for publication, I found myself in an argument about the placement of an apostrophe. There were two diagnoses in this case: aphasia from a cardiac source embolism to the left cerebral hemisphere and hypercoagulability as a paraneoplastic syndrome. In my view, aphasia is a Trousseau syndrome[1] (i.e., the word "aphasia" was suggested by Trousseau), whereas hypercoagulability as a paraneoplastic syndrome was Trousseau's syndrome, because Trousseau both described and suffered from the disease. I am very much against the trend to remove eponyms from the names of diseases and syndromes as to do so strips medicine of its history.

History in medicine is not a mere avocation. In addition to the old saw of helping to prevent the same errors from being made again and again, it provides us with the perspective needed to approach diagnostic and scientific challenges in our own era. It also combats hubris. In carefully researching my CPCs I have never encountered an idea that had not evolved from those before it. In grand rounds, in medical journals, and particularly in the lay press, we are regaled with "revolutionary" ideas, but that they are completely new is an illusion. Throughout history, people have always been on the "cutting edge" and have always believed that they had some sort of huge advantage over prior generations. Technological advances have often provided the impetus for this belief, whether it be the light microscope, the electron microscope, genetics, or imaging. I am particularly amused by the students or residents who are shocked to learn what was known "back in the day," as they derisively call it.

In 1865, Armand Trousseau described *phlegmasia alba dolens*, painful white edema, caused by venous thrombosis related to an underlying occult cancer. He suspected that this was caused by a factor in the blood that enhanced coagulation. His hematologists could not find that factor. A century and a half later, we have very little to add. It is obvious from the tone of Trousseau's lecture that he considered himself superior to those around him. He believed that he had "discovered" a new phenomenon. It is very unlikely that this was the case. Like all of us in medicine before and after Trousseau, our ideas are a manifestation of the times in which we live. Now we talk about chronic disseminiated intravascular coagulation instead of the quaint-sounding phlegmasia alba dolens of Trousseau, but knowledge of the phenomenon remains and always will remain incomplete. It is likely that fewer than 1 percent of all physicians in the 21st century know what Trousseau knew about this phenomenon, despite the Internet.

Less than a year after Trousseau's lecture on the subject, he diagnosed the syndrome in himself. The touching story of his effort, as he lay mortally ill, to make contact with his estranged son, a doctor who was living in Hawaii, provides a poignant punctuation to this remarkable story. Did Trousseau sacrifice too much of his personal life for the profession of medicine? Looking back, it seems easy for us to believe that we will do better, but that's the way they did it "back in the day."

Martin A. Samuels

REFERENCE

1. Varki A. Trousseau's syndrome: multiple definitions and multiple mechanisms. Blood 2007; 15:1723–9.

A 77-Year-Old Man with Ear Pain, Difficulty Speaking, and Altered Mental Status

OTITIC BACTERIAL MENINGITIS

Martin A. Samuels, R. Gilberto Gonzalez, Arthur Y. Kim,
and Anat Stemmer-Rachamimov

CPC 34-2007

PRESENTATION OF CASE

A 77-year-old right-handed man was admitted to the hospital because of the recent onset of pain in the ear, difficulty speaking, and altered mental status. The patient had been well until the day before admission, when he awoke in the morning with nasal congestion and pain on the right side of his face. That evening, pain, accompanied by drainage, developed in the right ear; his wife administered ciprofloxacin eardrops. The next morning, the temperature was 37.8°C. At about 9 a.m., the patient's wife noted that his speech was slurred. The patient said he was tired and retired to nap. Ninety minutes later, his wife found him on the floor, unresponsive, and she called emergency medical services.

When the emergency medical technicians arrived, the patient was conscious, had incomprehensible speech, and could not walk. The blood pressure was 140/94 mm Hg, the pulse 160 beats per minute, and the oxygen saturation 100% while the patient was receiving supplemental oxygen; the respiratory rate was 20 breaths per minute. Dried blood was present in the nares and mouth. The pupils were equal and reactive to light, the facial expression was symmetrical, the right-hand grip was weak, and the torso leaned to the right. The patient did not move his feet when requested to do so. He was transported by ambulance to the emergency department of this hospital, arriving at 12:30 p.m.

Several days before admission, the patient had slipped on an icy sidewalk and struck his head. He did not lose consciousness and did not seek medical attention. He had hypertension, adenomatous colonic polyps, and a torn left medial meniscus; the baseline creatinine level was 1.3 mg per deciliter (115 μmol per liter). Lip swelling suggestive of angioedema had occurred after he consumed shellfish; there were no allergies to medications. Medications included omeprazole, diphenoxylate, lisinopril, chlorpheniramine, hydrochlorothiazide, and triamterene. The patient had been born in China and had immigrated to the United States in his third decade. He was a

N Engl J Med 2007;357:1957–65.

retired university professor who lived with his wife and traveled to Martha's Vineyard, Massachusetts, and China frequently. He drank wine daily, did not smoke, and had no recent exposure to animals. His father had died from a cerebral hemorrhage, and his mother had died from complications of diabetes.

In the emergency department, the blood pressure was 95/77 mm Hg, rising to 163/94 mm Hg within 5 minutes after arrival; the pulse was 147 beats per minute, the respiratory rate was 20 breaths per minute, and the oxygen saturation was 96% while the patient was breathing 5 liters of oxygen per minute by means of a nasal cannula. The temperature was 37.4°C. On examination by a neurologist, the patient could be roused with mild stimulation; he had aphasia and did not follow commands. The gaze was midline without deviation; the pupils were equal and each 4 mm in diameter, decreasing to 2 mm on direct illumination. There was no ptosis or facial droop. Dried blood was present in the right external ear canal, both nares, and the oropharynx. The neck was supple, and rhonchi were heard in both lungs. The heart sounds were normal, and the abdomen was distended and tender in the right upper quadrant, without bowel sounds. The patient moved both arms and legs purposefully in response to noxious stimuli. The reflexes were 1+ in the arms, trace at the patellar tendons, and absent at the Achilles' tendons; the plantar responses were flexor.

An electrocardiogram showed sinus tachycardia with first-degree atrioventricular block but was otherwise normal. Laboratory-test results are shown in Table 1. Urinalysis revealed few bacteria and three to five granular casts per high-power field. Thiamine and glucose were administered intravenously, followed by lorazepam (4 mg).

Computed tomography (CT) of the head performed 1 hour after the patient's arrival in the emergency department, without the administration of contrast material, revealed pneumocephalus, opacified right mastoid air cells, and age-related parenchymal changes. The initial interpretation suggested the presence of a longitudinal fracture of the right temporal bone. A chest radiograph was normal.

Ninety minutes after arrival, the temperature rose to 38.6°C, and blood specimens were sent for culture. Acetaminophen, ceftriaxone (2 g), metronidazole (500 mg), and vancomycin (1 g) were administered. Three hours after arrival, a lumbar puncture was performed; the opening pressure was 270 mm of water. The cerebrospinal fluid was xanthochromic; the results of laboratory tests are shown in Table 2. Specimens were sent for fungal, bacterial, and viral cultures; Gram's staining; and testing for cryptococcal antigen and for herpes simplex virus DNA. The closing pressure was 170 mm of water.

Four hours after arrival, CT of the temporal bones, performed without the administration of contrast material, revealed pneumocephalus in the right middle and anterior cranial fossae, fluid within the middle ear and mastoid air cells, and loss of the bony integrity of the tegmen tympani. There was no evidence of a fracture of the temporal bone.

The results of a diagnostic test were received.

Table 1 Results of Hematology and Serum Chemistry Tests*

Variable	Adult Reference Values†	Values on Admission
Hematocrit (%)	Males, 41.0–53.0	45.7
Hemoglobin (g/dl)	13.5–17.5	16.0
White-cell count (per mm³)	4,500–11,000	8,600
Neutrophils (%)	40–70	74
Band forms (%)	0–10	24
Myelocytes (%)	0	1
Reactive lymphocytes (%)	0	1
Platelet count (per mm³)	150,000–350,000	99,000
Mean corpuscular volume (μm³)	80–100	98
Prothrombin time (sec)	11.1–13.1	13.9
Prothrombin time (international normalized ratio)		1.3
Partial-thromboplastin time (sec)	22.1–35.1	28.6
Antithrombin III, functional (%)	80–130	74
Protein C, functional (%)	70–140	75
Activated protein C resistance	(>2.0)	2.5
Protein S, functional (%)	70–140	95
Fibrinogen		Elevated
Glucose (mg/dl)	70–110	202
Sodium (mmol/liter)	135–145	137
Potassium (mmol/liter)	3.4–4.8	3.1
Chloride (mmol/liter)	100–108	102
Carbon dioxide (mmol/liter)	24–30	24.5
Urea nitrogen (mg/dl)	8–25	20
Creatinine (mg/dl)	0.6–1.5	1.8
Total bilirubin (mg/dl)	0.0–1.0	1.3
Conjugated bilirubin (mg/dl)	0.0–0.4	0.5
Total protein (g/dl)	6.0–8.0	6.9
Albumin (g/dl)	3.1–4.3	3.2
Globulin (g/dl)	2.6–4.1	3.7
Phosphorus (mg/dl)	2.6–4.5	0.9, slight hemolysis
Magnesium (mmol/liter)	0.7–1.0	0.6
Calcium (mg/dl)	8.5–10.5	9.1
Alkaline phosphatase (U/liter)	45–115	93
Aspartate aminotransferase (U/liter)	10–40	56
Alanine aminotransferase (U/liter)	10–55	24

(continued)

Table 1 (Continued)

Variable	Adult Reference Values†	Values on Admission
Creatine kinase (U/liter)	60–400	139
Creatine kinase, MB fraction (ng/ml)	0.0–6.9	0.7
Troponin T (ng/ml)	0.00–0.09	0.02
Toxic screen panels 1–5		Diphenhy-dramine and quinine present

*To convert the values for glucose to millimoles per liter, multiply by 0.05551. To convert the values for urea nitrogen to millimoles per liter, multiply by 0.357. To convert the values for creatinine to micromoles per liter, multiply by 88.4. To convert the values for total and conjugated bilirubin to micromoles per liter, multiply by 17.1. To convert the values for phosphorus to millimoles per liter, multiply by 0.3229. To convert the values for magnesium to milliequivalents per liter, divide by 0.500. To convert the values for calcium to millimoles per liter, multiply by 0.250.

†The reference values are affected by many variables, including the population of patients and the laboratory methods used. The ranges used at Massachusetts General Hospital are for adults who are not pregnant and do not have medical conditions that could affect the results. They may therefore not be appropriate for all patients.

DIFFERENTIAL DIAGNOSIS

Dr. Martin A. Samuels*: Dr. Gonzalez, may we see the images?

Dr. R. Gilberto Gonzalez: CT of the head showed pneumocephalus (Fig. 1A) and opacification of the right middle ear and mastoid air cells. There was a question of a longitudinal temporal-bone fracture, and a dedicated temporal-bone CT scan was obtained, which showed opacification of the right middle ear (Fig. 1B). Sagittal images demonstrated loss of integrity of the tegmen tympani (Fig. 1C). There was no evidence of a fracture.

Table 2 Results of Cerebrospinal Fluid Testing*

Variable	Adult Reference Range of Value†	On Admission		
		Value	Value for Tube 1	Value for Tube 4
Glucose (mg/dl)	50–75	91		
Total protein (mg/dl)	5–55	322		
Red-cell count (per mm³)	0		316	317
White-cell count (per mm³)	0–5		371	183
Neutrophils (%)	0		58	64
Band forms (%)	0		36	36
Lymphocytes (%)	0		2	
Other hematic cells (%)	0		4	

*To convert the values for glucose to millimoles per liter, multiply by 0.05551.

†The reference values are affected by many variables, including the population of patients and the laboratory methods used. The ranges used at Massachusetts General Hospital are for adults who are not pregnant and do not have medical conditions that could affect the results. They may therefore not be appropriate for all patients.

*Currently Chair, Department of Neurology, Brigham and Women's Hospital.

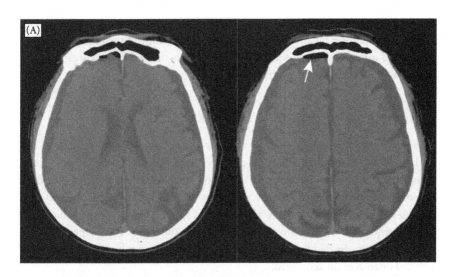

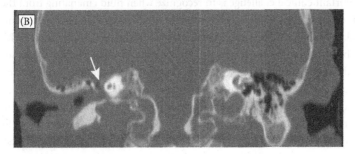

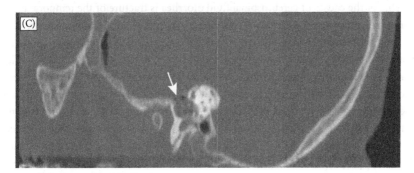

FIG 1 Radiologic Images of the Head.

CT of the head performed in the emergency department shows pneumocephalus, with air adjacent to the right frontal lobe (Panel A, arrow). Subsequently, dedicated temporal-bone CT, reformatted in the coronal plane, showed opacification of the right middle ear (Panel B, arrow). The sagittal image shows loss of integrity of the tegmen tympani (Panel C, arrow). There was no evidence of a fracture.

Dr. Samuels: Was the air in the epidural, subdural, or subarachnoid space?

Dr. Gonzalez: It appears to be subarachnoid. The air pocket in the middle cranial fossa is round, with an air–liquid level. If it were in the subdural or the epidural space, it would conform to the shape of the skull.

Dr. Samuels: Although this is clearly a case of otitic meningitis, it raises several important questions: the cause of the otorrhea, the meaning of the pneumocephalus, the risks of lumbar puncture, the cause of the aphasia, the likely causal organism, and the cause of the defect in the tegmen tympani.

OTORRHEA

This patient had drainage from his ear that was variously described as a discharge and as dried blood. Was this an infectious discharge from the external ear, or was it cerebrospinal fluid otorrhea? Cerebrospinal fluid otorrhea refers to the presence of cerebrospinal fluid in the external auditory canal due to an abnormal connection between the sub-arachnoid space and the tympanomastoid space. A rent in the tympanic membrane is required for the cerebrospinal fluid to enter the external ear. Otherwise, fluid accumulating in the middle ear is drained via the eustachian tube into the nasopharynx and often goes unrecognized.

An important clinical challenge is to recognize when fluid emanating from the ear is, in fact, cerebrospinal fluid. Cerebrospinal fluid otorrhea may be serosanguineous and mistaken for blood, as was probably the case in this patient. Otorrhea and rhinorrhea may be recognized as containing cerebrospinal fluid when a handkerchief soaked in the fluid does not stiffen when dry, because of the fluid's relatively low protein level (i.e., <2 g per liter). A fluid glucose level of greater than 40 mg per deciliter (2.2 mmol per liter) also suggests that the fluid is cerebrospinal fluid. The most accurate test is a measurement of β_2-transferrin, a protein that is found only in cerebrospinal fluid.[1] In this case, the otic discharge may well have been cerebrospinal fluid, but no test was obtained to document that fact.

One of the causes of cerebrospinal fluid otorrhea is fracture of the temporal bone. Temporal-bone fractures are classified as either transverse or longitudinal on the basis of their relationship to the otic capsule and the axis of the petrous ridge. In reality, many are oblique, with some features of both types. A longitudinal fracture, which was suspected in this case, may cause puncture of the tympanic membrane, producing otorrhea, whereas transverse fractures usually do not cause puncture of the tympanic membrane. In one study of 820 temporal-bone fractures,[2] 15% had cerebrospinal fluid fistulas, 85% of which involved the ear; 95% of the cerebrospinal fluid fistulas closed spontaneously within 14 days, and 7% of the patients contracted meningitis. Antibiotic prophylactic therapy administered until the fistula is closed may be helpful in preventing meningitis.[3]

PNEUMOCEPHALUS

Pneumocephalus, the accumulation of intracranial air, was seen on CT shortly after the patient's admission to the emergency department. It can be due to trauma, neoplasm, infection, or surgery. Otogenic pneumocephalus is not rare: among 59 consecutive patients with pneumocephalus, the cause was trauma in 36% of patients, otitis media in 31%, otic surgery in 31%, and congenital defects in 2%.[4] Rarely, pneumocephalus may be caused by brain abscess involving air-forming organisms,[5] but there is no evidence for such an infection in this case. In this patient, the presence of pneumocephalus is evidence of a cerebrospinal fluid fistula, which allowed cerebrospinal fluid to exit through the ear and air to enter from the mastoid air cells of pneumatized bone or from the external auditory canal.

PROS AND CONS OF LUMBAR PUNCTURE

The chance of increased intracranial pressure is substantial in the presence of otic infection. In the era before antibiotics, hydrocephalus in the presence of otic infection was termed "otitic hydrocephalus"; this was a misnomer in most cases, since it was usually increased levels of interstitial brain water (pseudotumor) related to poor venous drainage from the failure of one or more of the dural sinuses. However, in the presence of leptomeningitis, an authentic hydrocephalus may develop because of the slowing of cerebrospinal fluid flow and blockage of the resorption of cerebrospinal fluid into the venous system at the arachnoid granulations. The two processes (hydrocephalus and pseudotumor) could therefore coexist in this patient, producing increased intracranial pressure while leaving ventricular size relatively normal.

Fortunately, the neurologists caring for this patient were not afraid to perform a lumbar puncture, despite the risk of increased intracranial pressure. The risks of the procedure, though real, are generally overrated, and I believe it is likely that many more patients have had a deteriorating condition from the failure to perform the procedure than have had a complication or death resulting from the procedure. The presence of a mass, particularly near the midline or in the posterior fossa, probably increases the risks. If the clinician is concerned about performing the procedure in a patient in whom it is indicated because of the real threat of infection, rapid imaging of the brain should be performed before the procedure is undertaken.[6]

The cerebrospinal fluid in this patient was, indeed, under increased pressure (270 mm of water) and showed a neutrophilic pleocytosis, an elevated protein level, and a glucose level that was about 45% of the blood glucose level. All these findings strongly suggests a bacterial leptomeningitis. It is likely that the lumbar subarachnoid space, accessible with the use of the spinal needle, did not fully reflect the vigorousness of the inflammatory response around the brain, because the fluid was not flowing freely. The elevated cerebrospinal fluid protein level of 322 mg per deciliter may, in part, reflect stagnation of cerebrospinal fluid, known as Froin's syndrome.

APHASIA

One of the more interesting and cryptic aspects of this case is the aphasia. Disorders of speech and language are complex and often difficult to characterize accurately in the presence of generalized encephalopathy. I shall assume that the neurologist was correct in characterizing this patient's problem as aphasia, a disorder of language. For virtually all right-handed people and most left-handed people, the major systems for language are strongly lateralized to the left hemisphere. In general, aphasias are produced by disorders that affect the cerebrum, its subcortical connections, and the thalamus. It is uncommon, for example, to see aphasia with a subdural hematoma, a lesion on the surface of the brain, until the patient is so drowsy that the language problem is difficult to distinguish from a disorder of consciousness.

What disorder of the left hemisphere could have occurred in this patient? Septic dural sinus thrombosis is a common complication of infection of the tympanomastoid space,[7,8] but that should have affected the right transverse sinus, which should not produce aphasia. Dural sinus septic thrombophlebitis only rarely spreads to the opposite transverse sinus. Cerebritis or brain abscess in the left hemisphere could have occurred by hematogenous spread of infection in the right ear, but the imaging studies showed no such lesion.

The most likely explanation is cerebral vasospasm in reaction to the pus in the subarachnoid space. To produce aphasia, the middle cerebral arteries should be affected. Prolonged, severe vasospasm can lead to cerebral infarction, which may be the major sequela in survivors of bacterial, fungal, and tuberculous meningitis.

THE ORGANISM

What organism or organisms are responsible for this otitic meningitis? The most common bacteria are *Streptococcus pneumoniae* (about half of cases), *Neisseria meningitidis* (about one fifth of cases), *Listeria monocytogenes* (about one tenth of cases), and *Haemophilus influenzae* (about one tenth of cases).[9–11] If one hypothesizes that the infection in the ear actually caused the bony erosion that led to the cerebrospinal fluid fistula, one might favor more aggressive organisms such as *Staphylococcus aureus*, gram-negative organisms, and group A streptococcus. However, the relationship of the tegmen defects to the course of the ear infection is not known, so there is no way to predict the identity of the organism. The decision to treat the patient with broad-spectrum antibiotics, including coverage for anaerobic organisms, was well founded. The only additional intervention might have been intravenous high-dose corticosteroids, but the data supporting this approach are equivocal.[6]

DEFECTS OF THE TEGMEN TYMPANI

The final issue revolves around the defects of the tegmen tympani found on the temporal-bone CT. The tegmen tympani is the portion of the temporal bone that overlies the tympanic and mastoid cavities, forming the floor of the middle fossa. A few (less than five) defects in the tegmen are common and have been found in 15 to 34% of carefully examined temporal bones; however, five or more defects are rare (found in <1% of temporal bones). More than five defects are associated with an increased risk of neuro-otologic problems, including otorrhea and meningitis.[12] Tegmen defects may be congenital, leading to early and recurrent episodes of meningitis. Tegmen defects that arise late in life could be due to infection, trauma, or the long-term effect of a congenital defect. Chronic infection, with or without cholesteatoma, in the tympanomastoid space can lead to erosion of the tegmen. In the era before antibiotic treatment, this was probably a fairly common mechanism of otitic meningitis.

The arachnoid granulations (pacchionian granulations) are pockets of the suba-rachnoid space that project through the dura into the dural venous sinuses. Most of these are along the superior sagittal sinus, allowing for the return of cerebrospinal fluid to the venous system; however, aberrant arachnoid granulations can impinge on pneumatized bone in the posterior and middle fossa, erode the tegmen tympani, and lead to cerebrospinal fluid fistulas.[13] It is possible that minor head trauma could have exacerbated preexisting defects in the tegmen tympani.

SUMMARY

To synthesize the sequence of events in this case, there was chronic silent otitis media, and aberrant arachnoid granulations produced discontinuities in the tegmen tympani. Minor head trauma disrupted the fragile tegmen and, together with the chronic otitis media, produced a new rent in the tympanic membrane. Cerebrospinal fluid otorrhea, pneumocephalus, and bacterial meningitis ensued. The organism was aggressive, fur-ther eroding the tegmen tympani. Pus in the subarachnoid space caused cerebral vaso-spasm, producing aphasia. The dural sinuses, particularly the right transverse sinus, became incompetent, leading to increased intracranial pressure. The diagnostic tests were probably the blood culture and cerebrospinal fluid culture, as well as magnetic resonance imaging (MRI), angiography, and venography.

Dr. Nancy Lee Harris (Pathology): Dr. Caviness, you cared for this patient on the Neurology Service; can you comment on your thinking?

Dr. Verne S. Caviness, Jr. (Neurology): Dr. Alireza Atri was the neurologist called to see the patient in the emergency department. Aphasia was present before the patient's mental status deteriorated; we considered in retrospect that the patient might have had a seizure and that the aphasia and transient right hemiparesis might have been postictal. Dr. Atri immediately recognized that this was meningitis, instituted three-drug ther-apy, and performed the lumbar puncture. At that time, a temporal-bone fracture was considered and searched for but could not be identified. We considered a diastatic suture in the medial temporal bone. A defect in the tegmen tympani was not reported at the time.

Dr. Harris: Dr. Kim, what was the opinion of the consultants from the Department of Infectious Disease?

Dr. Arthur Y. Kim: We suspected bacterial meningitis from an otitic or a mastoid source or both.

CLINICAL DIAGNOSIS

Bacterial meningitis due to otitis or mastoiditis or both.

DR. MARTIN A. SAMUELS'S DIAGNOSIS

Otitic bacterial leptomeningitis, secondary to tegmen tympani defects caused by arach-noid granulations, possibly aggravated by minor head trauma.

PATHOLOGICAL DISCUSSION

Dr. Kim: The diagnostic test was Gram's staining of the cerebrospinal fluid specimen, which revealed moderate numbers of gram-positive cocci in pairs and chains, suggesting streptococcal species. Although *S. pneumoniae* remained a primary consideration, we also considered other organisms, including group A streptococci and enterococci. We recommended broad-spectrum antibiotics to cover these possibilities. Within hours, group A streptococci were grown on blood culture and cerebrospinal fluid culture.

Group A streptococci are a rare cause of bacterial meningitis, accounting for 0.5 to 1.5% of community-acquired cases[10,11,14]; the mortality rate (27%) is similar to that for pneumococcal meningitis (30%).[6] Otitis media due to group A streptococci is associated with high rates of local invasion, including tympanic perforation and mastoiditis, as was seen in this case,[15] and it is the most important risk factor for group A streptococcal meningitis among adult patients.[16] Most patients with group A streptococcal meningitis do not have the clinical features of septic shock associated with invasive group A streptococcal disease, and the incidence of the meningitis has not increased despite an increasing incidence of other forms of invasive disease.[16,17] After the culture results were received, additional imaging studies were performed.

Dr. Gonzalez: Brain MRI was performed before and after the administration of contrast material, as was magnetic resonance angiography and venography. In addition to the pneumocephalus, subtle areas of increased signal involved the cortex of the right temporal, parietal, and frontal lobes. Diffusion MRI did not show evidence of an acute ischemic event. The magnetic resonance venogram showed flow within all the major veins and sinuses. The angiogram was limited by the artifact of the technique, but it did not show good flow distal to the internal carotid arteries or distal to the basilar arteries. This can sometimes be seen in normal persons as an artifact, but we cannot rule out a process such as vasospasm.

Dr. Kim: Persistent hypotension and multiorgan failure ensued; vasopressor support was withdrawn, and death occurred 19 hours after admission to the emergency department. Permission for an autopsy was obtained.

Dr. Anat Stemmer-Rachamimov: At autopsy, multiple petechial hemorrhages were noted in the dura overlying the right middle fossa, and the underlying right mastoid bone was swollen, soft, and hemorrhagic. The venous sinuses were free of thrombi. The leptomeninges appeared cloudy, with small collections of white, thick fluid surrounding small meningeal vessels that were most prominent in the leptomeninges overlying the cerebral hemispheres (Fig. 2A).

Microscopical examination showed a dense inflammatory infiltrate in the subarachnoid space, which was composed of neutrophils and immature mononuclear cells (Fig. 2B). Fibrinoid necrosis and thrombosis were noted in some of the meningeal arterioles. In the brain parenchyma, inflammatory cells were clustered around cortical arterioles and scattered in the neuropil. The inflammation involved the left temporal lobe as well as other areas of the brain.

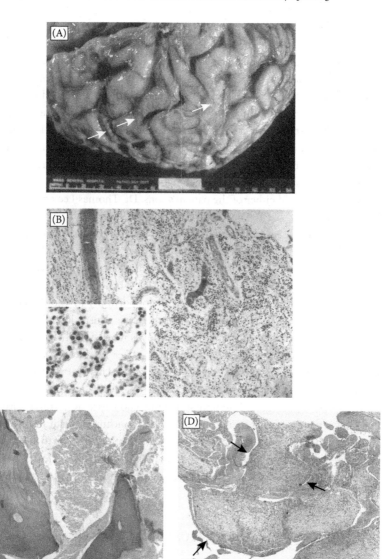

FIG 2 Pathological Examination of the Brain at Autopsy.
On gross examination, the leptomeninges were opaque and perivascular white exudate was present
(Panel A, arrows). Microscopical examination of the subarachnoid space showed an inflammatory
infiltrate (Panel B) composed of neutrophils and some immature myeloid cells (inset) (hematoxylin
and eosin). Examination of the right mastoid bone showed an inflammatory infiltrate in the mastoid
mucosa and mastoid air cells (Panel C). Aberrant arachnoid granulations (Panel D, arrows) are large,
necrotic, and inflamed.

Sections of the mastoid bone were reviewed with Dr. Saumil Merchant
(Massachusetts Eye and Ear Infirmary). There was no evidence of fracture, a preexisting chronic inflammatory condition (such as a cholesteatoma) in the middle ear,
or labyrinthitis in the semicircular canals. In contrast, the mastoid mucosal lining was
thickened by means of vascular engorgement, edema, and inflammatory-cell infiltrates

(Fig. 2C). Large inflamed and necrotic arachnoid granulations (>3 mm in diameter) were noted in sections of the mastoid bone (Fig. 2D), and aggregates of grampositive cocci were present in the subarachnoid space and in the mastoid air cells.

Arachnoid granulations may increase in size with age, and intermediate and large granulations (3.0 to 9.5 mm in diameter) may herniate through dural defects and erode bone (aberrant granulations).[12,13,18,19] The presence of large arachnoid granulations and the absence of fracture, preexisting middle-ear disease, and labyrinthitis suggest that a dural defect and bone erosion caused by aberrant arachnoid granulations are the most probable route for intracranial extension of the suppurative mastoiditis in this case, which then led to acute meningoencephalitis.

Dr. Harris: Would either of the patient's sons, Dr. Thomas Lee or Dr. Richard Lee, like to comment?

Dr. Thomas H. Lee, Jr. (Internal Medicine, Brigham and Women's Hospital): We learned from this case that the care of patients does continue after they die. The performance of the autopsy and the careful review of all aspects of this case for this conference provided us with two opportunities that I believe every family who loses a loved one would appreciate. The first was the opportunity to know what caused his death. During hospitalization, we knew that there was a suspicion of a fracture on the CT scan; after my father's death, we left the hospital believing that his fall on the ice had caused the fracture and therefore his death. After the autopsy, which showed no fracture, we realized that perhaps the fall had not caused his death. After the discussion at this conference, we now have a final answer.

The second opportunity is to have something good arise from tragedy. My brother and I know that our father, as a professor at the Massachusetts Institute of Technology, would have been completely in favor of having his death contribute to the education of physicians who will care for patients in the future. He would have joked that this was his final publication, and I would have said to him, "It is your first in a journal worth reading."

ANATOMICAL DIAGNOSIS

Acute bacterial meningoencephalitis, acute right otitis media and mastoiditis, and aberrant arachnoid granulations with erosion of the temporal bone.

REFERENCES

1. Oberascher G. Cerebrospinal fluid otorrhea—new trends in diagnosis. Am J Otol 1988;9:102–8.
2. Brodie HA, Thompson TC. Management of complications from 820 temporal bone fractures. Am J Otol 1997;18:188–97.
3. Brodie HA. Prophylactic antibiotics for posttraumatic cerebrospinal fluid fistulae: a meta-analysis. Arch Otolaryngol Head Neck Surg 1997;123:749–52.
4. Andrews JC, Canalis RF. Otogenic pneumocephalus. Laryngoscope 1986;96:521–8.

5. Parmar MS. Pneumocephalus associated with Bacteroides fragilis meningitis. J Postgrad Med 2004;50:272–3.

6. van de Beek D, de Gans J, Tunkel AR, Wijdicks EFM. Community-acquired bacterial meningitis in adults. N Engl J Med 2006;354:44–53.

7. Southwick FS, Richardson EP Jr, Swartz MN. Septic thrombosis of the dural venous sinuses. Medicine (Baltimore) 1986;65:82–106.

8. Stam J. Thrombosis of the cerebral veins and sinuses. N Engl J Med 2005;352:1791–8.

9. Schuchat A, Robinson K, Wenger JD, et al. Bacterial meningitis in the United States in 1995. N Engl J Med 1997;337:970–6.

10. Durand ML, Calderwood SB, Weber DJ, et al. Acute bacterial meningitis in adults: a review of 493 episodes. N Engl J Med 1993;328:21–8.

11. van de Beek D, de Gans J, Spanjaard L, Weisfelt M, Reitsma JB, Vermeulen M. Clinical features and prognostic factors in adults with bacterial meningitis. N Engl J Med 2004;351:1849–59. [Erratum, N Engl J Med 2005;352:950.]

12. Merchant SN, McKenna MJ. Neurotologic manifestations and treatment of multiple spontaneous tegmental defects. Am J Otol 2000;21:234–9.

13. Gacek RR. Arachnoid granulation cerebrospinal fluid otorrhea. Ann Otol Rhinol Laryngol 1990;99:854–62.

14. Swartz MN, Dodge PR. Bacterial meningitis—a review of selected aspects: general clinical features, special problems, and unusual meningeal reactions mimicking bacterial meningitis. N Engl J Med 1965;272:725–31.

15. Segal N, Givon-Lavi N, Leibovitz E, Yagupsky P, Lieberman A, Dagan R. Acute otitis media caused by Streptococcus pyogenes in children. Clin Infect Dis 2005;41:35–41.

16. van de Beek D, de Gans J, Spanjaard L, Sela S, Vermeulen M, Dankert J. Group A streptococcal meningitis in adults: report of 41 cases and a review of the literature. Clin Infect Dis 2002;34(9):e32–e36.

17. Sommer R, Rohner P, Garbino J, et al. Group A beta-hemolytic streptococcus meningitis: clinical and microbiological features of nine cases. Clin Infect Dis 1999;29:929–31.

18. Gacek RR. Evaluation and management of temporal bone arachnoid granulations. Arch Otolaryngol Head Neck Surg 1992;118:327–32.

19. Rosenberg AE, O'Connell JX, Ojemann RG, Plata MJ, Palmer WE. Giant cystic arachnoid granulations: a rare cause of lytic skull lesions. Hum Pathol 1993;24:438–41.

Perspectives and Updates

Mastoiditis was once a serious and common medical problem. One of the most feared complications was otitic meningitis. The antibiotic era changed all this. Otitis became a medically manageable disease and generations of physicians were trained without ever having seen a serious case. In this patient, an unusual organism, group A streptococcus, entered the meninges via an unusual route, erosion of the temporal bone by an aberrant arachnoid granulation. When the patient reached the emergency department, despite virtually immediate recognition of the syndrome of bacterial meningitis, broad-spectrum antibiotics were unable to prevent the fatal outcome. The case represents a warning regarding the virulence of the disease once the organism breaches the meninges. Whether a more favorable outcome would have occurred had the otitis media been recognized and treated earlier is, of course, unknown. Perhaps one lesson is for the clinician to be extremely cautious about infections near the meninges and to err on the side of caution by administering empiric treatment when this condition is seen in an immunocompromised or older person.

Another important lesson from this case stems from the extraordinary reaction of the family, as recorded in the CPC. This is a rare example in the Cabot Case series in which the identity of the patient was known. He was the father of two distinguished doctors, both members of the faculty of the Harvard Medical School. In a statement made at the end of the case discussion, Thomas H. Lee, speaking for himself and Richard Lee, his brother, makes a courageous statement about the enduring validity of the clinicopathological method. Despite the sad outcome, he said that the care of his father, even after his death, represented an important feature of medical care and that it gave the family some solace to know the cause of their father's death with certainty. Dr. Lee also had the grace and perspective to note that this exercise allowed something good to come from an otherwise tragic event. He noted that his father, an academic engineer, would have called this his last publication. In the final line of this CPC, Dr. Lee quips that he would have told his father that this was "his first in a journal worth reading." The use of humor combined with wisdom is indeed a mark of the Lee family.

Martin A. Samuels

A 49-Year-Old Man with Peripheral Neuropathy and Ascites

POEMS SYNDROME

Allan H. Ropper, Noopur S. Raje, Tara M. Lawrimore,
Sandra Camelo-Piragua, and Aliyah R. Sohani

CPC 7-2010

PRESENTATION OF CASE

Dr. Caron A. Jacobson (Medical Oncology): A 49-year-old man was admitted to this hospital because of ascites.

The patient had been well until approximately 4 years earlier, when paresthesias of both feet, weakness of the lower legs, and bilateral foot drop developed gradually. Three years before admission, he saw a neurologist at another hospital. Laboratory-test results, including testing for autoantibodies, were reportedly normal. Electromyography (EMG) reportedly showed prolonged F responses in both feet, normal motor and sensory responses in the distal segments of the arms, and no motor responses in the intrinsic foot muscles. A diagnosis of chronic inflammatory demyelinating polyneuropathy (CIDP) was made, and therapy with intravenous immune globulin was begun.

Two and a half years before admission, the patient was referred to the neurology clinic of this hospital. On examination, the Romberg test was markedly abnormal; there was bilateral foot drop, and the patient was unable to walk on his toes or heels. He was able to sign his name but not without visual control. Strength (on a scale of 0 to 5, where 5 is normal) in the ankle dorsiflexors measured 1 to 2; in the muscles of ankle eversion and inversion, 4–; in the extensor hallucis longus, extensor digitorum brevis, and toe flexors, 0; and in the plantar flexors, 4– to 4. The left hand was mildly weak, particularly the abductor pollicis brevis, and strength was normal in the proximal arms. Deep-tendon reflexes were absent. Perception of vibration was absent in both first toes, decreased in both ankles, and normal at the knees and fingers. Position sense was diminished in both first toes. There was no muscle atrophy or fasciculation, and the remainder of the neurologic examination was normal. As compared with the previous study, EMG and nerve-conduction studies showed decreased sensory responses, absent sural-nerve responses, prolonged F-wave latencies, and more prominent denervation in the tibialis anterior and medial gastrocnemius muscles, features consistent with a demyelinating polyneuropathy.

N Engl J Med 2010;362:929–40.

During the next 6 months, weakness in the patient's legs and arms increased, and intermittent stabbing pain in the lower legs developed. Intravenous immune globulin was stopped, and the administration of azathioprine and gabapentin was begun. Two years before admission, the patient reported difficulty inhaling when he was supine, as well as discoloration of his feet. Tests of liver and renal function and measurements of serum electrolytes, thyrotropin, glycated hemoglobin, and homocysteine and urinary methylmalonic acid were normal. Tests for rheumatoid factor; antineuronal nuclear antibodies; antibodies to *Borrelia burgdorferi*, gastric parietal cells, intrinsic factor, and myelin-associated glycoprotein; anti–double-stranded DNA antibodies; sulfatide autoantibodies; and GALOP (gait disturbance, autoantibody, late-age onset, and polyneuropathy) autoantibodies were negative, as was the co-GM1 triad antibody test (Athena Diagnostics), which tests for co-Asialo ganglioside antibodies, co-GD1b antibodies, and GM1 antibodies. Additional laboratory-test results are shown in Table 1. EMG testing showed further decreases in evoked motor responses and absent sensory responses in the right median and ulnar nerves. Spirometry showed a maximal inspiratory pressure of 23 cm of water while the patient was supine (20% of predicted) and a maximal expiratory pressure of 98 cm of water (45% of predicted); lung volumes were normal.

Plasmapheresis was begun. The patient's respiratory function improved; he thought that the strength in his arms and legs had improved somewhat, but intermittent edema of the legs developed. Eight months before admission, he was admitted to the hospital because of coagulase-negative staphylococcal bacteremia, which was treated with vancomycin; after treatment, he noted hearing loss and high-pitched tinnitus. Six months before admission, he began to have episodes of blurred vision, sometimes related to positional change, and intermittent peripheral-visual-field loss and scotoma. Approximately 2.5 months before admission, plasmapheresis was stopped and infusions of intravenous immune globulin were resumed. Leg edema and abdominal girth increased, associated with fatigue. Ophthalmologic and otolaryngologic examinations 2 months before admission revealed bilateral disk edema, enlarged blind spots, and sensorineural hearing loss.

Six weeks before admission, magnetic resonance imaging (MRI) of the brain with magnetic resonance angiography revealed pachymeningeal enhancement along the calvaria and the falx cerebri, enhancement of the dura and multiple cranial nerves, and arachnoid granulation that narrowed the right transverse sinus. A lumbar puncture was performed. The opening pressure was 120 mm of water; results of cerebrospinal fluid (CSF) analysis are shown in Table 1. Leg edema and abdominal discomfort and swelling increased. Furosemide was administered, with no improvement. Computed tomography (CT) of the abdomen performed at another hospital reportedly showed ascites and iliac and retroperitoneal lymphadenopathy, with lymph nodes up to 1.7 cm in diameter. The patient was admitted to this hospital.

The patient reported no neck, lower back, or joint pain or bladder or bowel symptoms. He had had erectile dysfunction for the past year, he had dyslipidemia and hypercholesterolemia controlled by diet, and he had had knee surgery in the past. He was allergic to penicillin and ondansetron. He lived with his wife and children, used leg braces and a walker to ambulate, and was a businessman. He drank alcohol rarely and did not smoke. There was no family history of diabetes, coagulopathy, or hematologic,

Table 1 Laboratory Data*

Variable	Reference Range, Adults†	2 Yr before Admission	6 Wk before Admission Blood or Serum	On Admission	4 Wk after Discharge	11 Wk after Discharge
Hematocrit (%)	41.0–53.0 (men)	47.1		29.0	34.1	34.6
Hemoglobin (g/dl)	13.5–17.5 (men)	16.7		10.0	11.8	11.5
White-cell count (per mm²)	4500–11,000	7500		3900	4800	7000
Differential count (%)						
Neutrophils	40–70	72		78	75	74
Lymphocytes	22–44	20		17	18	17
Monocytes	4–11	5		3	5	5
Eosinophils	0–8	2		1	1	3
Basophils	0–3	1		1	1	1
Platelet count (per mm³)	150,000–400,000	573,000 (ref 150,000–350,000)		408,000	447,000	330,000
Urea nitrogen (mg/dl)	8–25	19		31	29	19
Creatinine (mg/dl)	0.60–1.50	1.0		1.54	1.34	1.25
Estimated glomerular filtration rate (ml/min/1.73 m²)	>60			51	>60	>60
Protein (g/dl)						
Total	6.0–8.3	8.3		6.7	5.9	5.8
Albumin	3.3–5.0	4.5		3.5	3.1	3.1
Globulin	2.6–4.1	3.8		3.2	2.8	2.7
Vitamin B_{12} (pg/ml)	>250	191		163	443	
Antinuclear antibody	Negative at 1:40 and 1:160	Positive at 1:40 and 1:160, speckled pattern				

(Continued)

Table 1 (Continued)

Variable	Reference Range, Adults†	2 Yr before Admission	6 Wk before Admission Blood or Serum	On Admission	4 Wk after Discharge	11 Wk after Discharge
IgA (mg/dl)	69–309	96		36	51	54
IgG (mg/dl)	614–1295	1800		676	673	727
IgM (mg/dl)	53–334	117		81	131	111
IgG lambda M component (g/dl)‡		0.24		0.11	0.14	0.10
Free kappa light chain (mg/liter)	3.3–19.4			26.6		25.6
Free lambda light chain (mg/liter)	5.7–26.3			33.6		51.1
Ratio of free kappa to lambda light chains	0.3–1.7			0.8		0.5
Testosterone (ng/dl)	270–1070 (men)			86		
β_2-Microglobulin (mg/liter)	0.8–3.0				6.7	

	Cerebro-spinal Fluid	Ascitic Fluid
Color	Colorless (ref colorless)	Yellow (ref yellow)
Turbidity	Clear	Slight
Xanthochromia	None	
Red-cell count (per mm³)	None	Not done
White-cell count (per mm³)	4 (ref 0–5)	106
Differential count (%)		
Neutrophils	5	18
Lymphocytes	65	14
Monocytes	30	15
Nonhematic cells	0	53
Glucose (mg/dl)	68 (ref 50–75)	100
Protein (mg/dl)	112 (ref 5–55)	4200
Albumin (mg/dl)	61.0 (ref 11.0–50.9)	2600
IgG (mg/dl)	17.4 (ref 0–8.0)	
Agarose electrophoresis	Two bands (specimen concentrated 80 times)	
Lactate dehydrogenase (U/liter)		69
Serum ascites albumin gradient (g/dl)		0.9

(Continued)

Table 1 (Continued)

*Ref denotes reference range. To convert the values for urea nitrogen to millimoles per liter, multiply by 0.357. To convert the values for creatinine to micromoles per liter, multiply by 88.4. To convert the values for glucose to millimoles per liter, multiply by 0.05551.

†Reference values are affected by many variables, including the patient population and the laboratory methods used. The ranges used at Massachusetts General Hospital are for adults who are not pregnant and do not have medical conditions that could affect the results. They may therefore not be appropriate for all patients.

‡Values were from bands in the gamma region and were determined by means of serum protein electrophoresis and immunofixation.

autoimmune, ophthalmologic, or neurologic diseases. Medications included azathioprine (250 mg per day), gabapentin, duloxetine, and hydrocodone–acetaminophen.

On examination, the temperature was 36.3°C, the blood pressure 122/76 mm Hg, the pulse 72 beats per minute, the respiratory rate 20 breaths per minute, and the oxygen saturation 99% while the patient was breathing ambient air. There were crackles at the lung bases. Bowel sounds were present, and the abdomen was tense, distended, and nontender. There were contractures of the hands, 3+ pitting edema of the legs to the waist, and decreased strength in the arms and legs. Abdominal paracentesis was performed, 2 liters of ascitic fluid were removed, and abdominal discomfort decreased. Results of ascitic-fluid analysis are shown in Table 1. Ultrasonography of the abdomen revealed increased echogenicity of the liver, splenomegaly (span, 16.6 cm), and ascites; the portal and hepatic vasculature was patent. Urinalysis revealed a specific gravity of more than 1.040, 1+ albumin, a total protein level of 320 mg per liter (reference range, 0 to 135), and a ratio of total protein to creatinine of 0.18; it was otherwise normal.

Specimens from percutaneous, CT-guided fine-needle aspiration and core biopsy of a left retroperitoneal lymph node were obtained. Pathological examination of the biopsy specimens showed reactive hyperplasia; no malignant cells were identified. Flow cytometry identified normal B-cell and T-cell populations. Analysis of urine (concentrated 50 times) revealed small amounts of kappa Bence Jones protein and trace amounts of albumin; there was no Bence Jones protein in the serum. During the next week, multiple therapeutic paracenteses were performed; no malignant cells were seen. Tests for antibodies to the human immunodeficiency virus and human herpesvirus 8 (HHV-8) were negative, and levels of vascular endothelial growth factor (VEGF) and folate were normal. Tests of renal function returned to normal.

CT of the chest, abdomen, and pelvis after the administration of contrast material revealed scattered nodules (2 to 3 mm in diameter) in both lungs, diffuse lymphadenopathy (including a retroperitoneal paraaortic mass, 2.2 cm by 2.1 cm), ascites, a small pericardial effusion, and bilateral pleural effusions. Examination of a bone marrow–biopsy specimen and aspirate showed normocellular marrow with trilineage hematopoiesis; a stain for amyloid was negative. Immunohistochemical and flow-cytometric analyses showed no evidence of monoclonal B cells or plasma cells; the karyotype was normal. Congo red staining of a biopsy specimen of the abdominal fat pad was negative for amyloid. A radiographic skeletal survey showed lucency in the right tibial diaphysis. Azathioprine was discontinued, and the patient was discharged on the 11th day, returning for outpatient paracenteses one or two times weekly thereafter.

Three weeks later, MRI of the right lower leg showed heterogeneity of the marrow and an enhancing focal lesion within the medullary cavity of the midtibial diaphysis (3.7 cm in length) that was hypointense on T_1-weighted images and hyperintense on T_2-weighted images. A percutaneous, CT-guided biopsy showed bone with no evidence of a neoplastic process. Pathological examination of a biopsy specimen of the right antebrachial nerve revealed evidence of chronic demyelination and remyelination, with axonal degeneration affecting both myelinated and unmyelinated fibers.

Eleven weeks after discharge, CT of the neck, chest, and abdomen, performed in conjunction with positron-emission tomography (PET), showed intense uptake of ^{18}F-fluorodeoxyglucose (^{18}F-FDG) in a lytic lesion (5.4 cm by 3.8 cm) in the sacrum that had sclerotic margins and central soft-tissue components. Lymphadenopathy and pulmonary nodules were unchanged from previous CT examinations and not associated with increased ^{18}F-FDG uptake.

A diagnostic procedure was performed.

DIFFERENTIAL DIAGNOSIS

Dr. Allan H. Ropper[*]: May we review the imaging studies and the nerve biopsy?

Dr. Tara M. Lawrimore: CT of the abdomen after the administration of oral and intravenous contrast material revealed moderate ascites, soft-tissue anasarca, splenomegaly, and retroperitoneal lymphadenopathy that enhanced with contrast material (Fig. 1A). A radiographic skeletal survey showed a lucent lesion in the mid-diaphysis of the right tibia (Fig. 1B). MRI of the right lower leg confirmed the presence of a marrow-replacing lesion in the mid-tibia (Fig. 1 in the Supplementary Appendix, available with the full text of this article at NEJM.org). A combined PET–CT examination of the chest, abdomen, and pelvis revealed a marrow-replacing lesion with sclerotic borders that was centered within the sacrum and showed increased ^{18}F-FDG uptake (Fig. 1C and 1D). Extensive axillary, hilar, retroperitoneal, and pelvic lymphadenopathy was also present but did not show increased ^{18}F-FDG uptake.

Dr. Sandra Camelo-Piragua: Sections of the right antebrachial nerve that were stained with Gomori trichrome revealed a marked reduction in the number of myelinated fibers (Fig. 2A). Teased nerve-fiber preparations showed multiple segments of thinly myelinated axons; several shortened internodal lengths and occasional myelin ovoids were also noted (Fig. 2B). An Epon-embedded section that was 1 μm thick showed a severe decrease in thickly myelinated fibers, an increase in endoneurial and perineurial connective tissue, and scattered and clustered thinly myelinated fibers (Fig. 2C). Ultrastructural examination revealed a dramatic loss of thickly myelinated axons, scattered thinly myelinated axons, regenerative clusters of axons, and occasional small whorls of Schwann cells in an onion-bulb formation (Fig. 2D). In addition, several Schwann-cell stacks were present, indicating a loss of small unmyelinated axons. These features are consistent with chronic demyelination and remyelination, with axonal degeneration that affects both myelinated and unmyelinated fibers.

---

[*]Currently Vice-Chair, Department of Neurology, Brigham and Women's Hospital.

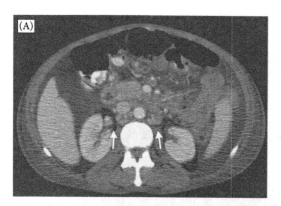

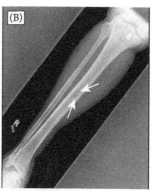

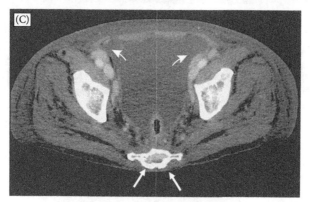

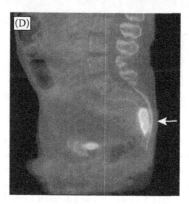

FIG 1 Radiographic Images.

An image of the upper abdomen from a CT scan obtained after the administration of contrast material (Panel A) shows findings of ascites and enhancing paraaortic lymphadenopathy (arrows). An anteroposterior radiograph of the right lower leg from a skeletal survey reveals a lucent lesion in the midtibial diaphysis (Panel B, arrows). An image of the lower pelvis from CT performed in conjunction with positron-emission tomography shows a sacral marrow-replacing lesion with sclerotic borders (Panel C, straight arrows) and lymphadenopathy of the pelvic sidewall (curved arrows). Increased uptake of 18F-fluorodeoxyglucose (FDG) is present in the sacral lesion (Panel D, arrow) on a fused midline sagittal reformation. The 18F-FDG activity anteriorly represents an accumulation of excreted tracer in the bladder.

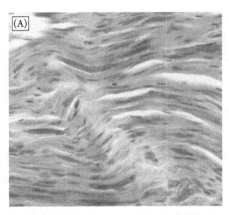

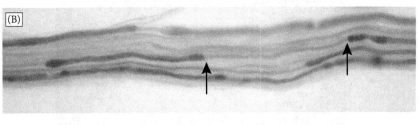

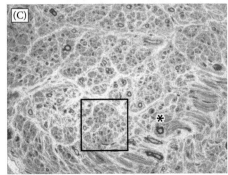

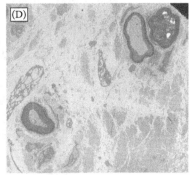

FIG 2 Nerve-Biopsy Specimen.

The nerve-biopsy specimen shows evidence of chronic demyelination and remyelination. Staining with Gomori trichrome (Panel A) shows severe reduction in the number of myelinated fibers. A teased-fiber preparation (Panel B) shows multiple segments of thinly myelinated fibers (one example is shown between two arrows) and shortened internodal distance. An Epon-embedded section that was 1 μm thick (Panel C) shows a marked decrease in thickly myelinated fibers (asterisk) and clusters of thinly myelinated fibers (rectangle). Electron-microscopical examination (Panel D) shows whorls of Schwann cells in an onion-bulb formation.

Dr. Ropper: This middle-aged man had progressive sensory and motor symptoms over a period of 4 years, as well as ascites, papilledema, limb edema, lymphadenopathy, and bone lesions. A neurologist discussing a patient with ascites is swimming in unfamiliar waters, and trying to make sense of these disparate findings requires an anchor. I will start with the neurologic aspects, trying to respect the time course of the disease as encountered by the patient's physicians.

Neuropathy as a Guide to Localization of Disease

Bilateral weakness and sensory loss in this patient make a lesion in the brain improbable. The absence of a sensory level, hyperreflexia, and Babinski signs rule out a spinal cord disorder. The usual pattern of root disease, polyradiculopathy, or multiple mononeuropathies is heterogeneously distributed motor and sensory loss (usually painful), which was not present. Instead, this patient had a prototypic polyneuropathy—symmetric distal sensory and motor features with absent reflexes.

Polyneuropathies can be classified as demyelinating or axonal. They can also be classified according to the diameter of the affected nerve fiber. Larger fibers are heavily myelinated and therefore most subject to processes that damage myelin. Most polyneuropathies, including the diabetic type, are axonal.

We are aided in this case by the findings of the loss of the perception of vibration and the decrease in the sense of joint position; both of these sensations are conducted by large fibers. The positive sensory symptom of paresthesia (in contrast to the negative symptom of numbness) is also a useful finding, since tingling is characteristic of acquired demyelinating neuropathies and is due to spontaneous firing of sensory nerves as a result of exposed sodium channels in denuded segments. The patient's Romberg sign and clumsiness that was corrected by visual guidance are additional typical features of large-fiber demyelinating neuropathy. In the distal legs, marked weakness with preservation of muscle bulk further signifies demyelination, because the preserved trophic influence of motor-nerve terminals on the muscle membrane maintains muscle size. Axonal neuropathies, in contrast, cause early atrophy. We can conclude that the process in this patient is a sensorimotor demyelinating polyneuropathy.

Demyelinating Polyneuropathy

The most common demyelinating polyneuropathy is CIDP, which was the initial diagnosis in this patient. However, demyelinating neuropathy has a fairly extensive differential diagnosis (Table 2). A large number of genetically determined conditions, broadly referred to as Charcot–Marie–Tooth disease, can result in demyelination but can be ruled out in this case because they are chronic. Exposure of this patient to drugs and toxins that can cause demyelination was not evident. Almost all the remaining demyelinating neuropathies are immune or inflammatory.

CIDP is an idiopathic multifocal inflammation of the nerves that can occur at any age in the form of a subacute sensorimotor polyneuropathy. It can be identified by the findings of electrical conduction block (segmental demyelination at areas of inflammation, as seen on nerve-conduction studies) and by a high level of protein in the CSF. CIDP is clinically similar to Guillain–Barré syndrome, except for the differing time course, and was at one time called chronic Guillain–Barré syndrome. CIDP is usually idiopathic but also can occur as a feature of some connective-tissue diseases. Corticosteroids, intravenous immune globulin, and plasma exchange (the last two were administered to this patient) are all effective treatments in most cases; if they are not effective, immunosuppressive drugs are added. Until a number of unusual systemic signs appeared in this patient 2 years before evaluation, all features had been compatible with CIDP.

Paraproteinemic Neuropathies

Another major category of immune demyelinating neuropathy is associated with a serum monoclonal gammopathy (also known as a paraprotein or an M component). In these paraproteinemic neuropathies, the abnormal protein may have antinerve antibody activity, usually directed against GM1, sulfatides, or myelin-associated glycoprotein (Table 2). The laboratory evaluation of demyelinating neuropathy therefore includes serum immunoelectrophoresis or immunofixation (protein electrophoresis alone is inadequate) and testing for antineural antibodies and connective-tissue disease.

The laboratory results in this case are not distinctive except for monoclonal IgG lambda paraprotein. The most common monoclonal gammopathy associated with polyneuropathy is monoclonal gammopathy of unknown significance (MGUS). Patients with MGUS have a paraprotein level of less than 30 g per liter, as this patient did, but kappa light chain is more common the lambda light chain seen in this patient. The low concentration of paraprotein in this case would be unusual for multiple myeloma, and examination of the bone marrow did not reveal neoplastic plasma cells. Waldenström's macroglobulinemia is characterized by the presence of an IgM paraprotein and by lymphoplasmacytic lymphoma in the bone marrow and sometimes in the lymph nodes; it may be associated with polyneuropathy. This patient's

Table 2 Causes of Demyelinating Polyneuropathy[*]

Cause	Example
Genetic	Charcot–Marie–Tooth disease, type 1
Toxic	
Natural	Diphtheria toxin, buckthorn toxin
Drugs	Amiodarone, taxol
Inflammatory	
Idiopathic	Chronic inflammatory demyelinating polyneuropathy†
With connective-tissue and other systemic disease	Sjögren's disease, lupus, sprue
Immune	
Paraproteinemic	Monoclonal gammopathy of unknown significance,† plasma-cell myeloma, Waldenström's macroglobulinemia, amyloidosis, the POEMS syndrome
Antineural antibodies	Mainly against sulfatides and myelin-associated glycoprotein
Paraneoplastic	Lymphoma
Parainfectious	Human immunodeficiency virus, Lyme disease, sarcoid

[*] POEMS denotes polyneuropathy, organomegaly, endocrinopathy, M protein, and skin changes.
†This is one of the more common causes of demyelinating polyneuropathy in general practice.

lymphnode–biopsy specimen showed no evidence of lymphoma. Amyloidosis, the result of deposition of abnormal light chains in tissues, may also be associated with neuropathy; amyloid neuropathy, however, is a small-fiber axonal sensory disturbance with prominent pain and relative preservation of the perception of vibration and the sense of joint position, which is the opposite pattern from the current case. No amyloid was identified on examination of a biopsy specimen of a fat pad.

The POEMS Syndrome

The combination of polyneuropathy and bone lesions has been called Crow–Fukase syndrome, because of early descriptions by Crow[1] and Fukase et al.[2] The acronym POEMS (polyneuropathy, organomegaly, endocrinopathy, M protein, and skin changes) was introduced by Bardwick et al.[3] and represents the elements they considered essential. Of these elements, only polyneuropathy and the monoclonal protein, both of which this patient has, are necessarily present in a given case (Table 3).[4] This patient had a low testosterone level and vitamin B_{12} deficiency, but he did not have other signs of endocrinopathy.

A moderately increased level of CSF protein in this patient is typical of the POEMS syndrome but does not distinguish it from CIDP. A low level of monoclonal IgG with lambda light chain is also characteristic of the POEMS syndrome. However, in contrast to multiple myeloma, the levels of other immunoglobulin subclasses are not reduced in the POEMS syndrome. This patient had discoloration of the skin of his feet (the color was not described) and edema of the legs. The characteristic skin changes in the POEMS syndrome include a purple hue, thickening, and hypertrichosis. The edema does not have the pitting quality that is associated with congestive heart failure and offers considerable resistance to digital pressure. The unusual systemic features in this patient have been recorded in other cases of the POEMS syndrome, specifically refractory ascites[5,6] and papilledema.[7–9]

In the POEMS syndrome, a clonal expansion of plasma cells occurs in association with sclerotic bone lesions (osteosclerotic myeloma). The syndrome may also involve lymph nodes in the form of angiofollicular hyperplasia, also known as Castleman's disease.

The mechanism of the POEMS syndrome is a puzzle. Why lambda light chain predominates, whereas kappa light chain predominates in MGUS, is unknown. Severe leg edema and ascites suggest a vascular leak. Organomegaly of the liver and spleen may indicate fluid extravasation in those organs, which has been attributed to elevated levels of circulating VEGF produced by the plasma cells.[10,11] Having conducted a trial of plasmid VEGF DNA for the treatment of diabetic polyneuropathy,[12] I can attest to the occurrence of local edema and hypertrichosis due to the protein, but I have not seen pigmentary changes or skin thickening. In the current case, serum levels of VEGF were not elevated but, nevertheless, elevated levels were suspected on the basis of clinical features, such as ascites, that are suggestive of a vascular leak. In some cases of the POEMS syndrome that are associated with the plasma-cell variant of Castleman's disease, HHV-8 has been found within plasmablasts.[13] Evidence of this viral infection was sought and not found in this patient. Several studies have shown elevated proinflammatory cytokines, including interleukin-1β, interleukin-6, and tumor necrosis factor α in some patients with POEMS.[14]

Diagnostic Procedure

I cannot endorse any diagnostic procedure in this case, because the diagnosis is certain and more information is not necessary for treatment. However, a biopsy of the sacral lesion would most likely reveal a plasmacytoma.

Dr. Nancy Lee Harris (Pathology): Could we have the medical students' diagnosis?

A Harvard Medical Student: After considering a broad differential diagnosis, our leading hypothesis was that this polyneuropathy was secondary to a plasma-cell

Table 3 Diagnostic Criteria for the POEMS Syndrome[*]

Major criteria
Polyneuropathy
Monoclonal plasma-cell proliferative disorder (almost always lambda light-chain–restricted)
Sclerotic bone lesions
Castleman's disease
Minor criteria
Vascular endothelial growth factor elevation
Organomegaly (splenomegaly, hepatomegaly, or lymphadenopathy)
Extravascular volume overload (edema, pleural effusion, or ascites)
Endocrinopathy (adrenal, thyroid,[†] pituitary, gonadal, parathyroid, or pancreatic[†])
Skin changes (hyperpigmentation, hypertrichosis, glomeruloid hemangiomata, plethora, acrocyanosis, flushing, or white nails)
Papilledema
Other symptoms and signs
Thrombocytosis[‡]
Polycythemia
Possible associated features
Clubbing, weight loss, hyperhidrosis, pulmonary hypertension or restrictive lung disease, thrombotic diatheses, diarrhea, and low vitamin B$_{12}$ level

[*]POEMS denotes polyneuropathy, organomegaly, endocrinopathy, M protein, and skin changes. Polyneuropathy and monoclonal plasma-cell disorder present in all patients; to make a diagnosis, at least one other major criterion and one minor criterion are required. Data are from Dispenzieri,[4] with permission from the publisher.

[†]Because of the high prevalence of diabetes mellitus and thyroid abnormalities, this diagnosis alone is not sufficient to meet this minor criterion.

[‡]Anemia and thrombocytopenia are distinctively unusual in this syndrome unless Castleman's disease is present.

disorder. CIDP is less likely in view of the systemic symptoms. We thought that the POEMS syndrome was the most likely diagnosis.

Dr. Harris: Dr. Jacobson, will you tell us what the clinical thinking was at the time of the diagnostic procedure?

Dr. Jacobson: This patient had peripheral neuropathy and a small monoclonal component restricted to a lambda light chain, two major criteria for the diagnosis of the POEMS syndrome; he had other features, including ascites, papilledema, hypogonadism, and thrombocytosis, that are considered minor diagnostic criteria for the POEMS syndrome (Table 3). However, an additional major criterion—increased serum levels of VEGF, Castleman's disease, or osteosclerotic bone lesions—was required.[4] The biopsy specimen of the lymph node did not show evidence of Castleman's disease, and the VEGF level was reported to be normal. For this reason, we requested the PET–CT scan to look for a sclerotic bone lesion that we could biopsy to confirm the presence of clonal plasma cells, which would warrant treatment for the POEMS syndrome. The diagnostic procedure was a biopsy of the sacral lesion.

CLINICAL DIAGNOSIS

POEMS syndrome.

DR. ALLAN H. ROPPER'S DIAGNOSIS

POEMS syndrome with demyelinating polyneuropathy.

PATHOLOGICAL DISCUSSION

Dr. Aliyah R. Sohani: Pathological examination of a specimen from a CT-guided needle biopsy of the sacral mass revealed sheets of mature-appearing plasma cells that showed lambda light-chain restriction (Fig. 3A, 3B, and 3C). In the context of no bone marrow involvement and a solitary bone lesion, the findings were diagnostic of a solitary plasmacytoma and confirmed the diagnosis of the POEMS syndrome.[4]

Unlike other forms of plasma-cell neoplasia that have systemic manifestations, the clinical symptoms of the POEMS syndrome are not related to tissue infiltration by plasma cells or to the deposition of immunoglobulins or amyloid but, rather, to high serum levels of VEGF.[11,15] In this case, staining of the plasmacytoma tissue with antibody to this cytokine revealed diffuse cytoplasmic reactivity within the clonal plasma cells (Fig. 3D).

The clonal plasma cells of nearly all patients affected by the POEMS syndrome show lambda light-chain restriction.[7] The light-chain variable-region gene of affected patients' clones is highly restricted to two genes of the Vλ1 subfamily, with a pattern of somatic hypermutation suggestive of antigen-driven selection.[16,17] Similar restricted usage of germ-line genes is not seen in other plasma-cell neoplasms that express lambda light chains, such as multiple myeloma and AL amyloidosis, suggesting an important

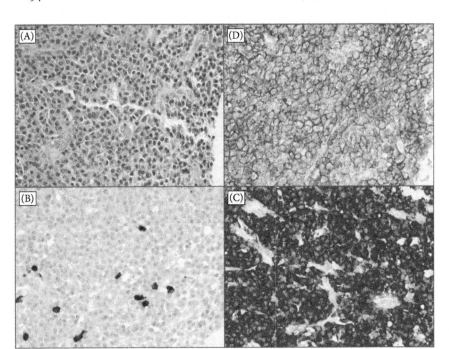

FIG 3 Biopsy Specimen of the Sacral Mass.

A specimen obtained by CT-guided needle biopsy of the sacral mass revealed sheets of mature-appearing plasma cells with eccentric nuclei, condensed nuclear chromatin, and moderately abundant eosinophilic cytoplasm containing paranuclear hofs (Golgi apparatus) (Panel A, hematoxylin and eosin). In situ hybridization shows that only rare plasma cells are positive for immunoglobulin kappa light chain (Panel B, in situ hybridization for kappa light chain) and that the majority of plasma cells are positive for lambda light chain (Panel C, in situ hybridization for lambda light chain). The plasma cells were strongly positive for the plasma-cell marker CD138, and they were negative for antibody to the latency-associated nuclear antigen of human herpesvirus 8 (not shown). Staining for an antibody to vascular endothelial growth factor (VEGF) shows diffuse cytoplasmic reactivity within the plasma cells (Panel D). (VEGF stain courtesy of Dr. Robert B. Colvin and Ms. Tricia Della Pelle, Department of Pathology, Massachusetts General Hospital.)

pathogenetic role for these specific lambda light chains in the POEMS syndrome, possibly related to interactions between the lambda light chains and VEGF.[16]

DISCUSSION OF MANAGEMENT

Dr. Noopur S. Raje: The POEMS syndrome is a chronic disease. Often, years can pass before all features manifest themselves and a diagnosis is made. While awaiting results of the bone biopsy, we also performed repeated testing for VEGF in our laboratory and found a VEGF level of 1005 pg per milliliter (reference range, 31 to 86).

Once the diagnosis was established, a management decision had to be made. Most patients survive longer than 10 years.[7] Typically, the number of features of the POEMS syndrome that a patient has does not influence the outcome, although extravascular volume overload and clubbing of the digits are associated with a poor outcome.

Treatment of the POEMS syndrome has generally been directed at the underlying plasma-cell neoplasm. This patient appears to have an isolated plasmacytoma. Radiation in patients with the POEMS syndrome and isolated plasma-cytomas has been associated with a response rate of over 50%. Thus, radiation would definitely be an option for this patient. Other therapies include the administration of corticosteroids, alkylatorbased chemotherapy, and high-dose chemotherapy with autologous stem-cell rescue. Although stem-cell transplantation offers the best response rate and rate of overall survival, it is associated with a high risk of complications[18,19]; despite this, more than two thirds of patients with neuropathy and other associated paraneoplastic features show improvement.

In view of the role of VEGF in the pathogenesis of the POEMS syndrome, thalidomide, lenalidomide, and bevacizumab are being administered to patients.[20–23] Thalidomide and lenalidomide are immunomodulatory agents that have antiangiogenic effects; thalidomide can cause neuropathy and therefore may not be the best choice for this patient. Bevacizumab is a monoclonal antibody against VEGF. Because of this patient's very high VEGF levels, we elected to begin treatment with bevacizumab.

The patient received bevacizumab (10 mg per kilogram of body weight) every 4 weeks for four cycles. By the end of the bevacizumab therapy, he no longer needed large-volume paracentesis, which previously had to be performed every 5 days; however, his neuropathy was unchanged. He then underwent stem-cell mobilization and harvest, followed by external-beam radiation (50 Gy) to the sacral lesion. During and after the radiation, his hemodynamic status continued to improve and he noted decreased paresthesias and increased strength, enabling him to walk with a cane. Nine months after the diagnosis of plasmacytoma, he was admitted to the hospital for high-dose melphalan therapy and stem-cell rescue, which was accomplished without major complications. Six months after the high-dose therapy, his motor strength continues to improve, his respiratory function is nearly normal, and he has no lymphadenopathy, organomegaly, edema, or ascites.

Dr. Ropper: I am skeptical that VEGF is the cause of the neuropathy, because in experimental models the protein does not cause axonal damage, myelin edema, or separation of myelin lamellae; in fact, it rescues myelin from taxol, platinum, and probably from the microvascular disorder of diabetes.

ANATOMICAL DIAGNOSIS

POEMS syndrome, with demyelinating neuropathy and solitary plasmacytoma of bone.

Presented at the Medicine Grand Rounds, February 19, 2009.

Financial and other disclosures provided by the authors are available with the full text of this article at NEJM.org.

REFERENCES

1. Crow RS. Peripheral neuritis in myelomatosis. Br Med J 1956;2:802–4.

2. Fukase M, Kakimatsu T, Nishitani H, et al. Report of a case of solitary plasma-cytoma in the abdomen presenting with polyneuropathy, and endocrinologic disorders. Clin Neurol 1969;9:657. abstract.

3. Bardwick PA, Zvaifler NJ, Gill GN, Newman D, Greenway GD, Resnick DL. Plasma cell dyscrasia with polyneuropathy, organomegaly, endocrinopathy, M protein, and skin changes: the POEMS syndrome: report on two cases and a review of the literature. Medicine (Baltimore) 1980;59:311–22.

4. Dispenzieri A. POEMS syndrome. Blood Rev 2007;21:285–99.

5. Higuchi M, Kamijo H, Koyama T, et al. POEMS syndrome caused refractory ascites in a polycystic disease patient undergoing hemodialysis. Clin Exp Nephrol 2003;7:301–5.

6. Loeb JM, Hauger PH, Carney JD, Cooper AD. Refractory ascites due to POEMS syndrome. Gastroenterology 1989;96:247–9.

7. Dispenzieri A, Kyle RA, Lacy MQ, et al. POEMS syndrome: definitions and long-term outcome. Blood 2003;101:2496–506.

8. Miralles GD, O'Fallon JR, Talley NJ. Plasma-cell dyscrasia with polyneuropathy: the spectrum of POEMS syndrome. N Engl J Med 1992;327:1919–23.

9. Nakanishi T, Sobue I, Toyokura Y, et al. The Crow-Fukase syndrome: a study of 102 cases in Japan. Neurology 1984;34:712–20.

10. Hashiguchi T, Arimura K, Matsumuro K, et al. Highly concentrated vascular endothelial growth factor in platelets in Crow-Fukase syndrome. Muscle Nerve 2000;23:1051–6.

11. Watanabe O, Maruyama I, Arimura K, et al. Overproduction of vascular endothelial growth factor/vascular permeability factor is causative in Crow-Fukase (POEMS) syndrome. Muscle Nerve 1998;21:1390–7.

12. Ropper AH, Gorson KC, Gooch CL, et al. Vascular endothelial growth factor gene transfer for diabetic polyneuropathy: a randomized, double-blinded trial. Ann Neurol 2009;65:386–93.

13. Bélec L, Mohamed AS, Authier FJ, et al. Human herpesvirus 8 infection in patients with POEMS syndrome-associated multicentric Castleman's disease. Blood 1999;93:3643–53.

14. Feinberg L, Temple D, de Marchena E, Patarca R, Mitrani A. Soluble immune mediators in POEMS syndrome with pulmonary hypertension: case report and review of the literature. Crit Rev Oncog 1999;10:293–302.

15. Watanabe O, Arimura K, Kitajima I, Osame M, Maruyama I. Greatly raised vascular endothelial growth factor (VEGF) in POEMS syndrome. Lancet 1996;347:702.

16. Abe D, Nakaseko C, Takeuchi M, et al. Restrictive usage of monoclonal immunoglobulin lambda light chain germline in POEMS syndrome. Blood 2008;112:836–9.

17. Soubrier M, Labauge P, Jouanel P, Viallard JL, Piette JC, Sauvezie B. Restricted use of Vλ genes in POEMS syndrome. Haematologica 2004;89(4):e4–e5.

18. Dispenzieri A, Kyle RA, Lacy MQ, et al. Superior survival in primary systemic amyloidosis patients undergoing peripheral blood stem cell transplantation: a case-control study. Blood 2004;103:3960–3.

19. Dispenzieri A, Moreno-Aspitia A, Suarez GA, et al. Peripheral blood stem cell transplantation in 16 patients with POEMS syndrome, and a review of the literature. Blood 2004;104:3400–7.

20. Badros A, Porter N, Zimrin A. Bevacizumab therapy for POEMS syndrome. Blood 2005;106:1135.

21. Dietrich PY, Duchosal MA. Bevacizumab therapy before autologous stem-cell transplantation for POEMS syndrome. Ann Oncol 2008;19:595.

22. Dispenzieri A, Klein CJ, Mauermann ML. Lenalidomide therapy in a patient with POEMS syndrome. Blood 2007;110:1075–6.
23. Kuwabara S, Misawa S, Kanai K, et al. Thalidomide reduces serum VEGF levels and improves peripheral neuropathy in POEMS syndrome. J Neurol Neurosurg Psychiatry 2008;79:1255–7.

Perspectives and Updates

This was the most recent case I discussed and the general approach to demyelinating neuropathy that appears in the table is up to date. The patient carried an initial diagnosis of chronic inflammatory demyelinating polyneuropathy (CIDP) but the diagnosis of POEMS was fairly obvious once the laboratory features were fully displayed, particularly the monoclonal gammopathy with a lambda light chain component.

Ascites is indeed an uncommon early feature of the disease but can be viewed as a type of vascular leak that leads to another characteristic feature of POEMS, the "O," or organomegaly. I escaped with a small joke: "A neurologist discussing a patient with ascites is swimming in unfamiliar waters." The Cabot exercises are typically surgically expunged of these comments and I had been thwarted over the years in many other CPC discussions from displaying my comic cleverness.

A clinical point that comes to mind regarding demyelinating neuropathies is that stabbing pains do occur and implicate a small-fiber disturbance buried within this predominantly large-fiber disease. Of course none of the polyneuropathies related to systemic diseases, including POEMS and CIDP, can be assumed to be either purely large- or small-fiber processes.

My comments regarding the absence of need for further diagnostic testing were considered provocative at the rounds, but they were meant to bring forth the issue of whether it is necessary to do a bone biopsy to document an osteosclerotic myeloma (plasmacytoma) once a focal bone lesion has been discovered by imaging. The problem of biopsy arises because of a reluctance of radiotherapy services to treat a bone lesion without confirmation of neoplasia, and that is a fair point. It is fascinating that the biopsied tissue stained diffusely for VEGF (Fig. 3D) despite the ostensible absence of circulating VEGF.

The main biological interest in this case is the role of VEGF in causing human disease. There has been more emphasis on antagonizing the effects of this protein in order to reduce the neovascularization in various tumors, including glioblastoma. In contrast, my colleagues and I have found that the neuropathies caused by thalidomide and cisplatin can be prevented and reversed by VEGF in experimental models.[1,2]

In the case of thalidomide, this is not surprising, as the drug is used as an antiangiogenic factor in the treatment of renal cell cancer. In fact, the VEGF blocker bevacizumab was chosen initially for treatment in this CPC patient, rather than the traditional approach of focused radiation. The patient later improved after radiation but ultimately underwent autologous stem cell rescue so that high-dose melphalan could be used to obliterate all the myeloma cells. This more aggressive approach to

POEMS has been published but, in this rare disease, it has proven difficult to carry out trials to gauge the effectiveness of bone marrow transplantation.

The other possible therapeutic role of VEGF in neuropathy may be in diabetes, but a randomized blinded trial that I conducted with colleagues gave ambiguous results, although it achieved its primary goal and some secondary endpoints. [3]

As I commented at the end of the case discussion, the immediate cause of the polyneuropathy of POEMS remains unclear, and I expressed skepticism that VEGF was solely responsible. This is based largely on the above-mentioned experiments with thalidomide and cisplatin neuropathy, which were rescued by VEGF, and by our clinical trial in diabetic neuropathy. In animal safety experiments with administration of VEGF, a polyneuropathy did not emerge, but we may not have explored this deeply enough.

A high circulating level of VEGF solves the mystery of organomegaly in POEMS; it is probably due to a vascular leak caused by the protein and associated tissue edema. Meningiomas, which are highly vascular tumors, contain very high concentrations of VEGF, and antiangiogenic drugs have been tried as therapy, mainly for anaplastic tumors.[4] It is likely that the edema surrounding these tumors is also due to the vascular leak caused by local VEGF production.[5] Perhaps myelin becomes edematous in POEMS and causes a demyelinating process. This would be a new biological mechanism for neuropathy.

Allan H. Ropper

REFERENCES

1. Kirchmair R, Tietz AB, Panagiotou E, et al. Therapeutic angiogenesis inhibits or rescues chemotherapy-induced peripheral neuropathy: Taxol-and thalidomide-induced injury of vasa nervorum is ameliorated by VEGF. Mol Ther 2007; 15:69–75.

2. Kirchmair R, Walter DH, Il M, et al. Antiangiogenesis mediates cisplatin-induced peripheral neuropathy. Circulation 2005; 111:2662–70.

3. Ropper AH, Weinberg D, Gooch C, et al. Vascular endothelial growth factor gene transfer for diabetic polyneuropathy: a randomized, double-blinded trial. Ann Neurol 2009; 65:386–93.

4. Puchner MJ, Hans VH, Harati A. Bevacizumab-induced regression of anaplastic meningioma. Ann Oncol 2010; 21:2445–6.

5. Schmid S, Aboul-Enein F, Pfisterer W, et al. Vascular endothelial growth factor: the major factor for tumor neovascularization and edema formation in meningioma patients. Neurosurgery 2010; 67:1703–8.

A 54-Year-Old Woman with Dizziness and Falls

PHEOCHROMOCYTOMA

Martin A. Samuels, Benjamin J. Pomerantz,
and Peter M. Sadow

CPC 14-2010

PRESENTATION OF CASE

Dr. Emily P. Zeitler (Medicine): A 54-year-old woman was admitted to this hospital because of episodes of dizziness resulting in falls.

Approximately 2 months earlier, while walking to work, the patient had the sudden onset of dizziness and the sensation of falling to the left, associated with diaphoresis and palpitations. She sat down, and the symptoms improved, although she continued to feel as though she would fall to the left. She was taken by ambulance to another hospital and admitted. She had a history of borderline hypertension and intermittent atrial fibrillation but had been otherwise well. Medications included metoprolol (25 mg three times daily), furosemide, and propafenone. On examination, the vital signs reportedly showed orthostatic changes in the pulse and blood pressure, and the neurologic evaluation was normal. Fluids were administered intravenously. Furosemide and propafenone were discontinued, the dose of metoprolol was decreased (25 mg twice daily), and she was discharged.

During the next 6 weeks, additional episodes of dizziness occurred and increased in frequency; the patient fell several times. She consulted a neurologist and was admitted twice to the other hospital. Magnetic resonance imaging (MRI) of the brain and carotid ultrasonography were reportedly normal. Treatment with meclizine was begun, without improvement, and a 5-day course of levofloxacin was administered.

On the day of admission, an episode of dizziness occurred, with the sensation of almost passing out. The patient was brought to the emergency department of this hospital by a friend. On arrival, she reported continued dizziness as well as a generalized headache. She reported that the episodes of dizziness occurred only when standing, never when sitting or supine, and were associated with a sensation of falling, diaphoresis, weakness in the legs, and occasionally, palpitations. During the episodes, she could hear coworkers speak but did not feel fully alert, and she had to hold on to a support to avoid staggering or falling. She did not sense the room spinning, and she did not have visual changes, loss of consciousness, fever, chills, urinary retention, or a change in bowel habits.

N Engl J Med 2010;362:1815–23.
Copyright © 2010 Massachusetts Medical Society

Fifteen years earlier, the patient had had several episodes of vertigo, with a sensation that the room was spinning, which lasted up to 3 to 4 days, were not related to position or associated with tinnitus or hearing loss, and were different from her current symptoms. The symptoms resolved without treatment and did not recur.

A diagnosis of atrial fibrillation had been made 2 years before admission, after an episode of palpitations. One year before admission, transthoracic echocardiography and a cardiac stress test had reportedly been normal. She had chronic ptosis of the left eyelid and mild peripheral edema. She had had three cesarean sections. She was widowed, worked as a waitress, and had been unable to work for 3 weeks because of her symptoms. She did not smoke, drink alcohol, or use illicit drugs. Her mother had had hypertension and cardiac arrhythmia and had died at 76 years of age, a sister had occasional supraventricular tachycardia, and a son had epilepsy; her other children and grandchildren were healthy. Her paternal family history was not known. Medications on admission included metoprolol, meclizine, and acetylsalicylic acid. She was allergic to penicillin and sulfa drugs.

On examination, the temperature was 36.7°C, the blood pressure 145/63 mm Hg, the pulse 60 beats per minute, the respiratory rate 18 breaths per minute, and the oxygen saturation 99% while she was breathing ambient air. There was slight ptosis of the left eye, with no nystagmus, and no dysmetria on finger-to-nose or heel-to-shin testing. There was a mild intention tremor in the right arm. There were no symptoms or signs of vertigo on head-turning maneuvers. The gait was slightly ataxic, more prominently so with tandem gait, and she reported feeling as if she were falling forward and to the left. There was nonpitting edema (+) of the legs; the remainder of the general physical and detailed neurologic examination was normal.

The complete blood count, the white-cell differential count, urinalysis, tests of coagulation and renal function, and serum levels of sodium, potassium, chloride, glucose, calcium, phosphorus, and magnesium were normal. Toxicologic screening of urine was negative. An electrocardiogram revealed a sinus rhythm of 53 beats per minute, with evidence of clockwise rotation, left-axis deviation, left anterior hemiblock, left atrial enlargement, and minor nonspecific ST-segment and T-wave abnormalities. MRI and magnetic resonance angiographic (MRA) scans of the head and neck obtained after the administration of gadolinium revealed a few nonspecific ovoid foci of hyperintensity, 5 to 6 mm in diameter, on T_2-weighted imaging and on fluid-attenuated inversion recovery sequences in the subcortical white matter in the right frontal lobe and both parietal lobes, without associated abnormal enhancement or decreased diffusion on diffusion-weighted imaging; these were thought to represent old subcortical infarcts. No intracranial mass, hemorrhage, or midline shift was identified. MRA showed no evidence of aneurysm or hemodynamically significant stenosis. The patient was admitted to the hospital.

Initial measurement of orthostatic vital signs revealed changes in blood pressure and pulse (Table 1) that were associated with light-headedness. Normal saline (a total of 1500 ml) was administered intravenously; the level of plasma urea nitrogen decreased from 20 mg per deciliter (7 mmol per liter) to 11 mg per deciliter (4 mmol per liter), but light-headedness and unsteadiness on standing persisted. Cardiac monitoring showed sinus tachycardia during the episodes of light-headedness. Repeated measurements of orthostatic vital signs on the second day are shown in Table 1.

A transthoracic echocardiogram showed a left ventricular ejection fraction of 76%, without wall-motion abnormalities, and mild tricuspid insufficiency.

Cardiac monitoring for 24 hours revealed sinus rhythm with sinus arrhythmia, with rates ranging from 77 to 144 beats per minute; there were 83 isolated premature ventricular contractions, 147 atrial premature contractions, and one run of supraventricular tachycardia (7 beats at a rate of 158 beats per minute) that coincided with symptoms of dizziness and palpitations. Meclizine and metoprolol were discontinued. The levels of electrolytes, vitamin B_1, vitamin B_{12}, and folate were normal, and testing for thyroid peroxidase antibodies and screening for syphilis were negative. Serial testing of cardiac enzymes showed no evidence of myocardial infarction. Enoxaparin and aspirin were begun.

On the fourth day, the patient reported the sudden onset of palpitations, without chest pain or shortness of breath. Measurements of the pulse and blood pressure are shown in Table 1. An electrocardiogram showed a supraventricular tachycardia with a ventricular rate of 150 beats per minute and a 2:1 conduction block, consistent with atrial flutter, and left-axis deviation. Metoprolol was administered intravenously (10 mg) and orally (25 mg), with a return of sinus rhythm at 80 beats per minute and a blood pressure of 140/50 mm Hg. The plasma cortisol level at 4 a.m. was 3.6 μg per deciliter (99 nmol per liter) (reference range, <10 μg per deciliter [<276 nmol per liter]), and levels of free thyroxine, thyrotropin, and total triiodothyronine were normal. The administration of fludrocortisone (0.1 mg daily) and metoprolol (25 mg daily) was begun, and a highsalt diet was instituted. When she was evaluated by the physical therapy staff, she had difficulty standing (necessitating posterior support), was unable to stand with her feet together and eyes open for more than 10 seconds, and used a stepping strategy to avoid falling. Vital signs are shown in Table 1. She was given a cane for stability, and exercises were prescribed to improve balance. On the sixth day, no further ectopy was seen on cardiac telemetry, and she was discharged.

Table 1 Blood Pressure and Pulse Measurements

Variable	On Admission Blood Pressure mm Hg	Pulse beats/ min	2nd Day Blood Pressure mm Hg	Pulse beats/ min	4th Day Blood Pressure mm Hg	Pulse beats/ min	5th Day Blood Pressure mm Hg	Pulse beats/ min
Supine	133/64	58	137/89	76	141/76	83	136/68	71
Sitting	151/73	85	143/78	84	148/75	76	126/76	78
Standing	103/69	103	139/78	103	129/89	90	132/89	81
Standing during supraventricular tachycardia					179/86	180		
Standing after walking 30 m							132/82	79
Standing after walking 90 m							126/78	77

At follow-up 5 days after discharge, she reported frequent episodes of light-headedness, dizziness, and unsteadiness, associated with palpitations.

A diagnostic test result was received.

DIFFERENTIAL DIAGNOSIS

*Dr. Martin A. Samuels:** This 54-year-old woman with a history of borderline hypertension and intermittent atrial fibrillation has worsening orthostatic intolerance that is resistant to treatment with volume expansion and mineralocorticoids. She had chronic left-lid ptosis, and an attack of vertigo 15 years earlier resolved spontaneously and never recurred. The current symptoms do not resemble those of the attack of vertigo.

Causes of Sensations of Dizziness

The initial symptom of the current illness was dizziness, one of the most challenging and common problems that doctors encounter in their patients. Dizziness is a lay term that reflects one of four syndromes: vertigo, defined as an illusion or hallucination of motion due to a disorder in the vestibular system; near-syncope, a feeling of faintness caused by inadequate cerebral perfusion; disequilibrium, caused by a disorder of gait; and ill-defined light-headedness, a common manifestation of anxiety (Table 2). Complicating the evaluation of patients with dizziness is the fact that there is frequently more than one cause. The clinical challenge is to recognize the dominant cause on which secondary or collateral symptoms may be superimposed. This patient's current problem is not vertigo, because there is no description of environmental movement and the patient clearly distinguishes the current symptom from the vertigo she had 15 years earlier.

Table 2 Conditions Producing a Sensation of Dizziness

Condition	Pathophysiology	Causes
Vertigo (an illusion of motion)	Vestibular disorder	Vestibular neuritis
		Labyrinthitis
		Meniere's disease
Near-syncope (feeling of faintness)	Reduced cerebral perfusion	Volume depletion
		Neurocardiogenic syncope
Dysequilibrium (gait disorder)	Factors affecting gait	Peripheral neuropathy
		Myelopathy
		Hydrocephalus
Light-headedness (ill defined)	Anxiety	Phobias
		Anxiety disorders
		Depression

*Currently Chair, Department of Neurology, Brigham and Women's Hospital.

Near-Syncope

The major cause of dizziness in this patient is near-syncope (the feeling of impending faint), occurring exclusively in the upright posture. The associated symptoms of diaphoresis and tachycardia are secondary phenomena, resulting from the sympathetic autonomic reactions to decreased cerebral perfusion. Near-syncope is distinguishable from a transient ischemic attack—a transient ischemic attack occurs in a particular vascular territory, whereas near-syncope is due to global cerebral hypoperfusion. This patient could relieve the symptoms by lying down, which suggests that the dizziness is caused by orthostatic (postural) intolerance. Causes of near-syncope are summarized in Table 3.

Tachycardia without hypotension that occurs exclusively in the upright posture is called the postural orthostatic tachycardia syndrome; this may be a manifestation of

Table 3 Causes of Near-Syncope and Underlying Conditions or Factors

Failure to maintain adequate cerebral perfusion in the upright posture (orthostatic dizziness)

Volume depletion

High ambient temperature

Peripheral nervous system alpha-blockade

Use of tricyclic drugs

Use of alpha-receptor antagonists

Blood pooling in the lower part of the body (prolonged crouching followed by standing)

Postural orthostatic tachycardia syndrome

Down-regulation of peripheral alpha receptors from exposure to catecholamines (e.g., pheochromocytoma)

Cerebral vasoconstriction

Hyperventilation

Reversible cerebral vasoconstriction syndrome (Call–Fleming syndrome)

Cryptogenic

Use of catecholaminergic agents (e.g., diet pills, cold remedies [pseudoephedrine], cocaine, methamphetamine)

Decreased cardiac output

Aortic stenosis

Asymmetric cardiac septal hypertrophy

Ischemic heart disease (i.e., angina equivalent)

Cardiac arrhythmias

Valsalva maneuver (straining)

Neurocardiogenic (neurally mediated) near-syncope

Overactive baroreceptor reflex (e.g., triggered by episodic hypertension caused by fright)

Systemic vasodilatation (vasodepressor)

Increased vagal tone (vasovagal)

mild orthostatic intolerance or simply a manifestation of anxiety while in the upright posture. Dizziness during or immediately after exercise is suggestive of a cardiac cause (e.g., aortic stenosis, asymmetric cardiac septal hypertrophy, or coronary ischemia), but this was not the case in this patient. Various cardiac arrhythmias may be a cause of dizziness, but in this case, dizziness had an inconsistent relationship with the presence of the arrhythmias and occurred only when the patient was in the upright posture. This meant that the major cause of the dizziness was probably orthostatic hypotension and that the arrhythmias were a collateral phenomenon, possibly produced by the same underlying disorder but not the cause of the symptom. Hypoglycemia produces a similar set of symptoms but would not be symptomatic in only the upright posture.

Superimposed on the major problem of orthostatic intolerance may be some degree of gait disorder, but the absence of unequivocal signs of neurologic disease (e.g., parkinsonism, cervical spondylosis, myelopathy, neuropathy, or cerebellar-system dysfunction in any position other than the upright one) leads me to conclude that the minor degree of gait dysfunction was secondary to the severe orthostatic intolerance. The bradykinesia of parkinsonism; the spasticity, hyperreflexia, Babinski signs, and proprioceptive problems of cervical spondylosis and other myelopathies (e.g., cobalamin or copper deficiency); and the sensory difficulties and areflexia of neuropathy all should be evident when a patient is in the sitting and prone positions. However, this patient's symptoms occurred only when she was in the upright posture. Some forms of purely midline degeneration of the cerebellum (e.g., alcoholic cerebellar degeneration) are manifested in patients who are in the upright position only, but such patients do not have orthostatic hypotension. This patient was found to have orthostatic hypotension, defined as a drop in systolic pressure of more than 20 torr or a drop in diastolic pressure of more than 10 torr on arising from the prone to the upright posture. Almost all measurements of blood pressure in this patient were lowest when she was upright, highest when she was sitting, and intermediate while she was lying down. The heart rate rose as the patient stood, except when metoprolol was present. She also had a history of atrial fibrillation and other documented episodes of supraventricular tachycardia, sometimes associated with the core symptom of dizziness.

Cerebral Perfusion and Orthostatic Intolerance

Maintenance of cerebral perfusion when a person is in the upright posture is a unique feature of the human nervous system, since no other animal that repeatedly lies down and stands up faces the challenge of having its head so far above its heart. To properly analyze this patient's symptoms, one must consider the mechanism that is responsible for maintenance of cerebral perfusion in the upright posture—normal function of the sympathoadrenal system. The sympathetic limb of the autonomic nervous system is represented by sympathetic nerves, which use norepinephrine as their neurotransmitter, and the adrenal medulla (a sympathetic ganglion that also acts as a gland), which secretes epinephrine into the blood.[1] Orthostatic intolerance results when the sympathoadrenal system is unable to maintain cerebral perfusion pressure in the upright posture. The causes of this inability to maintain cerebral perfusion pressure include volume depletion, autonomic neuropathy, pharmacologic blockade of receptors used by the sympathoadrenal system, and down-regulation of these same receptors because of chronic exposure to the natural agonists (epinephrine and norepinephrine).

This patient's orthostatic vital signs improved after the administration of fluids, an outcome suggesting the presence of a component of volume depletion. Diseases of the nervous system (e.g., Parkinson's disease or multiple-system atrophy) and neuropathies such as diabetic neuropathy may be associated with autonomic failure leading to orthostatic hypotension, but this patient had no evidence of any of these diseases. Furthermore, she was not taking any drugs that would block the action of epinephrine or norepinephrine. This leaves us with a diagnosis of chronic exposure to epinephrine and norepinephrine, which may be a consequence of overproduction of these agents by tumors of chromaffin cells in the adrenal medulla (pheochromocytoma) or in extraadrenal sites (extraadrenal paraganglioma).

Although the patient's blood pressure was not impressively elevated, there is no doubt that she had chronic hypertension. She had a history of borderline hypertension and was taking furosemide, metoprolol, and propafenone, presumably prescribed to control her blood pressure and atrial fibrillation. Hypertension is also suggested by the white-matter abnormalities that were noted on the MRI scan of the brain that was obtained at this hospital but that were not noted on an MRI scan obtained elsewhere a few weeks earlier. I was unable to compare the two scans, but if these lesions had accumulated over a period of a few weeks, it would indicate acceleration of the hypertension. This patient's blood pressure was often higher in the sitting position than in the standing and supine positions, a feature suggesting that compression of the abdomen caused a rise in the blood pressure. This constellation of findings strongly suggests the presence of a catecholamine-secreting tumor in the abdomen, namely, an adrenal pheochromocytoma.

In reviewing the case history, we can assume that the remote episode of vertigo was probably an attack of vestibular neuritis or benign paroxysmal positional vertigo unrelated to the current symptoms. The ptosis could represent partial Horner's syndrome caused by an extraadrenal catecholamine-secreting tumor, but this is very unlikely given the longevity of the finding. Furthermore, the other features of Horner's syndrome (meiosis and anhidrosis) are not described.

Pheochromocytoma

Pheochromocytoma (from the Greek, meaning dusky-colored tumor) is a neoplasm of chromaffin cells, first described and named by Ludwig Pick in 1912. Most chromaffin-cell tumors arise in the adrenal gland and are known as pheochromocytomas. The 10% that are extraadrenal are known as paragangliomas and arise from chromaffin cells in extraadrenal locations, including the organ of Zuckerkandl, the urinary bladder, and the carotid sheath. About 90% of pheochromocytomas produce some degree of hypertension, which may be joined over time with orthostatic hypotension. Orthostatic hypotension in patients with pheochromocytoma is probably the result of down-regulation of catecholamine receptors due to long-term exposure to the neurotransmitter, as well as volume depletion caused by inhibition of the renin–angiotensin system.[2] A few patients with pheochromocytoma have only orthostatic hypotension, with no evidence of hypertension.[3-7] Most patients with pheochromocytoma have signs of hypertension in the brain, as evidenced by MRI scans, even those in whom the measured blood pressures are not very elevated, as in this patient.

The diagnosis of pheochromocytoma is made by measuring levels of catecholamines in the serum and levels of catecholamine metabolites in the plasma and urine. Abdominal images usually show the adrenal mass. In patients with elevated catecholamine levels and a normal computed tomographic (CT) scan of the abdomen, a radionuclide scan with ^{123}I-metaiodobenzylguanidine may detect a paraganglioma.

The number of patients with a defined genetic cause for pheochromocytoma is increasing as more genes that cause the tumor are being found. Patients with pheochromocytoma should be tested for mutations in these four genes: the von Hippel–Lindau (VHL) gene, the rearranged during transfection (RET) proto-oncogene, the succinate dehydrogenase subunit B (SDHB), and the succinate dehydrogenase subunit D (SDHD).[8] The neurofibromatosis type 1 (NF1) gene is also associated with pheochromocytoma. There is no clinical evidence that this patient's pheochromocytoma has a genetic cause, but the patient does have family members with arrhythmias; the discovery that she harbors one of the genes known to produce the tumor could be important for future management of the disease and for family counseling. In one study, 24% of patients with nonsyndromic pheochromocytoma had mutations in one of these genes; the patients were 59 years of age or younger, and the tumors were unilateral in the majority of the patients.[9]

Summary

An adrenal pheochromocytoma is the most likely diagnosis in this case. The diagnostic test should have been measurement of serum levels of catecholamines (epinephrine, norepinephrine, and dopamine) and serum and urine studies of catecholamine metabolites (metanephrines and normetanephrines). A CT scan of the abdomen probably revealed an adrenal mass, which subsequently would have been removed, probably endoscopically, after appropriate preoperative catecholamine-receptor blockade.

Dr. Nancy Lee Harris (Pathology): May we have the medical students' diagnosis?

A Harvard Medical Student: We thought this patient had three major problems: autonomic dysfunction; dysfunction of the posterior column, causing ataxia and impaired proprioception; and an abnormal cardiac rhythm. Pheochromocytoma could explain her orthostatic intolerance and arrhythmias, and possibly posterior column dysfunction. Postural orthostatic tachycardia syndrome could explain her orthostatic intolerance and palpitations but is a diagnosis of exclusion. We also considered multiple-system atrophy as a cause of her primary autonomic failure, but most patients with this disease have gastrointestinal motility problems, which this patient did not have; this is also a diagnosis of exclusion. Our diagnosis is pheochromocytoma.

Dr. Harris: Dr. Rhee, you cared for this patient; would you tell us your thinking?

Dr. Eugene P. Rhee (Medicine): We thought that the changes in the patient's vital signs that occurred with changes in posture were dominated by excursions in heart rate. Aside from her initial set of vital signs, which preceded an intravenous bolus of fluids, there was no other set of measurements that met the technical definition of orthostatic hypotension. However, although in cases of orthostatic hypotension the heart rate typically does not rise, there were often marked increases in our patient's heart rate on standing, a feature that meets the criteria for the postural orthostatic tachycardia syndrome (an increase of more than 30 beats per minute or a heart rate of more than 120 beats per minute on moving from a supine to a standing position).[10] Pending the results of diagnostic studies obtained during her hospitalization, the patient was discharged with a diagnosis of postural orthostatic tachycardia syndrome.

Dr. Zeitler: Five days after discharge, a measurement of catecholamines in a 24-hour urine specimen showed 276 μg of metanephrine (reference range, 30 to 180) and 1649 μg of normetanephrine (reference range, 128 to 484). I ordered a CT scan of the abdomen and referred the patient for consultation with the endocrine service.

Dr. Benjamin J. Pomerantz: In the upper abdomen, there is an ovoid, avidly enhancing mass within the superior aspect of the left adrenal gland (Fig. 1A), which is better appreciated on the coronal reformatted image (Fig. 1B). No other abnormalities were noted in the abdomen or pelvis. Differential considerations for a solitary enhancing adrenal mass include adenoma, metastasis, primary adrenal cortical carcinoma and myelolipoma, and pheochromocytoma.

Dr. Marie B. Demay (Endocrinology): We measured plasma catecholamine levels to confirm that the elevated levels in the urine reflected abnormal plasma levels; we found 0.32 nmol of metanephrine per liter (reference range, <0.50) and 5.65 nmol of normetanephrine per liter (reference range, <0.9). The patient was already taking a betablocker (metoprolol). Since unopposed alpha-adrenergic actions can lead to complications, we recommended alpha-blockade with phenoxybenzamine. However, this drug was not approved by her insurance company, so we treated her with 1 mg of prazosin three times daily, with a rapid escalation to 5 mg three times daily. Calcium-channel blockers may also be used if alpha-blockade or beta-blockade cannot be undertaken. Volume expansion is required to prevent the orthostatic hypotension that often accompanies alpha-blockade, so we continued fludrocortisone and prescribed a high-salt diet. Shortly thereafter, a laparoscopic left adrenalectomy was performed by Dr. Antonia Stephen.

CLINICAL DIAGNOSIS

Postural orthostatic tachycardia syndrome.

DR. MARTIN A. SAMUELS'S DIAGNOSIS

Pheochromocytoma.

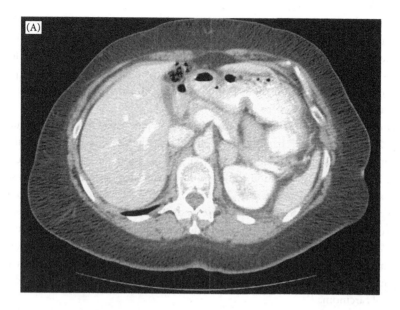

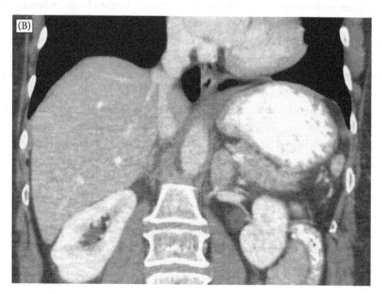

FIG 1 Abdominal CT Scans.
After the administration of contrast material, an axial image (Panel A) and a coronal reformatted image (Panel B) show a well-circumscribed, avidly enhancing ovoid mass (arrows) in the left adrenal gland.

PATHOLOGICAL DISCUSSION

Dr. Peter M. Sadow: The left adrenal gland and surrounding periglandular adipose tissue weighed 23.2 g (normal, 4 to 6). On sectioning, there was a tannish gray nodule, measuring 3.4 cm in greatest dimension, arising from the adrenal medulla. Intraoperative frozen-section examination confirmed the diagnosis of pheochromocytoma. In our case, the gross examination of the lesion is essential, since paraganglia reside directly adjacent to the adrenal gland and it is important to distinguish whether the lesion arises from the adrenal gland or adjacent to it. Intraadrenal paragangliomas (pheochromocytomas) are almost always benign, whereas extraadrenal paragangliomas may be malignant up to 20% of the time.[11–13]

On histologic examination, the lesion is well-circumscribed but not encapsulated (Fig. 2A). There are nests and cords of plump cells that have large nuclei, clumped chromatin, occasionally prominent nucleoli, and occasional intranuclear inclusions (Fig. 2B and inset), a common feature in endocrine neoplasms. The cytoplasm is pink and filled with neurosecretory granules, which are evident on electron microscopical examination. Surrounding these nests of cells are sustentacular cells, also derived from the neural crest. Immunohistochemical analysis showed that the neuroendocrine cells of the pheochromocytoma stained for the neurosecretory markers chromogranin A and synaptophysin (Fig. 2C and 2D). This staining, particularly for chromogranin A, may be useful in distinguishing pheochromocytoma from adrenal cortical carcinoma.[14]

There are no morphologic features that distinguish benign from malignant pheochromocytomas—even capsular or vascular invasion may be seen in benign tumors. Although several groups of investigators have tried to develop panels of immunostains that could be used to predict malignant behavior,[11–13,15,16] they have not proved reliable. The only reliable marker of malignant behavior, as for many endocrine tumors, is the presence of distant metastasis. Among the germline mutations found in patients with pheochromocytoma, mutations in the *SDHB* gene are associated with a 50% malignancy rate. The traditional "rule of 10" for pheochromocytomas (10% extraadrenal, 10 percent bilateral, 10% malignant, 10% without hypertension, and 10% hereditary) is changing with our increasing knowledge of the molecular biology of these tumors, and approximately 25% are now thought to have known associated mutations.[9,11,17]

Dr. Harris: Dr. Zeitler, how is the patient now?

Dr. Zeitler: I last saw her 10 months after the adrenalectomy. She had had a prompt and dramatic improvement in her symptoms of dizziness and palpitations; however, she continues to have brief sensations of unsteadiness and palpitations when standing, which resolve with sitting. These do not interfere with her life, and she has returned to work full time. The level of plasma normetanephrine decreased markedly but remained slightly elevated at 4 and 6 months of follow-up (1.55 and 1.04 nmol per liter, respectively). Genetic testing was not performed.

ANATOMICAL DIAGNOSIS

Pheochromocytoma.

Dr. Samuels reports receiving consulting fees from MC Communications. No other potential conflict of interest relevant to this article was reported. Disclosure forms provided by the authors are available with the full text of this article at NEJM.org.

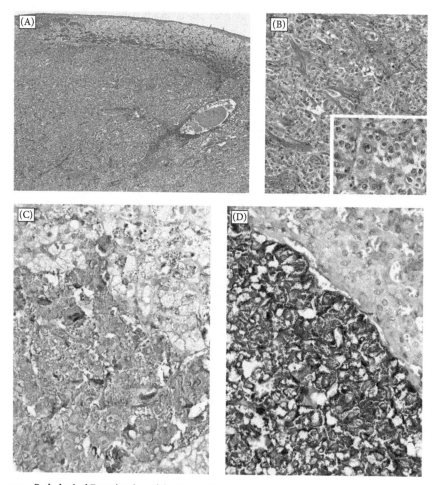

FIG 2 **Pathological Examination of the Resected Left Adrenal Gland.**
At low magnification, a cellular tumor is seen (Panel A, arrows; hematoxylin and eosin), with overlying normal adrenal cortex. At higher magnification, the tumor cells are arranged in the characteristic nested pattern ("zellballen") of pheochromocytomas (Panel B, hematoxylin and eosin); they have large, pleomorphic nuclei, with prominent nucleoli and eosinophilic, granular cytoplasm (inset). Immunohistochemical staining for chromogranin A is positive in the neuroendocrine secretory granules (Panel C), which is specific for paragangliomas and pheochromocytomas. A stain for synaptophysin is also positive in the neuroendocrine secretory tumor cells (Panel D).

REFERENCES

1. Carmichael SW, Winkler H. The adrenal chromaffin cell. Sci Am 1985;253:40–9.
2. Streeten DH, Anderson GH Jr. Mechanisms of orthostatic hypotension and tachycardia in patients with pheochromocytoma. Am J Hypertens 1996;9:760–9.
3. Daga Calejero B, Guitierrez Ibáñez E, Carmona Ainat A, et al. Orthostatic hypotension and syncope in a patient with pheochromocytoma. In: Garcia-Civera R, Barón-Esquivas G, Blanc J-J, et al., eds. Syncope cases. New York: Wiley-Blackwell, 2006:151–5.
4. Bortnik M, Occhetta E, Marino P. Orthostatic hypotension as an unusual clinical manifestation of pheochromocytoma: a case report. J Cardiovasc Med (Hagerstown) 2008;9:839–41.

5. Hamrin B. Sustained hypotension and shock due to an adrenaline-secreting phaeochromocytoma. Lancet 1962;2:123–4.

6. Richmond J, Frazer SC, Millar DR. Paroxysmal hypotension due to an adrenaline-secreting phaeochromocytoma. Lancet 1961;2:904–6.

7. Ueda T, Oka N, Matsumoto A, et al. Pheochromocytoma presenting as recurrent hypotension and syncope. Intern Med 2005;44:222–7.

8. Adler JT, Meyer-Rochow GY, Chen H, et al. Pheochromocytoma: current approaches and future directions. Oncologist 2008;13:779–93.

9. Neumann HP, Bausch B, McWhinney SR, et al. Germ-line mutations in nonsyndromic pheochromocytoma. N Engl J Med 2002;346:1459–66.

10. Low PA, Sandroni P, Joyner M, Shen WK. Postural tachycardia syndrome (POTS). J Cardiovasc Electrophysiol 2009;20:352–8.

11. World Health Organization classification of tumours: pathology and genetics of tumours of endocrine organs. Lyon, France: IARC Press, 2004.

12. Linnoila RI, Keiser HR, Steinberg SM, Lack EE. Histopathology of benign versus malignant sympathoadrenal paragangliomas: clinicopathologic study of 120 cases including unusual histologic features. Hum Pathol 1990;21:1168–80.

13. Tischler AS. Pheochromocytoma and extra-adrenal paraganglioma: updates. Arch Pathol Lab Med 2008;132:1272–84.

14. Lloyd RV, Sisson JC, Shapiro B, Verhofstad AA. Immunohistochemical localization of epinephrine, norepinephrine, catecholamine-synthesizing enzymes, and chromogranin in neuroendocrine cells and tumors. Am J Pathol 1986;125:45–54.

15. Eisenhofer G, Bornstein SR, Brouwers FM, et al. Malignant pheochromocytoma: current status and initiatives for future progress. Endocr Relat Cancer 2004;11: 423–36.

16. Sadow PM, Rumilla KM, Erickson LA, Lloyd RV. Stathmin expression in pheochromocytomas, paragangliomas, and in other endocrine tumors. Endocr Pathol 2008;19:97–103.

17. Dluhy RG. Pheochromocytoma—death of an axiom. N Engl J Med 2002; 346:1486–8.

Perspectives and Updates

The case was that of a patient who presented with the ubiquitous complaint of dizziness, which proved to be caused by orthostatic hypotension induced by downregulation of catecholamine receptors due to chronic catecholamine exposure from a pheochromocytoma. It is a very interesting and instructive case but involves an extremely unusual cause of dizziness.

Dizziness is the bane of the existence of the general physician, emergency physician, and neurologist. The problem is that in most cases this very common complaint arises from benign and often quite banal causes. But buried within the morass of dizziness are the occasional patients with serious and even life-threatening disorders. In the emergency department, the specter of cerebrovascular disease affecting the posterior circulation is often raised, particularly in older patients. This inevitably leads to expensive imaging (e.g., CT angigragraphy, MR angiography). If these examinations are normal, only money is lost, but an even greater problem revolves around the "incidentaloma," the finding that does not explain the complaint but has now come to light. For example, many older people have atherosclerosis of the verterbral and basilar arteries. If a patient complaining of dizziness is found to have these abnormalities, do they account for the problem? Now that interventions are available (e.g., angioplasty, stents, tissue plasminogen activator), it is actually dangerous and even a possible threat to life to treat an imaging finding that may not be the cause of the problem.

For this reason I have emphasized, over the years, that it is important for the clinician to determine by history and careful examination the nature of the dizziness. The four major types—vertigo (an illusion or hallucination of motion), near-syncope (the feeling of faintness), disequilibrium (various gait disorders), and anxiety—can often be teased apart by the astute clinician using the techniques of careful history taking combined with a focused medical and neurological examination. A salient feature of dizziness is that many patients suffer from more than one type, making it even more important for the doctor to carefully determine which type underlies the current complaint. There is a trend in emergency departments to apply algorithms to this problem in order to rapidly separate benign (usually peripheral) problems from serious (usually central) ones. For example, David Newman-Toker has shown that the application of three simple tests (the horizontal head impulse maneuver, an analysis of whether there is bidirectional nystagmus in a single position of the head, and the alternate eye-cover test looking for a vertical skew deviation) can accurately separate central from peripheral causes of vertigo. This three-step process has been cleverly labeled with the acronym HINTS (head impulse, nystagmus, test of skew). People with a peripheral problem (e.g., vestibular neuritis) have a positive head thrust maneuver (i.e., their vestibular ocular reflex is defective on one side); have nystagmus that beats in only one direction in a single position of the head; and, on alternate covering of the eyes, there is no vertical skew, recognized by a vertical corrective saccade of the eye when the occluder is moved from one eye to the other. The reverse is true for central processes, cleverly denoted by the acronym INFARCT (impulse normal or fast-phase alternating or refixation on cover test). This is indeed very useful; but, as this case shows, it is useful only when the cause of the dizziness is vertigo. When the cause is disequilibrium, anxiety, or, as in this case, near-syncope, this set of maneuvers simply doesn't apply.[1,2]

The key to the correct diagnosis in this case was the recognition that this patient meant by "dizziness" the feeling of faintness in the upright posture and not vertigo, disequilibrium, or anxiety. When the blood pressure was found to be highest with compression of the abdomen (i.e., on sitting up) and lowest on standing, it was a simple step to conclude that something in the abdomen was secreting catecholamines that, over time, had led to downregulation of catecholamine receptors on the high-resistance vessels, thus partially disabling the patient's ability to maintain cerebral perfusion pressure in the upright posture.

Martin A. Samuels

REFERENCES

1. Kattah JC, Talkad AV, Wang DZ, Hsich Y-H, Newman-Toker DE. HINTS to diagnose stroke in the acute vestibular syndrome. Stroke 2009; 40:3504–10.
2. Hansen CK, Joyce N, Carney E, Salciccioli JD, Vinton D, Donnino MW, Edlow JA. ED patients with vertigo: can we identify clinical factors associated with acute stroke? Am J Emerg Med 2011; 30: 587–91.

INDEX

Note: Page numbers followed by f or t indicate figures or tables, respectively.

Printed in the United States
By Bookmasters